Blackwell's Primary Care Essentials: Geriatrics

Second Edition

Blackwell's Primary Care Essentials Series

Second Edition

Blackwell's Primary Care Essentials: Geriatrics

Second Edition

Karen Gershman, MD, CMD, CAQ GERIATRICS

Associate Professor of Community and Family Medicine
Dartmouth Medical School
Faculty, Maine-Dartmouth Family Practice Residency Program
Augusta, Maine

Dennis M. McCullough, MD, CMD, CAQ GERIATRICS

Medical Director, Kendal at Hanover
Hanover, New Hampshire
Associate Professor and Chief Clinical Officer
Department of Community and Family Medicine
Dartmouth-Hitchcock Medical Center
Lebanon, New Hampshire

Series Editor

Daniel K. Onion, MD, MPH, FACP
Professor of Community and Family Medicine
Dartmouth Medical School
Director of Maine-Dartmouth Family Practice Residency Program
Augusta, Maine

Blackwell
Science

©2002 by Blackwell Science, Inc.

Editorial Offices:
Commerce Place, 350 Main Street, Malden, Massachusetts 02148, USA
Osney Mead, Oxford OX2 0EL, England
25 John Street, London WC1N 2BS, England
23 Ainslie Place, Edinburgh EH3 6AJ, Scotland
54 University Street, Carlton, Victoria 3053, Australia

Other Editorial Offices:
Blackwell Wissenschafts-Verlag GmbH, Kurfürstendamm 57, 10707 Berlin, Germany
Blackwell Science KK, MG Kodenmacho Building, 7-10 Kodenmacho Nihombashi, Chuo-ku, Tokyo 104, Japan
Iowa State University Press, A Blackwell Science Company, 2121 S. State Avenue, Ames, Iowa 50014-8300, USA

Distributors:
The Americas
Blackwell Publishing
c/o AIDC
P.O. Box 20
50 Winter Sport Lane
Williston, VT 05495-0020
(Telephone orders: 800-216-2522; fax orders: 802-864-7626)

Australia
Blackwell Science Pty, Ltd.
54 University Street
Carlton, Victoria 3053
(Telephone orders: 03-9347-0300; fax orders: 03-9349-3016)

Outside The Americas and Australia
Blackwell Science, Ltd.
c/o Marston Book Services, Ltd.
P.O. Box 269
Abingdon
Oxon OX14 4YN
England
(Telephone orders: 44-01235-465500; fax orders: 44-01235-465555)

Acquisitions: Nancy Anastasi Duffy
Development: Julia Casson
Production: Elissa Gershowitz
Manufacturing: Lisa Flanagan
Marketing Manager: Toni Fournier
Cover design by Leslie Haimes
Text design and typesetting by Graphicraft Limited, Hong Kong
Printed and bound by
    Edwards Brothers, Inc.

Printed in the United States of America
02 03 04 05 5 4 3 2 1

The Blackwell Science logo is a trade mark of Blackwell Science Ltd., registered at the United Kingdom Trade Marks Registry

Library of Congress Cataloging-in-Publication Data

Gershman, Karen.
  Blackwell's primary care essentials. Geriatrics / by Karen Gershman, Dennis M. McCullough. — 2nd ed.
      p. ; cm. — (Blackwell's primary care essentials series)
  Rev. ed. of: The little black book of geriatrics. c1997.
  ISBN 0-632-04521-3 (pbk.)
  1. Geriatrics.
  [DNLM: 1. Geriatrics. 2. Primary Health Care-Aged. WT 100 G381b 2002]
I. Title: Geriatrics. II. Title: Primary care essentials. III. McCullough, Dennis M. IV. Gershman, Karen. Little black book of geriatrics. V. Title. VI. Series.
  RC952 .G448 2002
  618.97—dc21   2001004550

To Miriam Axelrod, MD, and Melaine Gershman-Tewksbury, MD, who in kindling hope in their patients have given off a great light.

To my father, who thought I should be a physician, and to my mother and father whose excellent examples as teachers inspired me to be both.

K.G.

To Pamela Harrison, poet and partner, and our daughter Kate, who have always graciously supported my professional and personal journeys.

D.M.

Notice

The indications and dosages of all drugs in this book have been recommended in the medical literature and conform to the practices of the general community. The medications described and treatment prescriptions suggested do not necessarily have specific approval by the Food and Drug Administration for use in the diseases and dosages for which they are recommended. The package insert for each drug should be consulted for use and dosage as approved by the FDA. Because standards for usage change, it is advisable to keep abreast of revised recommendations, particularly those concerning new drugs.

Contents

Preface

In college, I had the habit of reading good literature in the bathtub late at night, sometimes until 2:00 or 3:00 in the morning. Lulled by the warm water and slumber, my eyelids and hands would go limp, and the book would inevitably tumble. Now most of my treasured library is a bit waterlogged, and the pages are bunched and wrinkled after having been hung up to dry.

I could attribute my novels' misadventures to my father, a professor of microbiology. It was he who insisted that the dreaded sciences of organic chemistry, comparative physiology, and physics be tackled early in the evening. "Save the humanities for later." My precious humanities were like dessert. They accompanied the reward of a tepid tub after an arduous day of classes.

In Herman Hesse's *The Glass Bead Game*, the main character of the book, the aged and esteemed master of the glass bead game, has taken on a young apprentice. The student is unfocused, inexperienced, and restless, yet the sage sees potential in him. So he sets about enticing his pupil down the difficult road of erudition. First he must create a bond with the youth. He will gain his trust by joining the student where the student is most comfortable and unthreatened: the tutor chooses an exhilarating walk in the early morning cold.

They come to a pond. The apprentice impulsively dives into its icy depths and begins swimming its length, preferring the physical challenge, one that he knows he can master. This is his escape for a time from the embarrassment of the ignorance he's apt to feel with his tutor in the cognitive realm. Left on the shore, the scholar gazes at his pupil, hoping that this is the place where they shall meet, where the bond will be created. Without pondering his own physical limitations, he plunges into the rough chill of the waters and drowns.

I still see myself in that silly bathtub, the water gone cold, blubbering over the death of a fictitious teacher and sharing with his pupil the remorse of a missed opportunity, the loss of a mentor.

Hesse's novel left me with a lasting admiration for the teacher who reaches more than halfway to capture the imagination of a novice and crosses the chasm, whether it be generational, cultural, class, or gender, to work together in shaping a discipline.

As I learn who my students are, it is each student's story that becomes the study and myself the pupil. Their uniqueness changes the nuance of the didactic, the approach to the patient. Family practice residents have contributed the writing of this book, enriching its repertoire.

In its earliest form this book was a collaborative effort among doctors and nurses. Its aim was to emphasize the geriatric patient's independence and individuality. Multiple disciplines working in concert with medicine are needed to achieve this, hence the "team management" sections of this book.

Dan Onion asked me to develop the next in a series of books based on the format he had used in his book *The Little Black Book of Primary Care*. Having learned a great deal from Dan's scientific approach to medicine, one that supplied references for current controversies, I could see the utility of such a geriatric manual. Dennis McCullough, a mentor since our first meeting at the Chapel Hill Family Practice Fellowship, has provided wise pearls of family practice experience. During the last legs of this book's production, I was diagnosed with breast cancer. Dennis' support and detailed review of the page proofs allowed for its timely completion.

One day this summer while sitting alongside my own pond, recuperating from chemotherapy, I was visited by a resident who had come to invoke a resurgence of my bone marrow. It was her notion that an exhilarating swim would do the trick. My fears of deep water made me an unwilling student and encumbered her cure. Eventually, she coached me across the pond and back, keeping me afloat as my colleagues have done these past months.

I hope you, the reader, whether you are a primary care provider, student, or resident, will find what we've put together useful, knowing all along that your patients will be most helped by what you bring of yourself to the patient encounter.

K.G.

ADDENDUM

My friend, colleague, and coauthor could not have fully realized how I have always relished the extra innings of the game, the tiebreaker, the overtime period. When I was asked to enter this process, I was awed by the quality and tone of Dr. Gershman's text, accomplished over months and months of hard labor—the first seven innings. Helping to bring Karen's work to print has been a thrill and a pleasure. I have enjoyed the opportunity to draw on my love of working with older folks and their families and with our healthcare team at Kendal at Hanover, a continuing care retirement community near the Dartmouth-Hitchcock Medical Center.

The perspectives that I have gained from trying to be a player on a geriatric team have substantially complemented my understanding of "diseases" in elderly people. Many answers to clinical situations are to be found in interdisciplinary discussions and in time-requiring "processing" with patients and their families—this book of information is only the starting point for this clinical work. I encourage the reader to listen, discuss, and work slowly over time in these wonderful and complicated partnerships to bring the very best care and caring to patients.

D.M.

Since the publication of the first edition, Karen has recovered from breast cancer, and lost a mentor whom she capriciously thought would live to be 100, her father. As with our parents, we are grateful to our patients for their enduring lessons.

Our patients, well into their 80s, foster an apprenticeship, continuing to parent generations younger than themselves, preparing us to do the same. So we have decided to dedicate this second edition to our respective children: Jackie, Abu, and Kate. They will always be our children no matter how old we get.

This book includes new topics such as hypothermia, liver failure, executive function testing of dementias, and family phases of adaption to chronic illness. There are expanded areas as well, eg, hospice management. Wherever possible we have used tables and decision trees to facilitate acquisition of disease entities. References have been updated and a pocket guide for screening in the elderly is folded into the cover for convenience.

K.G. & D.M.

Medical Abbreviations

5HIAA	5-Hydroxyindoleacetic acid
AA	Alcoholics Anonymous
AACD	Age-associated cognitive decline
AADLs	Advanced activities of daily living
AAMI	Age-associated memory impairment
ABG	Arterial blood gases
ABW	Actual body weight
Ac	Before meals
ACE	Angiotensin-converting enzyme
ACTH	Adrenocorticotropic hormone
ADLs	Activities of daily living
AFB	Acid-fast bacilli
afib	Atrial fibrillation
aflut	Atrial flutter
ALT	SGPT; alanine aminotransferase
ANA	Antinuclear antibody
ANP	Atrial natriuretic peptide
AP	Anterior-posterior
ARDS	Adult respiratory distress syndrome
AS	Aortic stenosis
As	Arsenic
ASA	Aspirin
ASCVD	Arteriosclerotic cardiovascular disease
ASHD	Arteriosclerotic heart disease
AST	SGOT; aspartate aminotransferase
asx	Asymptomatic
AV	Arteriovenous; or atrioventricular
avg	Average
bcp's	Birth control pills
BE	Barium enema

bid	Twice a day
BM	Bowel movement
BMD	Bone mass density
BMI	Body mass index
BP	Blood pressure
BPH	Benign prostatic hypertrophy
BSO	Bilateral salpingo-oophorectomy
BUN	Blood urea nitrogen
bx	Biopsy
CABG	Coronary artery bypass graft
CAD	Coronary artery disease
cal	Calories
CBC	Complete blood cell count
CEA	Carcinoembryonic antigen
chem	Chemistries
chemo rx	Chemotherapy
CHF	Congestive heart failure
CJD	Jakob-Creutzfeldt disease
CML	Chronic myelocytic leukemia
CN	Cranial nerve
CNS	Central nervous system
Complc	Complications
COPD	Chronic obstructive lung
CPAP	Continuous positive airway pressure
CPK	Creatine phosphokinase
Cr	Creatinine
CR	Controlled release
CRP	C-reactive protein
crs	Course
CSF	Cerebrospinal fluid
CT	Computed tomography
CVA	Cerebrovascular accident
CVP	Central venous pressure
CXR	Chest x-ray
d	Day
D_5S	Dextrose 5% in saline
DAT	Dementia, Alzheimer type
dB	Decibel

DI	Diabetes insipidus
DIC	Disseminated intravascular coagulation
DM	Diabetes mellitus
DNR	Do not resuscitate
DSM	Diagnostic and statistical manual
DTRs	Deep tendon reflexes
DVT	Deep vein thrombosis
dx	Diagnosis or diagnostic
ECT	Electroconvulsive therapy
EDTA	Ethylenediaminetetraacetate
EEG	Electroencephalogram
EF	Ejection fraction
EKG	Electrocardiogram
Epidem	Epidemiology
ETOH	Ethanol
ETT	Exercise tolerance test
FBS	Fasting blood sugar
Fe	Iron
FNA	Fine-needle aspiration
GFR	Glomerular filtration rate
GI	Gastrointestinal
GU	Genitourinary
HA	Headache
hgb	Hemoglobin
$HgbA_{1C}$	Hemoglobin A_{1C} level
HHNC	Hyperosmolar nonketotic coma
HIV	Human immunodeficiency virus
HMG-CoA	Hepatic hydroxymethylglutaryl-coenzyme A
h/o	History of
hs	At bedtime
HT	Hypertension
hx	History
Hz	Hertz
IADLs	Instrumental or intermediate activities of daily living
IBD	Inflammatory bowel disease

IBW	Ideal body weight
ICU	Intensive care unit
IHSS	Idiopathic hypertrophic subaortic stenosis
IL	Interleukin
im	Intramuscular
INH	Isoniazid
INR	International normalized ratio
IPG	Impedance plethysmography
IV	Intravenous
IVP	Intravenous pyelography
JVD	Jugular venous distension
L	Liter; or left
Lab	Laboratory tests
lb	Pound(s)
LBBB	Left bundle branch block
LBM	Lean body mass
LDH	Lactate dehydrogenase
LDL	Low-density lipoprotein
LFTs	Liver function tests
LH	Luteinizing hormone
LOC	Loss of consciousness
LP	Lumbar puncture
LS	Lumbosacral
LV	Left ventricle
LVH	Left ventricular hypertrophy
lytes	Electrolytes
M	Male
m	Meter
MCV	Mean corpuscular volume
Meds	Medications
METS	Metabolic equivalents
Mg	Magnesium
MI	Myocardial infarction; or mitral insufficiency
min	Minute
mL	Milliliter
MOM	Milk of magnesia
MPTP	Methylphenyltetrahydropyridine

MRA	Magnetic resonance angiography
MRSA	Methicillin-resistant *Staphylococcus aureus*
MS	Multiple sclerosis; mitral stenosis
musc-skel	Musculoskeletal
NAG	Narrow-angle glaucoma
neg	Negative
ng	Nanogram
NG	Nasogastric
NH	Nursing home
NIDDM	Non-insulin-dependent diabetes
nl	Normal
Nm	Nanometer
NNT	Number needed to treat
no.	Number
NPH	Normal-pressure hydrocephalus
npo	Nothing by mouth
NSAID	Nonsteroidal anti-inflammatory drug
NSR	Normal sinus rhythm
OTC	Over the counter
PAP	Pulmonary artery pressure
PAT	Paroxysmal atrial tachycardia
Pathophys	Pathophysiology
Pb	Lead
PCP	*Pneumocystis carinii* pneumonia
PCWP	Pulmonary capillary wedge pressure
PE	Pulmonary embolism
PET	Positron emission tomography
PFTs	Pulmonary function tests
PMNLs	Polymorphonuclear leukocytes
PMI	Point of maximal impulse of heart
PMR	Polymyalgia rheumatica
po	By mouth
POAG	Primary open-angle glaucoma
pos	Positive
postop	Postoperative
ppd	Packs per day
PPD	Protein derivative

pr	By rectum
preop	Preoperative
PSA	Prostate-specific antigen
PT	Prothrombin time
pt(s)	Patient(s)
PTH	Parathyroid hormone
PTSD	Post-traumatic stress disorder
PTT	Partial thromboplastin time
PUD	Peptic ulcer disease
PUVA	Psoralen + UVA light
PVC	Premature ventricular tachycardia
PVD	Peripheral vascular disease
PVR	Postvoid residual
px	Prognosis
q	Every
qd	Every day
qid	4 times a day
qod	Every other day
quad	Quadriceps
R	Right; or respirations
r/o	Rule out
RA	Rheumatoid arthritis
RBBB	Right bundle branch block
rbc	Red blood cell
rehab	Rehabilitation
REM	Rapid eye movement
ROM	Range of motion
RSD	Reflex sympathetic dystrophy
RV	Right ventricle
rx	Treatment
SAD	Seasonal affective disorder
s/p	Status post
sc	Subcutaneous
SD	Standard deviation
SE	Side effect(s)
sec	Seconds
sens	Sensitivity

si	Signs
SIADH	Syndrome of inappropriate antidiuretic hormone
sl	Sublingual
SLE	Systemic lupus erythematosus
SNP	Supranuclear-Palsy
soln	Solution
s/p	Status post
specif	Specificity
SPECT	Single-photon emission computed tomography
SPEP	Serum protein electrophoresis
SR	Slow release
SSRI	Selective serotonin reuptake inhibitor
SSS	Sick sinus syndrome
SVR	Systemic vascular resistance
SVT	Supraventricular tachycardia
sx	Symptoms
T_3	Triiodothyronine
T_4	Thyroxine
tab	Tablet
TAH	Total abdominal hysterectomy
TB	Tuberculosis
TCA	Tricyclic antidepressant
TENS	Transcutaneous electrical stimulation
TIA	Transient ischemic attack
TIBC	Total iron binding capacity
Tm/S	Trimethoprim/sulfa
TNG	Nitroglycerin
T°	Fever/temperature
TPA	Tissue plasminogen activator
TPN	Total parenteral nutrition
TSH	Thyroid-stimulating hormone
tsp	Teaspoon
TURP	Transurethral resection of prostate
UA	Urinalysis
UBW	Usual body weight
UGI	Upper gastrointestinal
UPEP	Urine protein electrophoresis
URI	Upper respiratory infection

US	Ultrasound
UTI	Urinary tract infection
UV	Ultraviolet
UVA	Ultraviolet A
UVB	Ultraviolet B
VDRL	Serologic test for syphilis (Venereal Disease Research Lab)
vfib	Ventricular fibrillation
vit	Vitamin
VRE	Vancomycin-resistant enterococci
vs	Versus
vtach	Ventricular tachycardia
w	With
w/o	Without
w/u	Workup
WBC	White blood cell
wk	Week
WPW	Wolff-Parkinson-White syndrome
yr	Year

Journals and Other Reference Abbreviations

(Journal abbreviation is followed by year, volume, and page or issue number)

ACP J Club	American College of Physicians Journal Club
Acta Neurol Scand	Acta Neurologica Scandinavica
Acta Psychiatr Scand	Acta Psychiatrica Scandinavica
Adv Wound Care	Advances in Wound Healing
Age Aging	Age and Aging
AHCPR	United States Agency for Health Care Policy and Research (Rockville, MD)
Alzheimer Dis Assoc Disord	Alzheimer Disease and Associated Disorders
Am Fam Phys	American Family Physician
Am Heart J	American Heart Journal
Am J Cardiol	American Journal of Cardiology
Am J Clin Oncol	American Journal of Clinical Oncology
Am J Gastroenterol	American Journal of Gastroenterology
Am J Ger Psychiatry	American Journal of Geriatric Psychiatry
Am J Hlth Syst Pharmacol	American Journal of Health-System Pharmacology
Am J Hosp Pharm	American Journal of Hospital Pharmacy
Am J Hypertens	American Journal of Hypertension
Am J Kidney Dis	American Journal of Kidney Disease

Am J Med	American Journal of Medicine
Am J Nurs	American Journal of Nursing
Am J Obgyn	American Journal of Obstetrics and Gynecology
Am J Phys Med Rehab	American Journal of Physical Medicine and Rehabilitation
Am J Psychiatry	American Journal of Psychiatry
Am J Pub Hlth	American Journal of Public Health
Am J Respir Crit Care Med	American Journal of Respiratory and Critical Care Medicine
Am Rev Respir Dis	American Review of Respiratory Diseases
Ann EM	Annals of Emergency Medicine
Ann IM	Annals of Internal Medicine
Ann LT Care	Annals of Long-Term Care
Ann Neurol	Annals of Neurology
Ann Oncol	Annals of Oncology
Ann Pharmacother	Annals of Pharmacotherapy
Ann Rheum Dis	Annals of the Rheumatic Diseases
Ann Rev Pub Hlth	Annual Review of Public Health
Ann Thorac Surg	Annals of Thoracic Surgery
Arch Fam Med	Archives of Family Medicine
Arch IM	Archives of Internal Medicine
Arch Ophthalm	Archives of Ophthalmology
Arch Phys Med Rehab	Archives of Physical Medicine and Rehabilitation
Arch Sex Behav	Archives of Sexual Behavior
Arch Surg	Archives of Surgery
Arth Rheum	Arthritis and Rheumatism
Aust NZ J Surg	Australia and New Zealand Journal of Surgery
Basic Res Cardiol	Basic Research in Cardiology
Biol Psychiatry	Biological Psychiatry
BJU Int	BJU International
BMJ	British Medical Journal
Bone Marrow Transplant	Bone Marrow Transplantation
Bone Miner	Bone and Mineral
Br J Cancer	British Journal of Cancer
Br J Clin Pract	British Journal of Clinical Practice

Br J Psychiatry	British Journal of Psychiatry
Br J Surg	British Journal of Surgery
Bull Rheum Dis	Bulletin on the Rheumatic Diseases
CA	CA: A Cancer Journal for Clinicians
Can J Psychiatry	Canadian Journal of Psychiatry
Can J Ophthalm	Canadian Journal of Ophthalmology
Cancer Causes Control	Cancer Causes and Control
Cancer Nurs	Cancer Nursing
Cancer Pract	Cancer Practice
Circ	Circulation
Clin Diabetes	Clinical Diabetes
Clin Endocrinol	Clinical Endocrinology (Oxford)
Clin Infect Dis	Clinical Infectious Diseases
Clin Gastroenterol	Clinics in Gastroenterology
Clin Ger Med	Clinics in Geriatric Medicine
Clin Gerontol	Clinical Gerontology
Clin Orthop	Clinical Orthopedics and Related Research
Clin Pharmacol Ther	Clinical Pharmacology and Therapeutics
Clin Symp	Clinical Symposia
Cmaj	Canadian Medical Association Journal
Conn Med	Connecticut Medicine
Consult Pharm	Consultant Pharmacist
Control Clin Trials	Controlled Clinical Trials
Convuls Ther	Convulsive Therapy
Crit Care Clin	Critical Care Clinics
Crit Care Med	Critical Care Medicine
Curr Concepts Cerebro Dis	Current Concepts of Cerebrovascular Disease
Curr Opin Neurol	Current Opinion in Neurology
Curr Probl Cancer	Current Problems in Cancer
Curr Probl Cardiol	Current Problems in Cardiology
Diabetes	Diabetes
Diabetes Metab Rev	Diabetes/Metabolism Reviews
Dis Mo	Disease-a-Month

Ear Hear	Ear and Hearing
Emerg Med Clin N Am	Emergency Medicine Clinics of North America
Endocr Rev	Endocrine Reviews
Eur J Cancer	European Journal of Cancer
Eur J Surg Oncol	European Journal of Surgical Oncology
Eur Respir J	European Respiratory Journal
Exp Aging Res	Experimental Aging Research
Fortschr Neurol Psychiatrie	Fortschritte der Neurologie-Psychiatrie
Gastroenterol Clin N Am	Gastroenterology Clinics of North America
Gastroenterol Int	Gastroenterology International
Gastrointest Endosc Clin N Am	Gastrointestinal Endoscopy Clinics of North America
Ger Clin N Am	Geriatric Clinics of North America
Ger Med Today	Geriatric Medicine Today
Ger Rev Syllabus	Geriatric Review Syllabus
Geriatrics	Geriatrics
Gerodontics	Gerodontics
Gerontol	Gerontologist
Gerontol Clin	Gerontologia Clinica
Heart Lung	Heart and Lung
Hlth Serv Res	Health Services Research
Horm Metab Res	Hormone and Metabolic Research
Hosp Pract	Hospital Practice
Inf Contr Hosp Epidem	Infection Control and Hospital Epidemiology
Int J Aging Hum Dev	International Journal of Aging and Human Development
Int J Epidemiol	International Journal of Epidemiology
Int J Psychiatr Med	International Journal of Psychiatry in Medicine
J Acoustic Soc Am	Journal of the Acoustical Society of America

J Acquir Immun Defic Syndr	Journal of the Acquired Immune Deficiency Syndromes and Human Retrovirology
Jama	Journal of the American Medical Association
J Am Acad Dermatol	Journal of the American Academy of Dermatology
J Am Board Fam Pract	Journal of the American Board of Family Practice
J Am Coll Cardiol	Journal of the American College of Cardiology
J Am Diet Assoc	Journal of the American Dietetic Association
J Am Geriatr Soc	Journal of the American Geriatrics Society
J Am Optom Assoc	Journal of the American Optometric Association
J Bone Joint Surg Am	Journal of Bone and Joint Surgery (American vol)
J Bone Miner Res	Journal of Bone and Mineral Research
J Chronic Dis	Journal of Chronic Disease
J Clin Endocrinol Metab	Journal of Endocrinology & Metabolism
J Clin Invest	Journal of Clinical Investigation
J Clin Oncol	Journal of Clinical Oncology
J Clin Psychiatry	Journal of Clinical Psychiatry
J Clin Psychopharmacol	Journal of Clinical Psychopharmacology
J Comm Health	Journal of Community Health
J Emerg Med	Journal of Emergency Medicine
J Endocrinol Metab	Journal of Endocrinology and Metabolism
J Endourol	Journal of Endourology
J Fam Pract	Journal of Family Practice
J Gen IM	Journal of General Internal Medicine
J Ger Psychiatry	Journal of Geriatric Psychiatry
J Ger Psychiatry Neurol	Journal of Geriatric Psychiatry and Neurology
J Gerontol	Journal of Gerontology

J Gerontol Med Sci	Journals of Gerontology. Series A, Biological Sciences and Medical Sciences
J Gerontol Nurs	Journal of Gerontological Nursing
J Hosp Infect	Journal of Hospital Infection
J Hypertens	Journal of Hypertension
J Hypertens Suppl	Journal of Hypertension Supplement
J Intern Med	Journal of Internal Medicine
J Midwife Women Hlth	Journal of Midwifery and Women's Health
J Natl Cancer Inst	Journal of the National Cancer Institute
J Neurol Sci	Journal of Neurological Science
J Neuropsychiatry Clin Neurosci	Journal of Neuropsychiatry and Clinical Neurosciences
J Optom Assoc	Journal of the American Optometric Association
J Psycho Nurs	Journal of Psychological Nursing
J Rheum	Journal of Rheumatology
J Trauma	Journal of Trauma
J Urol	Journal of Urology
Leuk Lymphoma	Leukemia and Lymphoma
Life Sci	Life Sciences
Maturitas	Maturitas
Mayo Clin Proc	Mayo Clinic Proceedings
Md State Med Assoc J	Maryland State Medical Association Journal
Mech Age Dev	Mechanisms of Ageing & Development
Med Aud Dig	Medical Audio Digest
Med Clin N Am	Medical Clinics of North America
Med Let Drugs Ther	Medical Letter on Drugs and Therapeutics
Milbank Q	Milbank Quarterly
Minn Med	Minnesota Medicine
Mmwr	CDC Morbidity and Morality Weekly Report

xxvi *Journals and Other Reference Abbreviations*

Mod Concepts Cardiovasc Dis	Modern Concepts of Cardiovascular Disease
Natl Ctr Hlth Stat	National Center for Health Statistics
Nejm	New England Journal of Medicine
Neuro Cln	Neurologic Clinics
Neurol	Neurology
Nurs Home Med	Nursing Home Medicine
Nurs Home Pract	Nursing Home Practice
Nutr Rev	Nutrition Reviews
Obgyn	Obstetrics and Gynecology
Oncology	Oncology
Ophthalm	Ophthalmology
Osteoporos Int	Osteoporosis International
Palliat Med	Palliative Medicine
Ped Derm	Pediatric Dermatology
Phys Postgrad Med	Physicians Postgraduate Medicine
Phys Ther	Physical Therapy
Prim Care	Primary Care
Prog Clin Biol Res	Progress in Clinical and Biological Research
Psych Ann	Psychiatric Annals
Psychiatr Clin N Am	Psychiatric Clinics of North America
Psychol Med	Psychological Medicine
Psychosom	Psychosomatics
Radiol Clin N Am	Radiologic Clinics of North America
Sci Am	Scientific American
Sci Am Med	Scientific American Medicine
Semin Oncol	Seminars in Oncology
Semin Spine Surg	Seminars in Spine Surgery
South Med J	Southern Medical Journal
Stroke	Stroke
Surg Clin N Am	Surgical Clinics of North America
Surv Ophthalmol	Survey of Ophthalmology
Urol Clin N Am	Urologic Clinics of North America

Acknowledgments

Several primary care providers and medical students have contributed to the writing of various sections of this book. They include:

Michelle Rebelsky, MD, MDFPR, Maine-Dartmouth Family Practice Residency	Ethics
Tom Bartol, RN-C, Richmond, ME	Diabetes Mellitus
James A. Schneid, MD, MDFPR	
Diana Berger, MD, Hanover, NH	Gout
Laura Chapman, Hanover, NH	Meningitis
Sandy Colt, GNP, Maine General Medical Center	UTIs/Constipation
Greg Feero, MD, MDFPR	Atrial Fibrillation
Rod Forrey, PA, MDFPR	Anxiety; NMS
Alicia Forster, MD, MDFPR	Prostate Cancer
James Glazer, MD, MDFPR	Enteral Feeding; Osteomyelitis; Hypothermia
Rick Hobbs, MD, MDFPR	Hospice & Palliative Care
Aubrey Ingraham, Hanover, NH	Syncope
Virginia Jeffries, MD, Concord, NH	Depression
Susan Wehry, MD, Burlington, VT	
Jonathan Kilroy, DO, MDFPR	Thrombolytics
Karen LeComte, MD, MDFPR	Hypertension
James MacDonald, MD, MDFPR	ETOH Abuse
Negean Mahoudi, Hanover, NH	HIV
Mark Rolfe, MD, MDFPR	
Kristin McDermott, DO, MDFPR	Dementia
Catherine Neilsen, MD, MDFPR	Pneumonia; Influenza; Elderly Abuse
Daniel K. Onion, MD, MDFPR	Cardiology
Rebecca Reeves, Albany, NY	Endocarditis
Rachael Solotaroff, Hanover, NH	CHF

Shannon Tome-Kenney, Biddeford, ME   Skin Infections
Stephanie Waecker, DO, MDFPR   Ovarian Cancer
Richard Wallingford, III, MD, MDFPR   TB

Special thanks to John Sutherland, MD, for reviewing the cardiology
chapter and Charles Alexander, MD, for reviewing the ethics chapter.
We would also like to thank Davene Fitch, Drew Travers, and especially
Bonnie Orr for their help in the preparation of the book.

We are indebted to James Glazer, MD, for his generous and
enthusiastic review of this entire second edition. His attention to detail,
salient inquiry, judgment, and respectful and lovely character made
working at deadline pace a pleasure.

1 Common Geriatric Problems

1.1 DYSFUNCTION IN THE ELDERLY

Cause: Loss of physical, mental, social function, excessive family burden (Gerontol 1980;20:649)

Epidem: In 1985, 20% of elderly were disabled; by 2060, 30% will be disabled (J Gerontol 1992;47:S253); among individuals 65 yr and older, >20% have difficulty walking a half mile, >30% have difficulty doing heavy housework, 50% have difficulty pulling or pushing large objects such as furniture; 30% community elders live alone: M/F ratio = 1:3; the remainder live in family settings: 54% w spouse, 13% w children, 3% w non-relatives (DHHS Pub. 1990;PF3029912900:d996)

50% of all long-term care payments come from individual and family finances, most of which are spent on NH care; Medicaid coverage during the first year of NH placement = 20%, but overall >90% of all public funds for NH care provided by Medicaid; Medicare pays for skilled home-care services, but only 3% of NH care; private long-term care insurance pays 2% of NH care (Gerontol 1990;30:7,21)

Sx: Loss of self-care/independent living skills; social, psychological, emotional isolation

Si: Inability to read 20/40; inability to hear and answer short, whispered question such as "What is your name?"; urinary incontinence; weight below acceptable range for height; inability to recall three objects after 1 min; often sad or depressed; cannot get out of bed, make own meals, do own shopping; trouble with stairs, bathtubs, rugs, lighting; doesn't know where to call in emergency or if ill (Ann IM 1990;112:699); inability to touch back of head with both hands, touch back of waist, or contralateral hip; inability to sit and touch toe of shoe; no grip strength (J Fam Pract 1993;17:429)

ADLs: Katz functional assessment (Gerontol 1970;10:20) records loss of independence in 6 skills (in the order in which they are lost: bathing, dressing, toileting, transferring, continence, feeding); usually they are regained in the reverse order; assess actual capacity, not reported performance (Nejm 1990;322:1207); Mahoney and Barthel ADL scale has more specific questions (Md State Med Assoc J 1965;14:61); speed and pain in performing ADLs in arthritis pts (J Chronic Dis 1978;31:557); use of rehabilitation for ADLs (Arch Phys Med Rehab 1988;69:337); falls and incontinence associated w lower and upper extremity impairment (Jama 1995;273:1348)

Instrumental activities of daily living (IADLs): more complex activities like shopping, seeking transportation, preparing food, climbing stairs, managing finances, housework, telephone, meds, and job (Fillenbaum IADLs; J Am Geriatr Soc 1985;33:698); mnemonic "SHAFT": shopping, housework, accounting, food preparation, transportation (Mayo Clin Proc 1995;70:891)

Other IADL scales: home assessment (Clin Ger Med 1991;7:677); nutrition (Am Fam Phys 1993;48:1395); driving (Clin Ger Med 1993;9:349), states where standard vision tests required for driver license renewal have fewer fatalities, whereas states requiring cognitive function test show no difference in fatalities (Jama 1995;274:1026); identify older pts at risk for functional decline after acute medical illness and hospitalization w scoring system based on Mini Mental State Exam (MMSE), IADLs, and age (J Am Geriatr Soc 1996;44:251); advanced ADLs (AADLs) helpful in community-dwelling elderly; predict functional decline in women by slow gait, long-acting benzodiazepine use, low exercise level, depression, basal metabolic index >29 J Am Geriatr Soc 2000;48:170)

Crs: For every 5 adults with 5–6 limitations in ADLs, 1 pt may be expected to improve in all ADLs in 2 yr (Milbank Q 1990;68:445); pts who have trouble performing IADLs have 12 times the baseline probability of developing dementia (J Am Geriatr Soc 1992;40:1129)

Cmplc: NH placement; Medicaid eligibility for NH admission requires a medical or behavioral dx, plus 2 impaired ADLs; caregiver burnout: 70% of primary caregivers are middle-aged, married women; 30% are elderly themselves (Gerontol 1987;27:616); prevalence of depression among caregivers is 30–50% (J Gerontol 1990;45:P181); measures of function strong predictors of 90-day and 2-yr mortality (Jama 1998;279:1163)

Lab: CBC, TSH, routine blood chemistries

Rx:

Team Management: Annual geriatric evaluation (Nejm 1995;333:184); rehab; change medical regimen so as not to inhibit function; solicit community services; be vigilant about underlying depression; PT, OT evaluation, instruction (Jama 1997;278:1321)

1.2 FALLS IN THE ELDERLY

Am Fam Phys 2000;61:2173; Rubenstein LZ, UCLA intensive geriatric review course, 1996; Nejm 1994;331:821; J Am Geriatr Soc 1995;43:1146; Ann IM 1994;121:442; Nejm 1990;322:1441; also see "Falls" in Chapter 2.

Cause:

Intrinsic:

- Visual: cataracts, acuity loss, glare, dark adaptation (J Am Geriatr Soc 1991;39:1194; Nejm 1991;324:1326)
- Vestibular: previous ear infection, ear surgery, aminoglycoside, quinidine, furosemide (Lasix)
- Proprioceptive: peripheral neuropathy, cervical degeneration; one-third of elderly have abnormal position sense (Jama 1988;259:1190)
- CNS: stroke, Parkinson, NPH, dementias (or Alzheimer disease, end stage)
- Cognitive: dementia, delirium
- Musc-skel: deconditioning, lower extremity weakness, eg, severe arthritis (Nejm 1988;319:1701); leg weakness imparts 5 times the risk of fall compared with balance or gait problem, which imparts only 3 times the risk of fall; knee extension (quads) and ankle plantar flexion (gastrocnemius and soleus) strength contribute to gait velocity and step length; foot problems like thick nails, calluses, bunions, toe deformities, ill-fitting shoes (J Am Geriatr Soc 1988;36:266)

- Drugs (>4 meds a risk factor) especially long-acting benzodiazepines (NH [J Am Geriatr Soc 2000;48:652]), psychoactive drugs (J Am Geriatr Soc 1999;47:30), tricyclics (Nejm 1998;339:875)

NH falls (Ann IM 1994;121:442): 20% are cardiovascular, eg, hypotension—drug-induced, postprandial, postural, bradycardia (J Gerontol 1991;46:M114); 5% due to acute illness like pneumonia, febrile illness, UTI, CHF (Am J Med 1986;80:429); only 3% falls from overwhelming intrinsic event, eg, syncope, seizure, stroke, psychoactive drugs (Nejm 1992;327:168)

Extrinsic:
- Environmental hazards >50%, eg, cords, furniture, small objects, optical patterns on escalators, stairs, floors (Clin Ger Med 1985;1:555); majority occur with mild–moderate activity, eg, walking, stepping up, stepping down, changing position; 70% at home, 10% on stairs (descending > ascending) (Age Aging 1979;8:251)
- *NH:* (Paradoxically) restraints (J Am Geriatr Soc 1999;47:1202; Ann IM 1992;116:369); higher fall rate during shift changes and when staffing ratios inadequate (J Am Geriatr Soc 1987;35:503)

Epidem: Accidents 5th leading cause of death in elderly; falls constitute two-thirds of accidental deaths; two-thirds of falls are preventable; 33% of elderly (>65) living in the community fall each year; females > males, whites > blacks (Nejm 1994;330:1555); active elderly at greater risk than frail elderly for injury (J Am Geriatr Soc 1991;39:46)

Over 50% of all NH pts fall during their stay (J Am Geriatr Soc 1995;45:1257) because of greater frailty, but rate may be high because better reporting (J Am Geriatr Soc 1988;36:266)

Pathophys: Fracture risk from falls increased in elderly because of decreased capability for energy absorption in tissue and impaired protective responses like reaction time, muscle strength, level of alertness, cognition (J Gerontol 1991;46:M164)

Falls from standing height provide sufficient energy to fracture hip (Jama 1994;271:128; Nejm 1991;332:1326); more likely to fracture a wrist than a hip when falling forward bracing a fall; falling backward more hazardous because of risk of breaking hip (J Am Geriatr Soc 1993;41:1226)

In old age the strategy for maintaining balance after a slip changes from weight shifting at hip when younger to rapid forward stepping when older (Rubenstein 1996)

Sx: H/o hypotensive sx posturally, postprandially, on micturition; may have h/o PAT, SSS, AS, hemiplegia, neuropathy, seizures, anemia, hypothyroidism, poor nutritional status, ETOH abuse, intercurrent illness (UTI, pneumonia, CHF); or use of antihypertensives, antidepressants, sedatives, hypoglycemics, phenothiazines, or carbamazepine

Si: Evaluate environment: stairs, floors (slippery from urine, high-polish linoleum, thick-pile rugs), low-lying furniture, pets, shower, lighting, stairway handrails, toilet grab bars, footwear, slippers

Tinetti Gait/Balance Assessment

Balance:
- Upon immediate standing (if abnormal, consider myopathy, arthritis, Parkinson, postural hypotension, deconditioning, hip disease, hemiparesis)
- With eyes closed and feet together (if abnormal, consider multisensory deficit or diminished proprioception)
- If unstable with sternal nudge or turning 360 degrees (consider Parkinson, NPH, CNS disease, back problems, cervical spondylosis); especially important to determine prior to beginning exercise classes
- While sitting (if abnormal, consider impaired vision, proximal myopathy, ataxia)
- When turning neck (if abnormal, consider cervical arthritis or spondylosis, vertebrobasilar insufficiency)
- When reaching up, bending down, standing on one leg are screening tests for higher-functioning individuals in the community; if unable to perform, at risk for falls at home (J Am Geriatr Soc 1986;34:119)

Gait: See Table 1-1. 6% of F >65, 38% >85; 63% NH residents have gait abnormality (J Am Geriatr Soc 1996;44:434); timed 8-foot walk and other lower extremity function tests predict mobility-related ADL disability in 4 yr (Nejm 1995;332:556); NH pt's self-selected gait speed and perception of physical disability are predictive of functional loss (J Am Geriatr Soc 1995;43:93); comfortable walking speed better predictor than treadmill test of cardiac status in pts w CHF; changes w normal aging: broader-based, smaller steps, diminished arm swing, stooped posture, slower turning

Step height:
- Frontal lobe gait: seen in vascular dementia, most common gait abnormality: wide-based, slightly flexed, small shuffling steps,

Table 1-1. Tinetti Gait Assessment

Gait Abnormality	Type of Gait	Description	Etiology	Dx/Rx
Step height/length	Spastic	Wide-based, slightly flexed, small shuffling steps, hesitant steps, can't initiate step, "glued to floor," Circumduction, scrape foot along floor, hand-arm spasticity	Vascular dementia Stroke	Trochanteric pads decrease hip fx Surgery
	NPH	Bilateral circumduction, sometimes increase urinary frequency and urgency Short steps, decreased velocity of stride length and associated shoulder movements, increased sway, poor balance, difficulty turning	Spinal stenosis	Surgery Shunt
	Parkinson's	Lacks arm swing, turn en bloc (moves whole body when turns), hesitation, gets stuck while walking especially in open spaces like doorways, festination		Front-wheeled walker
	Steppage	W foot slap	Seen in distal motor neuropathies	Foot orthotics
Path deviation	Vestibular	Broad-based foot stamping, pt looks at feet Unsteady on one side and then the other	Sensory ataxia Peripheral neuropathy	Pos Rhomberg/ position/ vibration sensitivity at ankle
	Weakness	Slow unsteady swagger, use furniture to grab onto when walking	Deconditioning	Atrophy, 2/5 strength
Postural sway	Cerebellar	Wide-based, irregular, unsteady, veering, truncal titubation	MS	
	Waddling	Broad based	Seen with severe arthritis, myositis, PMR	
	Antalgic	Seen with arthritis of hip when cane held incorrectly on same side Throwing trunk out over affected hip, resulting in stress on hip and low back		Analgesics, hip replacement
	Hysterical	Hemiparesis without circumduction, hemiparetic arm normal during walking, good strength lying down but ataxia when walking, staggering a long time to get to opposite wall, tightrope walking, pt drags person assisting them down to the ground		Reassurance

hesitant steps, can't initiate step; "glued to floor" (Nejm 1990;322:1441)

- Spastic gait: seen in stroke w circumduction, scrape foot along floor, hand–arm spasticity; also seen w cervical stenosis and myopathy w bilateral circumduction; sometimes increased urinary frequency and urgency (J Am Geriatr Soc 1996;44:434)
- Parkinsonian gait: lacks arm swing, turns en bloc (moves whole body when turns), hesitation, gets stuck while walking ("freezing"), especially in open spaces like doorways, festination (involuntary increase in speed of walking in attempt to catch up with displaced center of gravity forward), 4th most common gait abnormality
- NPH: short steps, decreased velocity of stride length and associated shoulder movements, increased sway, poor balance, difficulty turning; overlap between NPH and vascular etiologies, eg, hydrocephalus from stroke may account for similar gait abnormalities (J Am Geriatr Soc 1996;44:434)
- Steppage gait w foot slap: seen in distal motor neuropathies

Path deviation: observe from behind, one foot at a time in relation to midline; abnormal path deviation in:

- Vestibular gait: seen with sensory ataxia; 2nd most common gait abnormality, broad-based, foot stamping, pt looks at feet; and peripheral neuropathy gait; 3rd most common, unsteady on one side and then the other, Romberg (pt unable to maintain balance w eyes closed)
- Muscle weakness, slow unsteady swagger, grabs onto furniture when walking

Postural sway: observe from behind for truncal side-to-side motion; w:

- Cerebellar gait: 5th most common gait disturbance, wide-based, irregular, unsteady, veering, truncal titubation (shimmying of thorax with respect to the rest of the body)
- Antalgic gait: seen with arthritis of hip when cane held incorrectly on same side, throwing trunk out over affected hip resulting in stress on hip and low back (J Am Geriatr Soc 1996;44:434; Ger Med Today 1985;4:47)
- Waddling gait: broad-based, seen with severe arthritis, myositis, PMR
- Hysterical gait: hemiparesis without circumduction, hemiparetic arm normal during walking, good strength lying down but ataxia

when walking, staggering, takes a long time to get to opposite wall, gait resembles attempts at tightrope walking, pt drags person assisting them down to the ground, not known to occur in pts >70 yr (J Am Geriatr Soc 1996;44:434)

Cmplc: Clustering of falls associated with high 6-mo mortality (Age Aging 1977;6:201), 6% fracture some bone, of these one-fourth fx hip (J Am Geriatr Soc 1995;43:1146); 2% of injurious falls are fatal, of those 13% die from pulmonary embolus; white M 85 yr and older have highest rate of deaths attributable to falls, exceeding 180/100,000 population (Ann Rev Publ Hlth 1992;13:489); 5% serious soft tissue injury (Nejm 1988;319:1701)

Prolonged lies while waiting for help (<10% of falls) if >1 h may cause dehydration, pressure sores, rhabdomyolysis, pneumonia (Jama 1993;268:65)

25% of fallers subsequently avoid ADLs, IADLs, and AADLs for fear of falling again (J Gerontol 1994;49:M140; Nejm 1988;319:1701)

NH admissions (Nejm 1997;337:1279; Am J Publ Hlth 1992;82:395):

Increased use of health care services (Med Care 1992;30:587); approximately 50% pts that are hospitalized for falls may end up in NHs (Emerg Med Clin N Am 1990;8:309)

Lab: Routine w/u: CBC w differential, UA, chem screen, stool guaiacs, TSH, vit B_{12}, and ESR (r/o PMR), EKG, CXR, and/or CT as hx indicates

Noninvasive: No need for Holter monitor; prevalence of ventricular arrhythmia is 82% in both fallers and non-fallers; no sx reported with these arrhythmias (J Am Geriatr Soc 1989;37:430)

Rx:

Prevention:

Programs reduce falls by one-third (Jama 1997;278:557; Nejm 1994;331:821)

- Assessing falls in elderly (J Am Geriatr Soc 1993;41:309,315,479): Medicare allowable charges for the evaluation of falls: CBC, EKG, MRI, neurologic, orthopedic, physical therapy consultation, safety and functional evaluation of pt's home (Jama 1996;276:59); w questionnaire assess those at risk of immobility because of fear of falling (J Gerontol Med Sci 1995;45:239); patient education sheet (Am Fam Phys 1997;56:1815)
- Minimizing number of meds and using lowest possible doses

- Estrogen replacement: for treating osteoporosis (Am J Med 1993;95:75S; Nejm 1993;329:1141; also see 10.1 Osteoporosis)
- Exercise programs (Nejm 1994;330:1769; J Am Geriatr Soc 2001;49:10) to increase muscle strength and flexibility (J Am Geriatr Soc 1996;44:513; FICSIT trials, in Jama 1995;273:1341)
  - Resistance training: to improve weakness, which may be more of a limiting factor than endurance (J Am Geriatr Soc 1994;42:937)
  - Flexibility programs: to increase range of motion for tight hip flexors common in thoracic kyphosis, tightness in hip abductors and adductors
  - Balance and gait training: especially getting in and out of chairs, turning around; NH standard physical therapy is of moderate benefit (Jama 1994;271:519); perturbation training (pushes in different directions to stimulate postural responses) more useful in community setting
  - Endurance training: to help compensate for extra energy cost that gait dysfunctions impose; using crutches requires 60% more energy than normal walking; 3-wk bed rest decreases Vo_2 max by 27%
- Tai Chi: cardiorespiratory function better among older Tai Chi practitioners (J Am Geriatr Soc 1995;43:1222); Tai Chi decreases falls (Phys Ther 1999;77:371; J Am Geriatr Soc 1996;44:489,498)
- Assistive aids: 23% of noninstitutionalized elderly use assistive aids; of those who use assistive aids, 49% use a cane (70% use incorrectly), 24% use a walker, 12% use a wheelchair (Natl Ctr Hlth Stat 1992;217:1)
- Trochanteric pads: decrease hip fractures (Nejm 2000;343: 1506,1562; Jama 1994;271:128), facilitate compliance w graduated implementation; pts are more likely to wear them if the trochanteric pads are only worn at pt-specified limited time periods (J Am Geriatr Soc 1993;41:338)
- Neck collars for vertebral insufficiency (Rubenstein 1996)
- Proper shoes: high-heel shoes decrease balance in elderly women (J Am Geriatr Soc 1996;44:434)
- Chairs, toilet seats should have arm rests and increased seat height
- Obstacle-free, glare-free, adequately lit environment
- Avoid physical and pharmacologic restraints (Ann IM 1992;116:369; Jama 1991;265:468), fewer serious injuries in hospital without bedrails (J Am Geriatr Soc 1999;47:529); alternatives: special areas for walking, lower beds, floor pads, alarm systems (Am Fam Phys

1992;45:763), surveillance by staff; avoid sleep meds w potential for falls: instead tape player w headphones w tapes of favorite music, talking books, and family messages; table containing diversionary activity, eg, meal, playing cards, to encourage sitting instead of wandering (Ann LT Care 1999;7:17); hospital alternatives: use of family visitors, professional sitters, lower beds, "functional" ICUs

1.3 GERIATRIC PHARMACOLOGY

Mayo Clin Proc 1995;70:685

Underused Drugs: β-blockers s/p MI (Ann IM 1999;130:897; Jama 1999;282:113; Lancet 1999;353:955; Jama 1998;280:623; Nejm 1998;339:489; Jama 1997;277:115); HRT (Jama 1999;282:113; 1997;277:1140)

Overused Chronically Administered Drugs: TNG patches and paste, isosorbide dinitrate, sleeping meds, antipsychotics for dementia, antidepressants, digoxin, diuretics, antihypertensives, antiepileptics, laxatives and vitamins, NSAIDs, H_2 blockers, and sucralfate (Nurs Home Med 1995;3:254); 10% of all elderly hospitalizations are due to adverse drug reactions (Ann IM 1992;117:634); most common drug–drug interactions causing side effects leading to hospitalization are diuretics, benzodiazepines, ACE inhibitors (J Am Geriatr Soc 1996;44:944; Ann IM 1995;123:195); see Table 1-2 for other serious drug adverse reactions

Pharmacokinetics:

Absorption: Absorption of ciprofloxacin eliminated by concomitant administration of antacids or sucralfate; omeprazole inhibits cyanocobalamin absorption

Distribution: Pts taking interacting meds or with low albumin states such as renal failure, and malnutrition may show evidence of toxicity despite normal serum levels, eg, nystagmus w phenytoin; warfarin displaced and therefore potentiated by allopurinol, metronidazole (Flagyl), Tm/S (Bactrim); phenytoin (Dilantin) potentiated by INH, benzodiazepines, phenothiazine; increase in plasma B_1-acid glycoprotein leads to increased protein binding of basic drugs, thereby decreasing amount of free active drug, eg, lidocaine and propranolol

Table 1-2. Drugs Inappropriate for the Elderly

All new ORDERS or all NEW ADMITS: The physician is required to change the following drugs to alternate therapies OR document benefit vs risk.

Drug	Adverse Outcome	Alternate Therapy
Pentazocine	CNS effects (confusion/hallucinations)	Another narcotic analgesic
LA Benzos (1)	Sedation/increase falls/fx	SA benzodiazepines
Amitriptyline (2)	Anticholinergic (sedation, constipation, dry mouth . . .)	SSRI, Effexor, Serzone
Doxepin	" "	" " "
Meprobamate	Addictive, extremely sedating	Other anxiolytic/hypnotic
Disopyramide	Increased effect of heart contraction	Other antiarrhythmic
Dig >0.125 mg (3)	N/V, visual disturbances, CNS, fatigue	Low dose or monitor levels
Methyldopa	Bradycardia and depression	Other antihypertensives
Chlorpropamide	Increased risk of hypoglycemia	Other oral hypoglycemic
GI Antispas (4)	Highly anticholinergic	Use only if benefit > risk
Barbiturates	Addictive, extremely sedating	Trazodone
Meperidine	Not effective orally, resp. depression	Other narcotic
Ticlopidine (5)	Neutropenia, N/V, rash, not > ASA	Plavix

1. Flurazepam, Chlordiazepoxide, Clorazepate, Diazepam, Clonazepam
2. Amitriptyline OK to use for neurogenic pain—must document
3. Digoxin OK at higher doses if afib present
4. Dicyclomine, Hyoscyamine (Levsin), Propantheline, Belladonna Alkaloids, Clindinium, Chlordiazepoxide
5. Ticlodipine OK if pt has had previous stroke precursors (TIA); can't tolerate ASA

Adipose tissue proportion increases from 18% to 36% (M) and from 36% to 48% (F); total body water decreases by 15% from ages 20 to 80 yr; therefore, increase in volume of distribution of lipophilic drugs, eg, sedative hypnotics, and decrease in hydrophilic drugs, eg, digoxin, aminoglycoside, penicillins

Excretion: Decrease in renal blood flow 1%/yr after age 50, GFR decreased by 35% between 3rd and 10th decades of life
Creatinine Clearance:

Cr Clearance = [(140 − age) × weight in kg]/serum Cr × 72
(× 0.85 if woman)

If <30, cut the drug dose by half; digoxin toxicity not always recognized in the elderly so imperative to base dose on Cr clearance (J Am Geriatr Soc 1996;44:54); can either lengthen drug interval or decrease dose (Drugs 1994;48:380):

Drug interval = (nl Cr clearance/pt's Cr clearance) × nl interval

Drug dose = (pt's Cr clearance/nl Cr clearance) × nl dose

Measured Cr clearance may be better than estimated in higher-functioning elderly (J Am Geriatr Soc 1993;41:716); drug levels should be drawn just prior to scheduled dose after 3–5 half-lives of dosing; aminoglycoside may have same efficacy w once daily dosage (Clin Infect Dis 2000;30:433)

Metabolism:

Drugs requiring phase 1 (oxidation, reduction, hydrolysis), eg, diazepam (Valium), lidocaine, isosorbide, are affected by decreased enzymatic activity of P450 with aging (Med Let 1999;41:59); phase 2 (conjugation), eg, oxazepam (Serax), lorazepam (Ativan), metabolism is not affected by aging (Fig 1-1) (Med Let 1996;38:75)

More adverse drug interactions when renally excreted drugs used simultaneously, eg, digoxin not cleared when given with quinidine or verapamil; lithium not cleared when given with NSAIDs or thiazides; types of renal-drug interactions: 1) allergic is not dose-related and takes weeks to resolve, eg, methicillin, ACE

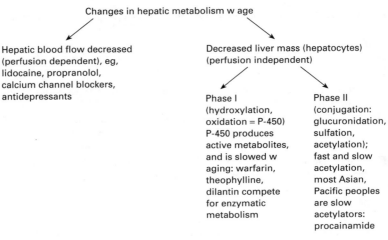

Changes in hepatic metabolism w age

Hepatic blood flow decreased (perfusion dependent), eg, lidocaine, propranolol, calcium channel blockers, antidepressants

Decreased liver mass (hepatocytes) (perfusion independent)

Phase I (hydroxylation, oxidation = P-450) P-450 produces active metabolites, and is slowed w aging: warfarin, theophylline, dilantin compete for enzymatic metabolism

Phase II (conjugation: glucuronidation, sulfation, acetylation); fast and slow acetylation, most Asian, Pacific peoples are slow acetylators: procainamide

Figure 1-1. Changes in hepatic metabolism with age.

inhibitors, NSAIDs, trimethoprim, cimetidine; 2) hemodynamic is dose-related and takes days to resolve, eg, anti-inflammatory drugs, ACE inhibitors; 3) toxic is dose-related and takes weeks to resolve, eg, gentamicin, phenacetin, lithium; 4) pseudo azotemia is dose-related and takes days to resolve, eg, trimethoprim, cimetidine (Am J Kidney Dis 1996;27:162)

Drug–Drug Interactions (Ger Rev Syllabus 1999–2001:33)
- Tricyclic antidepressants and type I antiarrhythmics have potentially fatal interactions
- Warfarin interacts with many drugs
- Erythromycin may raise levels of theophylline and digoxin
- IV contrast is contraindicated for patients who have taken metformin
- Quinidine raises serum levels of digoxin
- Selegiline taken with some antidepressants can cause severe delirium
- Statins may interact with other lipid-lowering drugs (eg, gemfibrozil, niacin) to cause rhabdomyolysis
- Sucralfate interferes with absorption of quinolones

Pharmacodynamics:
- Decreased receptor response: decreased effect of adrenergic medications, eg, α-adrenergic agonists, α-adrenergic blockers
- Increased receptor response: increased effect of opiates, eg, morphine, and increased effect of benzodiazepines, eg, diazepam; clonazepam 0.5 mg hs and increase by 0.5 mg q 1–2 wk (drug half-life 48 h) and assess pt's gait; alternative pain therapies: topical therapy: add capsaicin cream 0.25–0.75%, lower potency for first 2 wk then switch to higher potency, may tolerate better if applied w lidocaine ointment 2.5–5.0% for first few days of treatment, may interfere with substance P (Life Sci 1979;25:1273), reduces tenderness and pain with only adverse effect of localized transient burning (Ann IM 1994;121:133; J Rheum 1992;19:604); consider neural blockade after all else fails

Pain: (Management of cancer pain, AHCPR Pub. No. 94-0592, 1992; Storey P. Primer of palliative care. 2nd ed. Gainesville, FL: American Academy of Hospice and Palliative Medicine, 1996; "Pain management" in Kemp C. Terminal illness: a guide to nursing care. 2nd ed. Philadelphia: Lippincott, 1999:122
- Midrin, sumatriptan safer for migraines than ergots
- Acetaminophen <4 gm d can cause hepatotoxicity in the elderly (Ger Rev Syllabus 1999–2001:255)

Table 1-3. Dosage Conversion: Oral Morphine to Transdermal Fentanyl

Oral Morphine (mg/24 h)	Transdermal fentanyl (μg/h)
45–134	25
135–224	50
225–314	75
315–404	100
◆	◆
◆	◆
◆	◆
1035–1124	300

Source: Janssen Pharmaceutica.

- Postherpetic neuralgia with constant pain: nortriptyline or desipramine 12.5–25.0 mg increased q 2–3 d in 10-mg increments as tolerated and if no benefit switch to nortriptyline or maprotiline and if still no benefit, add anticonvulsant; lancinating pain: carbamazepine 150 mg/d or alternative anticonvulsant, may add antidepressant
- Opioids for severe pain (Med Let Drugs Ther 1993;35:1): See Tables 1-3 and 1-4; morphine sulfate for cancer or postop pain; pain despite >12 mg/d, switch to 10 mg liquid morphine sulfate q 4 h with rescue dose (one-half regular q 4 h dose q 2–3 h); slow-release morphine q 12 h must be accompanied by immediate-release morphine for breakthrough pain (one-sixth to one-third of slow-release dose (sl, po, or pr); drowsiness occurs within first few hours of therapy, onset unlikely after this period; tolerance requires weeks to months of continuous administration, and may not develop in some pts; respiratory depression unlikely to develop if none present in 2–3 d; monitor sleep respiratory rate, if does not fall below 12 breaths/min when dose increased, will not develop respiratory depression; physical or psychological dependence does not occur early in its administration; bisphosphonates good adjuvant analgesic; pts get equally confused after the administration of epidural or general anesthesia (Jama 1995;274:44)
- To convert oral narcotic to equivalent morphine sulfate po multiply by 0.15 for propoxyphene, 0.2 for meperidine, 0.3 for codeine, 0.5 for pentazocine, 2 for oxycodone, 3 for methadone, 8 for hydromorphone; to convert im narcotic to equivalent morphine sulfate po multiply by 1.5 for pentazocine, 6 for methadone, 40 for

Table 1-4. Commonly Prescribed Opioids (Oral and Transdermal)

Drug	Approximate Equianalgesic Dose	Usual Starting Dose for Moderate to Severe Pain
Opioid alone		
Morphine	30 mg q 3–4 h (repeat around the clock) 60 mg q 3–4 h (single dose or intermittent dosing)	0.3 mg/kg q 3–4 h
Morphine controlled release (MS Contin, Oramorph)	90–120 mg q 12 h	N/A
Transdermal fentanyl	25–75 µg/h q 72 h	N/A
Hydromorphone (Dilaudid)	7.5 mg q 3–4 h	0.06 mg/kg q 3–4 h
Combination opioid preparations		
Codeine (with aspirin or acetaminophen)	180–200 mg q 3–4 h	0.5–1 mg/kg q 3–4 h
Hydrocodone (in Lorcet, Lortab, Vicodin, etc.)	30 mg q 3–4 h	0.2 mg/kg q 3–4 h
Oxycodone (Roxicodone, also in Percocet, Percodan, Tylox, others)	30 mg q 3–4 h	0.2 mg/kg q 3–4 h

Adapted from Agency for Health Care Policy and Research. Management of Cancer Pain. Clinical Practice Guideline No. 9. AHCPR Pub No. 94-0592. March 1994:54.

hydromorphone, 3 for morphine sulfate, 0.8 for meperidine, 30 for butorphanol (Ger Rev Syllabus 1996:179)
- Ketamine IV for cancer patients unresponsive to morphine (Anesthesiology 1999;90:1528)

Management of Opioid-Induced Constipation (Nejm 1996;335:1124): *Prevention:* 100 mg docusate sodium plus 17.2 mg sennosides po bid; 10 mg bisacodyl po hs if no BM in past 24 hours, repeat in morning if no BM; *titration:* 100–200 mg docusate plus 34.4 mg sennosides po tid; 15 mg bisacodyl po tid; *obstipation:* 30–60 mL MOM + 30 mL mineral oil bid; 30–60 mL lactulose qid

Herbs: See Table 1-5.

Vitamins: 1–6 gm vit C reduces cold sx by 21% and shortens course by 1 d

Vitamin E boosts immune system response in elderly (Jama 1997;277:1380)

Table 1-5. Controversial Uses of Herbs

Potentially Beneficial Herbs	Potentially Dangerous Herbs
Chamomile: digestion	Chaparral: hepatitis
Echinacea: immunity booster	Comfrey: liver toxicity
Feverfew (0.2% parthenolide): migraine	Ephedra: raises BP, palpitations
Garlic: cholesterol	Lobela: acts like nicotine
Ginger: nausea, motion sickness	Yohimbine: weakness, nervous
Ginkgo biloba: helps w dementia (24% ginkgo flavone glycosides, 6% ginkgolides and bilobalide) 30–40 mg tid × 4–6 wk (Lancet 1992;340:1136)	stimulation
Hawthorn: HT and angina	
Mild thistle: liver damage	
Saw palmetto: enlarged prostate (Med Let 1999;41:15)	
Valerian: mild sedating and tranquilizing effect (Ann LT Care 1999;7:19)	

From Shimonura SK, UCLA Intensive course in Geriatric Medicine and Board Review 1/96.

Folic acid for vascular dementia prevention (Arch Neurol 1998; 55:1449)

Zinc improved cell-mediated response especially for chronic infection (J Am Geriatr Soc 1998;46:19)

Hormone Replacement Therapy (J Am Geriatr Soc 1996;44:1; Nejm 1997;336:1769; 1994;330:1062; Obgyn 1994;83:161; J Am Geriatr Soc 1993;41:426: also see 8.2 Coronary Artery Disease, 10.1 Osteoporosis)

Estrogen: Conjugated 0.625 mg/d or 0.5 mg/d micronized estradiol or 2.0 mg/d estradiol valerate or estropipate 0.625 mg or transdermal estradiol 0.05 or 5.0 qd plus cyclic medroxyprogesterone acetate 5.0–10.0 (d 1–12 or 1–14), or continuous w medroxyprogesterone acetate 2.5 or 5.0

Evaluation of postmenopausal bleeding: Endometrial bx for bleeding, manage by switching to continuous-combined regimen: increase progesterone by 2.5 mg until amenorrhea or adverse effects occur, if sx persist >10 mo (28% of pts), then perform bx (Ann IM 1992;117:1038); if no atypia on bx specimen, increase progesterone, eg, 10 mg/d for 14 d of the mo for 6 mo; if atypia present, dilatation and curettage indicated (Mayo Clin Proc 1995;70:803)

25% of estrogen prescriptions remain unfilled

Alternatives to Estrogen: Megestrol acetate (Megace): progesterone agent, decreases hot flashes (Nejm 1995;332:1638,1889; 1994;331:347); micronized progesterone helps w insomnia (Med Clin N Am 1995;79:1337); phytoestrogens (Obgyn 1996;87:897) in high-soy diet of Japanese women associated w infrequent hot flashes and other menopausal sx (Lancet 1992;339:1233); 1/2 cup soybeans = 200 mg isoflavone/d (~0.3 mg conjugated steroidal estrogen)

1.4 URINARY TRACT COLONIZATION/INFECTION

J Am Geriatr Soc 1996;44:927,1235; Ann IM 1990;150:1389; Clin Ger Med 1990;6:1

Cause: *Escherichia coli* predominant pathogen (50%) in elderly; instrumentation and institutionalization lead to *Proteus mirabilis, Klebsiella, Enterobacter, Serratia,* and *Pseudomonas aeruginosa*; 25% of elderly with urinary catheters have enterococci in urine; coagulase-neg staphylococci in ambulatory elderly; resistant organisms, eg, *Citrobacter freundii, Providencia stuartii*

Epidem: F/M = 2:1; UTIs cause 30–50% of all bacteremia and septicemia; catheter bacteriuria increases by 3–10%/d; bacteriuria increased in NH (33%) secondary to immobility, DM, fecal/urinary incontinence, deteriorating mental status

Pathophys: Attachment of bacteria to epithelial cells of the bladder is promoted by the changing hormonal status of the elderly pt, BPH, prostatic or renal stone formation, a decrease in bacteriostatic prostatic secretions, increased vaginal pH, decreased lactobacillus, anatomic weakening of pelvic floor; MS, DM, CVA, Alzheimer cause impaired bladder emptying, bacterial colonization; fecal incontinence causes retrograde colonization

Sx: Dysuria, fever, urinary urgency, frequency, hematuria, suprapubic discomfort are UTI-specific sx; nonspecific sx of UTI much more frequent, eg, change in mental status, change in functional capacity, acute-onset incontinence, decreased appetite, weakness, falls, hypotension, abdominal pain, nausea and vomiting, increased blood sugar in diabetics; must have specific or nonspecific sx before beginning treatment

Si: Foul-smelling urine more indicative of dehydration than UTI (Nurs Home Med 1997;5:101)

Crs:

Uncomplicated (first infection): Infrequent UTIs (separated by at least 2–3 mo) occurring in a functionally independent, community-based elder with no hx of gu complications and improving within 24–48 h of beginning therapy

Complicated: Hospitalized pt, or recurrent UTIs (separated by 4 wk), recent instrumentation, or GU complications; relapsing infection (separated by 2 wk; bacterial persistence) less common, r/o stones, chronic prostatitis (positive UA after prostatic massage), pyelonephritis, and fistulas

Cmplc: Sepsis, chronic pyelonephritis, incontinence

Lab: Clean-catch UA: combined pos reading for nitrates, leukocyte esterase highly predictive of a UTI; whether to culture if UA pos debatable; replace catheter to obtain fresh specimen

Xray: Bladder US for PVR; renal US if suspect chronic pyelonephritis, obstruction

Rx: Rx of asx bacteriuria not shown to decrease morbidity or mortality

Preventive: Indwelling catheter when:

1. Retention unmanageable surgically
2. Risk of wound infection from incontinence high
3. Terminally ill pt w pain on movement w change of clothes
4. Pt preference when not responding to other incontinence therapy
5. Bacteriuria 48 h after short-term catheter: rx as sx UTI

Cranberry juice 300 mL/d × 6 mo to acidify urine (Jama 1994;271:751), 2 gm vit C; separating patients w indwelling catheters in NH in different rooms reduces risk of UTI (J Hosp Infect 1997;36:147)

Suppress recurrent infections (>3/yr) or w h/o urosepsis: TMP/SM2 (1 tab qd in M and one-half tab in F) and continue as long as UA neg; may use nitrofurantoin in this setting as well; intravaginal estrogen decreases pH, reducing colonization w gram-neg bacilli (Nejm 1993;329:753)

Therapeutic: Treat symptomatic bacteriuria × 7–10 d in F, × 14 d in M; rx nonspecific sx at first occurrence; if sx do not respond to rx, sx may not be indicative of UTI; rx asymptomatic bacteriuria in pts with h/o short-term catheters, urinary manipulation, and instrumentation (Arch IM 1990;150:1389)

Uncomplicated: Tm/S or amoxicillin, if resistance is suspected or
drug allergy exists, use a quinolone (ciprofloxacin or levofloxacin
250–500 mg qd); replace catheter

Complicated: Stable outpatient or NH pt: start with a quinolone and
change to narrower-spectrum drug once sensitivities have returned;
× 14 d for T° > 101 degrees for upper UTI; replace catheter

Unstable: NH pt: ampicillin and ceftriaxone im q 12–24 h in NH,
remove and replace catheters; hospitalized pt: ampicillin and
gentamicin IV, vancomycin and gentamicin IV, fluoroquinolones
and ampicillin IV, 3rd-generation cephalosporin or aztreonam IV
(Nurs Home Med 1997;5:100); chronic bacterial prostatitis: Tm/S
or quinolone × 4 wk; linezolid (Zyvox) po bid × 10 d for VRE or
MRSA, vancomycin for MRSA

0.5 mg Estriol at hs × 2 wk, then 2/wk × 8 mo decreases recurrent
UTI without risk to endometrium (Nurs Home Med 1998;6:77)

Yeast usually represents colonization unless in acute care setting
(J Am Geriatr Soc 1998;46:849)

1.5 CONSTIPATION

Mayo Clin Proc 1996;71:81; J Am Geriatr Soc 1994;42:701;
1993;41:1130; Geriatrics 1989;44:53

Cause:

Primary: Slowed colonic transit; pelvic floor dysfunction (J Am Geriatr
Soc 2000;48:1142); decrease in large-bowel motility due to decreased
fiber, decreased fluid, immobility, laxative abuse

Secondary:
- Neurologic: CNS central lesions, Parkinson, CVA, dementia
- Obstructive (more common): colonic-anorectal disorders
  (diverticula, irritable bowel, megacolon, hemorrhoids, strictures,
  polyps, colorectal cancer)
- Metabolic: constipation can be first sign of DM, hypothyroid,
  hypercalcemia, heavy metal intoxication, hyper/hypoparathyroidism,
  hypokalemia
- Drugs: Fe-containing rx, anticholinergics, calcium channel blockers
  (verapamil), antipsychotics, diuretics, narcotics, antiparkinsonian
  medications

Epidem: Most common digestive complaint, subjective nature of the complaint makes accurate determination of the prevalence of true constipation difficult; 10% for those >75 yrs (Gerontol Clin 1972;14:56); 30–50% of elders use laxatives regularly

Pathophys:

Definitions:

- Functional constipation: for at least 12 not necessarily consecutive weeks: straining >25% of time, or hard stools >25% of time, or feeling of incomplete evacuation >25% of time, or <3 BMs/wk or sense of anorectal obstruction in >25% of BMs, or manual aid to facilitate >25% of BMs, or hard or lumpy stools >25% BMs; loose stool should not be present—no sx of irritable bowel syndrome
- Rectal outlet delay (prolonged defecation secondary to anorectal dysfunction): anal blockage and prolonged defecation or manual disimpaction needed (Gastroenterol Int 1991;4:99)

  Frail/institutionalized pts w increased total gut transit time develop colonic dilatation due to decrease in intraluminal pressures; increased gut transit time also caused by a disruption in coordinated segmental motion of the colonic circular smooth muscle, impaired rectal sensation and tone; also rectal dyschezia or increased rectal tone (irritable bowel syndrome); weakening of abdominal muscles and decreased external and internal anal sphincter tone

Sx: Change in usual bowel frequency (<3 BMs/wk); straining with evacuation and prolonged defecation (10 min or more for completion of BM); sense of incomplete defecation; fecal soiling and/or fecal incontinence; abdominal distension and discomfort; need for manual disimpaction

Si: Diminished bowel sounds; lax abdominal musculature; masses in sigmoid, transverse, and descending colon; decreased rectal tone; decreased perianal sensation and anal reflex; presence of hard stool in rectal vault (empty vault common and does not preclude a high impaction); soft stool impacted in rectal vault may indicate rectal dysfunction; masses, hemorrhoids, fissures, oozing stool (overflow diarrhea); distended abdomen; nausea/vomiting; hard stool in rectum or colon; chronic or semi-acute dehydration with tenting of skin

Crs: May be chronic or acute; r/o irritable bowel syndrome (usually associated with a long hx of bowel disorders, "gas problems," abdominal pain relieved by defecation, and alternation between constipation and diarrhea); colorectal cancer w obstruction, anal fissure, rectal ischemia, and anorectal tumor may be associated with rectal pain on defecation

Cmplc: Cardiovascular (angina, MI, arrhythmias); megacolon (volvulus of sigmoid, cecal rupture); rectal prolapse; fecal incontinence (UTIs and sepsis, decubitus ulcers); hemorrhoids; laxative abuse

Lab: Fasting glucose, TSH (r/o hypothyroidism), calcium, potassium, BUN, Cr, guaiac stool, urine specific gravity, heavy metal screen

Xray: Flat plate of abdomen to r/o impaction; barium studies not recommended due to barium retention; colonoscopy if colonic cancer is suspected (anemia, family hx, or guaiac-pos stools) (Mayo Clin Proc 1996;71:81)

Rx:

Preventive: Increase fluid intake to 1200–2000 mL/d; then increase fiber intake (dietary fiber or OTC supplements, eg, Citrucel; psyllium)— must take at least 1200 mL fluid/d if using fiber supplementation; begin regular exercise program; adjust toileting schedule to coincide with natural urge to defecate; consider morning coffee or tea; avoid meds that lead to constipation; avoid routine use of stimulant laxatives

Therapeutic: Initiate preventive regime, as above; increase fiber (Citrucel) 1 tsp up to tid except if pt is bedridden, has <1000 mL fluid intake/d, or has a hx of megacolon or volvulus

For slow transit: use laxatives in increasing order of strength as follows: sorbitol 15–30 mL qd to tid; MOM 15–30 mL qd or bid (contraindicated in moderate renal insufficiency); Senokot 1–2 qhs 3 ×/wk or qhs (for maintenance); bisacodyl 10-mg supplement up to 3 ×/wk; for rectal dyschezia: glycerin supplement 3 ×/wk or up to qd; tap water enema, 500 mL, as needed; mineral oil enema, 100–250 mL, qd

For fecal impaction: digital disimpaction followed by oil retention enemas and subsequent tap water enemas qd until clear; follow with cathartics to cleanse colon; senna 30 mg up to tid and sorbitol 30 mL up to tid; if large fecal load still present (but without obstruction) give 1–2 L polyethylene glycol (GoLYTELY)

When abdominal xray is clear of impaction, begin maintenance bowel regime as above; stool softeners, eg, docusate sodium (Colace), only when straining is to be avoided (post-MI, angina, hemorrhoids, post-surgery); always avoid use of highly irritant laxatives, eg, phenolphthalein (Ex-Lax, Correctol)

Team Management: Nursing staff, family assist pt to upright commode when urge to defecate occurs; osteopathic maneuvers: sacral rocking (gentle pressure on sacrum w inspiration while pt prone)

1.6 MALNUTRITION

Ger Rev Syllabus 1996:145–151; Rueben D, Nutritional problems and assessment, UCLA intensive geriatric review course, 1/19/96; Nurs Home Med 1994;2:206; J Am Geriatr Soc 1995;43:415; Geriatrics 1990;45:7

Cause: Inadequate intake, inadequate dentition, poverty and inadequate range of food groups, malabsorption, nutrient–drug interactions, chronic disease, or acute insult; taste decreased secondary to decreased olfaction w age (J Gerontol 1986;41:460)

Dehydration: reduced access to fluids, decreased thirst perception, reduced response to serum osmolality, decreased ability to concentrate urine following fluid deprivation

Epidem: Malnutrition occurs in 37–40% of community elderly, 35–65% of hospitalized elderly, 19–58% of institutionalized elderly (Nurs Home Med 1994;2:206)

Sx: Nutritional hx from the pt or caregiver regarding eating preferences, restrictions, and allergies; use of mineral/vit supplements and nonprescription meds; taste change, chewing, swallowing problems, nausea/vomiting/diarrhea

Si: D-E-N-T-A-L Screening Survey (J Am Geriatr Soc 1996;44:980):
Dry mouth
Eating difficulty
No recent dental care
Tooth or mouth pain
Alteration or change in food selection
Lesions, sores, or lumps in the mouth
Changes seen in nutritional deficiencies may be mistaken for changes occurring with aging on screening exam (brittle hair and nails, sunken eyes, pale sclerae, prominence of the bony skeleton, especially the extremities and chest); may also see cracked lips, sores around the mouth, poor dentition, magenta tongue, muscle wasting, peripheral edema, blunted mental status

Height and weight most reliable of the anthropomorphic measurements; assess ability to self-feed; when intake is difficult to assess or is obviously poor, obtain a 24–72 h calorie count (in NH 2 wk after admission, allowing the pt to settle into environment)

Meds that interfere w vits:

Trimethoprim and phenytoin interfere w folate

Cholestyramine, mineral oil, and neomycin interfere w vit A absorption, causing night blindness

Hydralazine is a vit B_6 antagonist; INH increases vit B_6 urinary excretion

Lab: Assess the severity of weight loss by determining the ratio of the pt's ABW to IBW; for M calculated at 106 lb for the first 5 feet and 6 lb for each inch above 5 feet; for F it is 100 lb for the first 5 feet and 5 lb for each inch above 5 feet

Knee height measurements, arm span, or summation of body part measurements may be used to accurately assess height in pts who are unable to stand erect (Gottschlich M, Matavese L, Shronts EP, eds. Nutrition support dietetics core curriculum, 2nd ed. Silver Spring, MD: American Society of Parenteral and Enteral Nutrition, 1993:44); take into account ethnic variation and compare to other family members; ABW is affected by hydration status and thus dehydration should be r/o before other causes of weight loss investigated

Significant weight loss: 2% in 1 wk or 5% in 1 mo; 7.5% in 3 mo; 10% decrease in weight from the UBW in 6 mo

Crs: Vit B_1, vit C become deficient over wk to mo while fat-soluble vit (A, D, E, K) take longer because of enterohepatic circulation; obesity about the waist and abdomen increases free fatty acids in the portal system leading to increased lipid production and CAD

Cmplc: Pressure sore formation, compromised immune function, increased rate of infection, longer recuperation periods, and consequent loss of independence

Rx:

Prevention: Older pts trying to gain weight require 30–35 kcal/kg IBW; check lytes prior to aggressive nutritional support; if tube feeding indicated, start at 20 kcal/kg IBW and slowly advance to 30–35 kcal/kg IBW; energy needs for pts whose weight is <76% of IBW should be calculated using ABW, not IBW which could result in an overestimate of caloric requirements, extreme fluid, and lyte shifts

Estimate protein needs using albumin levels; albumin has half-life of 21 d, reflects previous protein expenditure due to a number of causes, eg, liver disease, infection, nephrotic syndrome, postop states, inadequate intake and malabsorption; dehydration may falsely elevate albumin; albumin levels of 3.1–3.5 gm/dL indicate mild depletion; 2.6–3.1 gm/dL moderate depletion; and <2.6 gm/dL severe depletion; low albumin a predictor of mortality as well (Jama 1994;272:1036); single best predictor of death in malnourished NH pt is cholesterol below 150 mg/dL (J Am Geriatr Soc 1996;44:37)

NH pts require 1 gm/kg IBW/d of protein; this increases to 1.2 gm/kg IBW in presence of infection or pressure sores and to 1.5 gm/kg IBW with overwhelming infection and after major surgery; protein provides 20% of the energy from regular diet, therefore 1800-cal diet furnishes 90 gm of protein; most dietary supplements provide 10 gm of protein/can (240 mL); protein food sources expensive for elderly in poverty

Restrictive diets: 3 gm Na, ADA diet not likely to improve the status of CHF or DM in old age, more likely to cause protein-energy malnutrition

Poor wound healing, consider vit C 500 mg/d and zinc sulfate 220-mg tid (Ann IM 1988;109:890)

Treatment:

- Dehydration: fluid requirements of 1500 mL/d; can consider subcutaneous fluid infusion for dehydration (J Am Geriatr Soc 2000;48:795)

- Hypernatremia: require 30-mL free water/kg body weight, or replace 25–30% of deficit/d:
  Free water deficit = 0.6 × IBW × (1 − 140/Measured serum Na) (Nejm 1977;297:1444)

- Hypodermoclysis: sc fluids when IV access difficult, for acute illness (J Am Geriatr Soc 1996;44:969; Jama 1995;274:1552); useful in NH

  Vitamin Supplementation: Low-dose multivitamin enhances lymphocyte proliferation, IL-2 production, decreases infection risk in elderly

- W aging skin vit D synthesis from sunlight decreased, thus supplement those at risk for osteoporosis; especially important in institutionalized elderly; vit K also helps w bone metabolism

- Vit B_6 helps maintain glucose tolerance, cognitive function; enhances aging immune system, but decreases the effectiveness of L-dopa in treatment of Parkinson
- Vit B_{12} protects against high homocysteine levels associated w stroke; neither vit B_{12} nor folic acid absorbed well in atrophic gastritis; screen for vit B_{12} deficiency (J Am Geriatr Soc 1995;43:1290; Am J Clin Nutr 1997;66:741); oral B_{12} (1000–2000 gm/d) effective in absence of intrinsic factor
- Increased consumption of leafy vegetables rich in retinoids decreases risk of age-related macular degeneration (Jama 1994;272:1413)
- Antioxidant vit C, E, and β-carotene may reduce risk of cancer, cataracts, and heart disease (Nutr Rev 1994;52:S15) vs β-carotenes not shown to help (Nejm 1996;334:1145,1150)
- Fiber: psyllium-containing products also lower cholesterol when given w meals; phytate (cereals, legumes, vegetables) can impair calcium, zinc absorption

1.7 VISION

CATARACTS

Ger Rev Syllabus 1996:138–144

Cause: Sun exposure, age, trauma, uveitis, retinitis pigmentosa, intraocular malignancies, DM, hypoparathyroidism, hypothyroidism, steroids (topical as well as systemic), congenital, environmental/UV radiation, smoking, diets low in antioxidants

Epidem: 18% of those age 65–74 yr and 46% age >75 yr; leading cause of reversible blindness in the U.S.; second leading cause of overall blindness in the U.S.; cataract extraction is the most frequently performed surgical intervention on the Medicare population (12% of the 1995 Medicare budget)

Pathophys: Water-insoluble proteins increase w age, leading to brown pigmentation of lens:
- Nuclear cataract (most common): sclerosis of fibers in the lens w increased refractive index secondary to color changes
- Anterior subcapsular: usually iritis leads to adherence to the lens, forming posterior synechiae and eventually, w epithelial cell

proliferation, a subcapsular connective tissue plaque; lens is opacified and liquefied until the entire lens cortex is involved, forming a "mature" cataract
- Posterior subcapsular: formed by epithelial cells that migrate beneath the posterior capsule and enlarge

Sx: Reduced visual acuity although may report improved near vision (nuclear), distant or increased glare (posterior subcapsular)

Si: Opacities often visible on ophthalmoscopic exam; difficult to visualize fundus

Crs: Develop after age 40, almost anyone who lives long enough will develop them; painless progressive variable loss of vision

Cmplc: R/o normal changes of aging: dark adaptation, decreased peripheral vision, diminished perception of low-contrast objects; advanced cataract may swell and the capsule may become leaky, causing secondary glaucoma

Rx:
- 90% of extractions are extracapsular, leaving the posterior capsule in place, providing an anchor for the intraocular lens
- Phacoemulsification (ultrasonic wave) used to pulverize the lens so it can be aspirated prior to placement of implant; less valuable for pts w hard sclerotic nuclear cataracts
- Lens replaced by eyeglass, contact lens or, preferably, implant
- Complications of treatment: opacification of posterior capsule (50% over 3-yr period)—can use laser to correct this w improvement in 90% of pts
- Pts w macular degeneration, also related to sun exposure, may also have cataracts; thus do not repair cataracts when there is coexistent severe macular degeneration (sometimes difficult clinical decision)
- Complication rates of surgery low: faulty wound closure w aqueous humor leakage and intractable secondary glaucoma; explosive choroidal hemorrhage which can cause blindness; endophthalmitis requiring hospitalization for IV antibiotics and corticosteroids (Beers MH, et al., eds. The Merck manual of geriatrics. 3rd ed. Whitehouse Station, NJ: Merck Research Laboratories, 2000)
- Second eye cataract surgery improves functional outcome, eg, reading normal print, engaging in activities previously precluded by vision impairment (Lancet 1998;352:925)

GLAUCOMA

Cause: Primary open-angle glaucoma (POAG): 70% of cases due to impaired aqueous drainage through the trabecular meshwork; POAG accounts for 90% of glaucoma in the elderly in the U.S.; narrow-angle (NAG): steroid-induced, traumatic, inflammatory, neovascular, low tension

Epidem: Risk factors: increased age, female; weaker association with HT, cardiovascular disease, diabetes, smoking, UV light exposure, and diet; POAG: 6 times more common in blacks whereas NAG more prevalent among Asians, especially Chinese

Pathophys:

POAG: anatomically normal outflow channels but increased resistance to aqueous humor outflow from gradual meshwork occlusion

NAG: as lens thickens, anterior chamber is made more shallow, especially in farsighted pts w smaller eyes; elevated intraocular pressure occurs when the base of the iris is pushed forward, sealing off trabecular meshwork outflow; aqueous humor continuously produced by the eye circulating through the anterior chamber cannot leave through outflow channels, producing intraocular pressure of 50–60 mmHg in hours (nl intraocular pressure = 20 mmHg), irreversible changes in 48–72 h

Crs: POAG: 2% visual field loss/yr (Nejm 1993;328:1097)

Sx: *POAG:* asx till very late, gradual loss of visual fields over years; *NAG:* acute pain, blurred vision, halos from corneal edema, nausea

Si: POAG: diagnosis depends on the presence of optic nerve excavation (cupping), visual field defects, w or w/o intraocular pressure elevation (common but not a diagnostic feature); if intraocular pressure <21 mmHg but no visual field deficit, then only ocular HT

Rx:

POAG:

Preventive: Yearly intraocular pressure measurement w Schiøtz tonometer and ophthalmoscopic exam for optic head excavation increases detection rate to 80%, usually done by optometrist or ophthalmologist; stereoscopic equipment and formal visual field testing increase the accuracy of diagnosis

Therapeutic: Management falls largely to ophthalmologist and is directed toward lowering intraocular pressure (does not always stop progression of visual loss)

Topical:
- β-Blockers reduce the secretion of aqueous humor; watch for systemic side effects of β-blockers (bradycardia, CHF)
- Adrenergics, eg, epinephrine, decrease aqueous humor production and increase its outflow through the trabecular meshwork
- Miotics, eg, pilocarpine, carbachol, constrict pupil-stimulating longitudinal muscle fibers of the ciliary body, thereby opening the trabecular meshwork pores

Oral:
- Carbonic anhydrase inhibitors, eg, acetazolamide, decrease production of aqueous humor, numerous adverse effects in the elderly—confusion, paresthesias, drowsiness, anorexia, calcium phosphate renal stones; prostaglandin analogue does not exacerbate asthma or cardiovascular sx (Gen Rev Syllabus 2001:129)

Surgical:
- Filtration procedures designed to create drainage between the anterior chamber and the subconjunctival space; follow q 6 mo

NAG:

Therapeutic: Emergency pilocarpine 2–4% q 5 min × 6, or acetazolamide 250 mg

Surgical: Laser iridotomy within 24 h, expect cure

MACULAR DEGENERATION

Am Fam Phys 2000;61:3035

Epidem: The leading cause of irreversible blindness in U.S. elderly; among people >55 yr in the U.S., 2.2% are blind in one eye from macular degeneration; increased w age, whites, females; weaker association with HT, cardiovascular disease, diabetes, smoking (Jama 1996;276:1141,1147), UV light exposure

Pathophys: Degenerative changes in the macula lead to loss of fine central vision, but not peripheral vision; as macular changes such as pigment mottling and the appearance of drusen also occur in all older retinae, the label of acute macular degeneration is only used when there is accompanying loss of visual acuity; for both of these conditions the anatomic changes lie on a continuum; so the criteria for defining a diseased vs healthy eye in an older person is difficult

Sx: Sudden or recent central vision loss, blurred vision, distortion, new scotomata indicate neovascularization; Amsler grid facilitates monitoring

Si: Hard yellow-white pinhead-size drusen is localized disorder of retinal pigmented epithelium vs soft drusen w more widespread damage; 3 forms: dry or atrophic (80–90% w central loss of vision), subretinal neovascular membrane, retinal pigment epithelial detachment with drusen

Rx:

- Low vision aids: magnifying devices, eg, magnified TV, special lighting (Geriatrics 1995;50:51; J Am Optom Assoc 1988;59:307)
- Photocoagulation (Arch Ophthalm 1994;112:489): indicated for symptomatic choroidal neovascularization outside foveal avascular zone (minority of pts), postpones visual loss; complc: scar if "runoff" beyond intended area of treatment
- Photodynamic rx w verteporfin (Vis dyne) for patients w age-related classic subflaval choroidal neovascularization (wet) (Med Let 2000;42:81)

Team Management: Low vision aids, support group; improve function in bathroom for low-vision persons using contrasting colors of cup, soap, and soap dish; install wall-mounted soap dispenser, mirror w extension arm; alphabetize medicine cabinet; keep cabinets closed; mark positions of cold and hot on faucet so same temperature settings can be selected each time; shampoo and other items in distinguishable shaped bottles; mark desired water level in bathtub (Am Fam Phys 2000;61:3035)

DIABETIC RETINOPATHY

Cause: Diabetes neovascularization and hemorrhage

Epidem: Third leading cause of adult blindness (7% of all blindness); increased prevalence (3%) with greater longevity, positively correlated with the duration of diabetes

Pathophys: Selective loss of mural cells in the basement membrane of retinal capillaries; when glucose is converted by aldose reductase to sorbitol, water moves into the mural cells and they rupture; mural cells have contractile properties and their loss results in capillary dilatation, leading to increased volume of blood flow and resultant microaneurysms, which hemorrhage and lead to exudate formation

Sx: Loss of vision, glaucoma in end stages

Si:

Non-proliferative: Hemorrhages in both the nerve fiber and mid retinal layers, cotton wool spots (nerve fiber layer infarcts), vascular dilatation and tortuousness, microaneurysms, macular edema

Proliferative: Neovascularization at the disc and, elsewhere, preretinal/vitreous hemorrhage, traction retinal detachment, posterior retinal breaks, glaucoma, macular edema

Crs: Early (3–5 yr) first see minimal visual loss from macular edema or clouding of vision from small vitreous hemorrhage, microaneurysms (>5 in each eye); then nonproliferative changes; then proliferative changes

Rx:

Preventive: Annual ophthalmologic exam; correlation between ACE inhibitor and postponement of diabetic retinopathy (Am J Med Sci 1993;305:280); tight diabetic control reduces progression

Therapeutic: Aldose reductase inhibitor (Epalrestat) to decrease sorbitol; proliferative: laser photocoagulation early slows down visual loss; w nonproliferative, vitrectomy w impending retinal detachment

1.8 HEARING PROBLEMS

Ger Rev Syl 2001:123–126

Cause:

- Sensorineural (most common): cochlea or auditory nerve damage due to loud noise (usually bilateral); ototoxic drug effects may be delayed in onset; aminoglycoside dose-related, hearing loss less common than vestibular disturbance and tinnitus; vestibular disturbance and tinnitus are often first signs, taking as long as 2 wk to abate after drug discontinued; aging (presbycusis: high-frequency loss); unilateral causes include trauma, infection, acoustic neuroma, Ménière's—also associated w peripheral vertigo
- Conductive (uncommon): cerumen impaction, middle ear disease, otosclerosis

- Central hearing loss: impaired speech discrimination beyond what would be expected based on threshold change (10% of cognitively impaired)

Epidem: Prevalence increases with age; in the Framingham cohort 41% >65 yr had some level of impairment, only 10% had tried hearing aids; 80% of men between 85 and 90 yr reported having trouble hearing; in NHs prevalence ranges from 50–100%

Si: Whisper test from behind pt; observation of lip-reading ("intentness index"); types of hearing loss:
- Conductive: bone thresholds > air thresholds
- Sensorineural: both air and bone thresholds are elevated

Crs: Declines 2 times faster in M than F; F have more sensitive hearing above 1000-Hz frequency, while M have more sensitive hearing at lower frequencies (J Acoustic Soc Am 1995;97:1196)

Cmplc: Social isolation/withdrawal from conversations, frustration/resentment; mislabeled with dementia, depression; greater risk of falling, impaired mobility, cognitive impairment

Lab: Audiometry tests and interpretation: measured in decibels at which the stimulus can be heard 50% of the time; test ability to understand words (speech discrimination)

Rx:

Conductive:
- Amplification: improvement in social function, emotional well-being, communication function, less depression; hearing aids are most helpful for understanding speech and listening to TV or movies, not as helpful in crowded or noisy situations; barriers: cost (largest obstacle, >1000); self-perceived handicap; difficulties with the small controls due to arthritis; excessive feedback from ear-mold fittings; if loss >80 dB, only limited improvement w hearing aid
- Involvement of a hearing aid specialist for identification of appropriate equipment and training and counseling; adjustment may take wks to mos and is strongly influenced by motivation; cochlear implants w profound sensorineural deafness if conventional hearing aid not feasible (Nejm 1993;329:1092)

Team Management: Physician–patient relationship: minimize background noise as much as possible; use good lighting; face the person at eye level; encourage pts to wear their hearing aids to an office visit; speak clearly from closer range and lower pitch if possible rather than shouting; use gestures and write down important instructions

1.9 INCONTINENCE

URGE INCONTINENCE

Ann IM 1995;122:438; Lancet 1995;346:94; AHCPR Pub. No.
92-0039, 1992; Nejm 1998;280:1995;320:1; 1985;313:800; Urol
Clinics of NA 1998;25:625; AFP 1998;57:2675

Cause: Decreased CNS inhibition common in many normal elders;
accentuated in dementia (voiding dysfunction in NPH results from
paraventricular compression of frontal inhibitory centers leading to
urge incontinence), Parkinson, CVA, or cervical stenosis; or with
parasympathomimetic drugs, eg, bethanechol (Urecholine), cisapride;
or irritation from cystitis, prostatitis, BPH, bladder tumor

Epidem: One-third have urge incontinence (common in community-
dwelling elderly)

Pathophys: Detrusor overactive instability may be due to CNS lesion,
detrusor hyperreflexia, or aging (Urol Clin N Am 1996;23:55)
Detrusor instability w (most common form in the elderly) or w/o
impaired contractility (J Urol 1993;150:1668)

Sx: Little warning; volume of urine lost may be large or small; stained
clothing; asking about diapers or accidents is insulting (Geriatrics
1999;54:22); inquire about degree of control

Lab: Cystometrics show spastic contractions; office cystometry
(Am Fam Phys 1998;57:2675)

Rx:
- Antibiotics for any infection
- If minimal in community-dwelling elderly: planned voiding, avoid
  caffeine, alcohol, carbonated drinks
- Biofeedback (Ann IM 1985;103:507); pelvic exercises; extend
  voiding intervals by half-hour increments once dry (J Am Geriatr
  Soc 1999;47:309; JAMA 1998;280:1995; 1991;265:609); prompted
  voiding q 2 h helps cognitively impaired pts (J Am Geriatr Soc
  1990;38:356) and is 25–40% effective (Dis Mo 1992;38:65)
- Behavioral plus meds added benefit in treating urge incontinence
  (J Am Geriatr Soc 2000;48:370)
- Oxybutynin (Ditropan) 5 mg po tid (anticholinergics, ie,
  parasympathetic inhibition), adding oxybutynin to prompted
  voiding more effective (J Am Geriatr Soc 1995;43:610), or

propantheline 7.5–30.0 mg po tid; tolterodine (Detrol) 1–2 mg po bid (Med Let 1998;40:101)

- Imipramine 25–50 mg po hs (α-stimulation, parasympathetic inhibition)
- Flavoxate not effective
- Trial of bladder relaxants; if urinary retention >150 mL, suspect detrusor hyperreflexia coexisting w mild urinary outflow obstruction in males, or detrusor overactivity w impaired contractility; in pts w detrusor hyperreflexia and impaired contractility in which involuntary contractions are only provoked at higher bladder volumes, catheterize hs, avoid bladder relaxants (Jama 1996; 267:1832)
- Estrogen may be useful in women w urge incontinence; also ameliorates dyspareunia and reduces the frequency of recurrent cystitis (Nejm 1993;329:753); local therapy better (S. Cummings AMDA annual conference Mar 2000, Osteoporosis), caution regarding systemic absorption
- Refer for further urologic w/u if recurrent UTIs (Ann IM 1995;122:749), microscopic hematuria, failure to respond to pharmacologic or behavioral treatment, diagnostic uncertainty

OVERFLOW INCONTINENCE

Cause: Bladder outlet obstruction, eg, BPH, uterine prolapse, large cystocele, ureteral stenosis (associated w atrophic vaginitis), constipation (up to 10% in hospitalized pts), stimulant drugs, neuropathy (impaired sensory input to sacral micturition center); or diminished detrusor strength (flaccid due to lower motor neuron disease); or herpes zoster (from pain); or neurosyphilis which causes detrusor sphincter dyssynergy (Urol Clin N Am 1996;23:11); or meds (anticholinergics, calcium channel blockers, smooth muscle relaxants, opiates)

Epidem: Overflow incontinence less common than other forms of incontinence

Sx: Obstructive w diminished urinary stream; leakage of urine, usually small amounts; frequency; if neuropathic, will have no sensation of bladder fullness

Si: Prostate's palpated size correlates poorly w actual size; suprapubic and abdominal exam for distended bladder

Lab: PVR >200 mL (easy office procedure); in women w large cystoceles, urine may "puddle" below catheter's reach, giving falsely low value for PVR; obtain renal function tests (Ouslander 1996, UCLA Intensive Geriatric Review Course, 1/96) and refer for cystometrics or voiding cystourethrogram; cystometrics show no contractions w 400+ mL when due to diminished sensation

Rx:

- Stool softeners for constipation
- Rx prolapse or BPH; finasteride modest and delayed benefits (Nejm 1992;327:1185); rx for 4 yrs reduced probability of surgery and led to less extensive resection of prostate w local anesthesia in frail elderly men (Nejm 1998;338:557)
- Block sphincter constriction (α-blockade) w prazosin (Minipress)
- 1–2 mg po tid or terazosin (Hytrin); finasteride (5α-reductase inhibitor decreases BPH) not as effective (Ann IM 1995;122:438)
- Bladder neuropathy from cobalamin deficiency reversible w vit B_{12} replacement (J Intern Med 1992;231:313); 60% of diabetics w incontinence do not have neuropathic bladder, they have constipation from autonomic neuropathy (J Am Geriatr Soc 1993;41:1130)
- Self-catheterization (J Am Geriatr Soc 1990;38:364) may be impractical in frail elderly (Ouslander 1996, UCLA Intensive Geriatric Review Course, 1/96); long-term catheters indicated in 1–2% pts
- Increase detrusor strength w bethanechol (Urecholine) 10+ mg po tid, mostly useful in the setting of anticholinergic agents that can't be discontinued; or phenoxybenzamine (Dibenzyline) 10 mg po qd (parasympathomimetics); monitor PVR
- Wood pulp–containing absorbent undergarments superior to polymer gel; garments for F and M differ because different target zone of urinary loss (Urol Clin N Am 1996;23:11); substantial out-of-pocket expense (Geriatrics 1999;54:22)
- Indwelling catheter care: do not irrigate or clamp; leakage may be due to bladder spasm, so use smaller catheter; treat only symptomatic UTIs and do not use prophylaxis; consider acidification if no urea-splitting organisms and silicon catheter if obstruction occurs frequently
- Refer for urologic w/u if large cystourethrocele, markedly enlarged prostate (check PSA first), symptoms or signs of obstruction, and pt is a surgical candidate

STRESS INCONTINENCE

Urol Clinics NA 1998;25:625; AFP 1998;57:2675

Cause: Estrogen deficiency effect on urethral mucosa; or pelvic relaxation after childbirth or urologic surgery; neuropathies
Epidem: One-third have mixed stress and urge incontinence
Pathophys: Sphincter insufficiency
Sx: Loss of urine w cough, sneeze, laugh
Si: Cystocele on physical exam if due to pelvic relaxation
Lab:

- Voiding record kept for 48–72 h useful; milder form of intrinsic sphincter deficiency occurs in older F resulting from urethral atrophy, they leak urine at higher amounts of bladder capacity (200 mL); thus if incontinent in morning after full night's sleep, then probably have volume-dependent stress incontinence
- Urinary stress test: pt should tolerate 300–500 mL before becoming very uncomfortable; if tolerates <250 mL, need further evaluation for interstitial cystitis (pain related to voiding without objective evidence of disease, which may be due to deficiency in bladder lining, autoimmune phenomena, r/o carcinoma-in-situ w cystoscopy) (Waxman J. "Hemorrhagic cystitis" in Ellsworth, R. Primary Care Essentials: Urology. Malden: Blackwell, 2001:55)

Rx:

- Kegel exercises 20–200 daily (J Gerontol 1993;48:M167); postural maneuvers (Obgyn 1994;84:770); pre-contractions can reduce cough-related urine (J Am Geriatr Soc 1998;46:870); vaginal weights better than Kegel's; pessaries (J Am Geriatr Soc 1992; 40:635)
- Oral estrogen unless worried about breast cancer risk, in which case can take intermittently po or try vaginal administration 0.5–1.0 gm of Premarin cream 1–2 mo, then taper; most can be weaned to 2–4 ×/mo (Urol Clin N Am 1996;23:55); if chronic therapy necessary, consider adding progestational agent in pts who still have uterus; need to treat concurrently w exercises to be effective (Ouslander 1996, UCLA Intensive Geriatric Review Course, 1/96); estrogen vaginal ring therapy superior to systemic therapy (J Am Geriatr Soc 1999;47:1383); worse = estrogen plus progesterone (Obstet Gynecol 2001;97:116)

- For neuropathic types, imipramine 25+ mg hs (α-stimulation, parasympathetic inhibition), or phenylephrine (α-stimulation), or biofeedback (Ann IM 1985;103:507)
- Surgery (bladder neck suspension safe and effective, AP repair, sphincter repairs)
- Pessaries: foldable-recreate the urethrovesicular angle (Smith-Hodge); no incontinence but prolapse-use space occupying-doughnut, inflatable

FUNCTIONAL INCONTINENCE

Cause: Can't get to toilet
Si: All normal
Rx: Schedules plus reinforcement of prompted voiding w 25–40% response rate can be identified during a 3-d trial period (Jama 1995;273:1366)

1.10 FEMALE SEXUAL DYSFUNCTION

Br J Obstet Gynaecol 1997;104:87

Cause: Uterus not necessary for orgasm; radical procedures to remove part of the vagina do not affect ability to have orgasm (Obgyn 1993;81:357); quality of first sexual experience after breast cancer treatment strongly influences later sexual recovery (CA 1988;38:154); women receive less sexual counseling after acute MI than do men; in couples who do not resume sexual activity there is deterioration of their emotional relationships (Heart Lung 1987;16:154); any major illness in self or partner can become watershed point
Epidem: Young people, especially physicians, underrate the extent of sexual interest of older people
Pathophys: Androgens derived largely from the adrenal gland and a small amount from the ovaries sustain libido; however, coital activity not correlated w blood levels of estradiol, testosterone, androstenedione, FSH, or LH (Maturitas 1991;13:43)

Sx: Key screening questions: Are you sexually active? Do you have a healthy partner? Is there a change in your level of desire? Is there any discomfort w sexual activity? Is vaginal dryness a problem? Is there difficulty achieving orgasm?; dyspareunia (in 33% of F >65 yr) associated w postmenopausal urogenital atrophy including a feeling of dryness, tightness, vaginal irritation, burning w coitus, and postcoital spotting and soreness; w very old, explore from perspective of sexual feelings, thoughts, always ask about self-stimulation, masturbation; can be useful to start with "Sexual feelings continue to be important for many people during aging—this can sometimes surprise people as they get older—how would you describe this part of you?"

Si: Look for signs of vaginitis (erythema introitus), atrophy (thinned, pallorous mucosa), depression

Crs: Most significant determinant of sexual activity is unavailability of partner; rate of sexual activity earlier in life persists into old age; orgasm usually survives most illness and treatments; sexual touching almost always continues to be pleasurable; most couples have resumed sexual activity 7 mo after acute MI; risk of death during sexual intercourse very low

Rx:

Prevention: Let older women know that sexual fantasies, desires are normal, but be nonjudgmental about those who are satisfied w abstinence; open discussion of body image w couples (after breast removal, w placement of ostomy bags, incontinence, stroke); assumption of heterosexuality leads to a reluctance of older lesbians to interact w health system (J Gerontol Nurs 1990;16:35); staff attitudes and beliefs central problem for NH elderly who are categorized as having sexual problems (Arch Sex Behav 1994;23:231; J Am Geriatr Soc 1987;35:331); β-blocking agents decrease vaginal lubrication; ACE inhibitors and calcium channel blockers do not cause sexual dysfunction; all psychotropic drugs associated w inhibition of sexual function; antidepressants can cause anorgasmia (J Clin Psychiatry 1991;52:66); alcohol causes sexual dysfunction, though very small amounts may help some people

Therapeutic: Formal sex education yields more permissive attitudes (Int J Aging Hum Dev 1982;15:121); estrogen therapy reverses atrophic changes but may take as long as 6–12 mo; water-based lubricants better, eg, Astroglide, Replens; vaginismus (involuntary vaginal muscle contractions because of painful intercourse) responds to estrogen and voluntary contraction and relaxation of introitus w finger in the introitus, then w partner penetration in stages; androgen controversial (give progestational agent to avoid endometrial hyperplasia); masturbation (manual or w mechanical device); Silverstone B, Hyman HK. Growing older together: a couple's guide to understanding and coping with the challenges of later life. Thorndike, ME: Thorndike, 1998

1.11 MALE SEXUAL DYSFUNCTION (IMPOTENCE)

J Am Geriatr Soc 1997;45:1240; Ger Rev Syllabus 1996:310; Jama 1993;270:83; Arch IM 1989;149:1365; J Am Geriatr Soc 1998;36:57; 1997;35:1015

Cause:
- Decreased libido due to psychological, social, physical (decreased testicular perfusion), and endocrine
- Decline in androgen production secondary to testicular failure as well as hypothalamic hyporesponsiveness and excessive binding of testosterone in the plasma; morning peak of testosterone much lower in the elderly
- Decreased erectile rigidity (hypothalamic-pituitary-testicular-autonomic dysfunction, penile arterial occlusive disease, Peyronie disease causing venous leakage)
- Decreased orgasm (decreased testosterone, retrograde ejaculation secondary to damage of proximal sphincter s/p TURP or from DM)

Epidem: 29% M >80 yr have sex 1 ×/wk; probability of erectile dysfunction in men >70 yrs = 67% (Arch Sex Behav 1993;22:545); there may be multiple causes, vascular or neurologic (48%), diabetes (17%), psychological problems (9%), drugs (4%), low testosterone (3%)

Pathophys: Atherosclerosis, clot, or vascular surgery lead to decreased arterial supply to penis; venous leakage; trauma to nerves of the penis from lumbar disc disease, rectal surgery, prostatectomy; diabetic neuropathy; alcoholic peripheral neuropathy; drugs, eg, β-blockers, alcohol, cimetidine, antipsychotics, antidepressants, lithium, sedative hypnotics, hormones

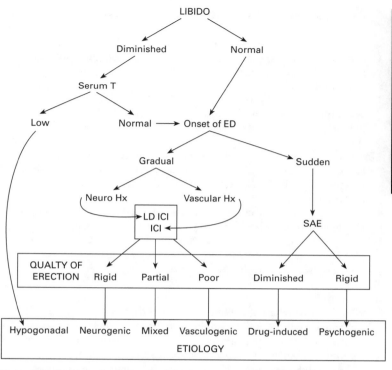

Figure 1-2. Algorithm for the evaluation of erectile dysfunction (ED). ICI = intracavernosal injection; LD = low dose; SAE = sleep-associated erections; T = testosterone. (Reproduced by permission from Godschalk MF, Sison A, Mulligan T. Management of erectile dysfunction by the geriatrician. J Am Geriatr Soc 1997; 45:1240–6.)

Sx: Erectile dysfunction or lack of interest or decreased mobility; failure to reach ejaculation is very common and can be missed if not asked about (Fig 1-2)

Si: Gynecomastia, diminished male-pattern hair suggests endocrine etiology; abdominal/femoral bruits suggest vascular disease; penile size may prevent effectiveness of suction device; fibrous bands or plaques on penis suggest Peyronie disease; penile-brachial index after 3–5 min bicycling w legs in air to dx pelvic steal; nocturnal tumescence not reliable; testicular atrophy suggests hypogonadism; absence of vibratory sense or neural reflex arcs suggests neuropathy; review meds; couple discussion helpful

Crs: Intermittent course suggests psychogenic origin while progressive suggests organic; however, chronic illness course may cause intermittency also

Lab: Lipid profile, HbA1c, testosterone level (3 morning samples 30 min apart for pooled assay; J Clin Endocrin Metab 1995;80:3025), LH if hypogonadal, urine zinc level, prolactin level, liver function

Xray:

Noninvasive: Nocturnal penile tumescence suggests psychogenic etiology; duplex Doppler US delineates arterial, sinusoidal venous insufficiency; all usually not necessary, dx gleaned by asking about nighttime erections

Dx: Intracavernosal injection of vasodilator papaverine or prostaglandin E_1 (PGE1). If neurogenic etiology suspected, 15 mg papaverine or 5 mg PGE1. If vascular etiology suspected, 30 mg papaverine or PGE1—28 gauge needle inserted into side of penis 30–60 sec, response in 15 min w 20–40 min erection.

Rx:

Therapeutic:

- Avoid drugs w adverse effects of sexual dysfunction: calcium channel blockers and ACE inhibitors have the least effect of the antihypertensive meds; phenothiazine causes retrograde ejaculation; minor tranquilizers affect the limbic system, decreasing libido; MAO inhibitors, tertiary amine tricyclics, cimetidine, digoxin, progestational agents, heparin, estrogen
- Treat hypothyroidism, diabetes
- Mechanical: have spouses of COPD pts assume the superior position in sexual intercourse
- Low testosterone: treat w testosterone im q 2 wk or testosterone patches; replacing testosterone in men increases strength, libido, well-being, reduces osteoporosis (Androderm patch) (Geriatrics 1995;50:52); side effects of therapy: BPH, painful gynecomastia, polycythemia, HT, CHF; Testoderm must be worn on scrotum, less rash than w Androderm (Med Let 1996;38:47); if trial of testosterone fails, check prolactin
- Replace zinc in pts w hyperzincuria: 70 mg elemental zinc/d (J Am Geriatr Soc 1988;36:57)

- Vascular or neurologic etiology: alprostadil (Nejm 1997;336:1; 1996;334:873); topical prostaglandin E_1 (Clin Diabetes 1996;14:111; J Urol 1995;153:1828); if unsuccessful, try penile prostheses (80% success rate): self-contained hydraulic (Flexi-Flate and Hydroflex models) or cable spring (OmniPhase); low satisfaction w intracavernosal prostaglandin injection, avoid pain w slow injection PGE1, pellets (rx prolonged erection >4–6 hrs w aspiration 10–20 mL blood from corpora cavernosum, then inject phenylephrine); angioplasty disappointing results; vacuum erection devices: 70–90% satisfaction rate
- Oral phosphodiesterase inhibitor for mixed sildenafil (Viagra), increases penile response to sexual stimulation and well tolerated (Nejm 1998;338:1397)
- Yohimbine, trazodone, Vit E not proven to help
- L-arginine, alpha blocker (Moxisylyte)
- Discussion of adaptation over time is warranted since many men come to understand that sexuality and sexual intimacy do not depend on capacity to perform intercourse alone

1.12 HYPOTHERMIA

Geriatrics 1999;54:51; Conn Med 1995;59:515

Cause:

Accidental: Spontaneous decrease of core temperature to lower than 35°C (95°F) usually in a cold environment, or *dysfunction of hypothalamic thermoregulation* from underlying illness (hypothyroidism, myxedema, hypoglycemia, hypoadrenalism, pancreatitis) or drugs; variety of age-related physiologic factors and disease states predispose older patients to hypothermia:
- Malnutrition
- Infections (most frequently missed)
- Social factors (isolation, poverty)
- Alcohol toxicity (Geriatrics 1999;54:51)

Autonomic Dysfunction: Inability to vasoconstrict peripheral vessels or increase heart rate in response to cold; reduced ability to perceive cutaneous temperature changes; decrease in metabolic rate heat production and shivering response is reduced (Conn Med 1995;59:515)

Epidem: Age 75+ yrs are 5 times as likely to die from hypothermia (Geriatrics 1999;54:51); 33% of elderly patients developed hypothermia in warm months; with sepsis, hypoproteinemia, cachexia, neuroleptic medication (most commonly thioridazine) (Arch IM 1989;149:1521); 74% mortality rate (Conn Med 1995;59:515)

Pathophys: Decrease in O_2 delivery to tissue occurs due to increase in blood viscosity, decreased cardiac output and leftward shift of oxyhemoglobin dissociation curve, respiratory alkalosis; depressed renal blood flow with a decrease in GFR by 50%, renal inability to resorb water, cold-induced diuresis leading to intravascular volume depletion (Geriatrics 1999;54:51)

Sx: Decreased cold perception

Mild hypothermia may mimic cognitive decline, cerebral vascular accident, and hypothyroidism or myxedema coma; cerebral metabolism decreases 7% for each 1°C decline in temperature (Geriatrics 1999;54:51)

Temperature <32°C (89.6°F): skin is cold, violent shivering, chills, fatigue, confusion, hallucinations

<28°C (82.4°F): unconscious; pronounce death if K^+ >10 or no spontaneous cardiac activity after rewarmed to 34°C (93°F)

Si: Hypothermia defined as core body temperatures lower than 35°C (95°F) by esophageal or rectal measurement of temperature; hypothermia may be classified as:

- *Mild*, 32.2–35°C (90–95°F): cerebral dysfunction begins to manifest with confusion, disorientation, introversion, and amnesia; tachycardia progressing to bradycardia; increased BP; bronchospasm; cold diuresis; shivering; ataxia
- *Moderate*, 28–32.2°C (82.4–90°F): depression-level consciousness; pupil dilatation; paradoxical undressing; pulse decrease of 50%; afib, aflutter, ventricular ectopic beats, T wave inversion, prolongation of PR/ST segments, Osborne J waves (Fig 1-3); hypoventilation; no insulin activity; hyporeflexia; diminished shivering; rigidity
- *Severe/profound*, <28°C (82°F): coma; loss of ocular reflexes; decreased BP; ventricular dysrhythmias, asystole; apnea; extreme oliguria; peripheral areflexia
- At 19°C (66.2°F): EEG flat

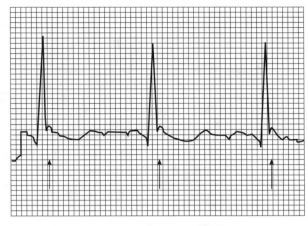

Figure 1-3. On EKG, one-third of patients with hypothermia will exhibit a J wave (Osborne wave), a slow positive deflection at the end of the QRS segment.

Cmplc: Ventricular fibrillation, hypoglycemia, hyperkalemia, impaired drug clearance, acute renal failure, DIC, upper GI bleed, respiratory failure; late cardiomyopathy due to multiple micro infarcts. Adverse reactions occur with rewarming:
1. Rewarming shock—sudden deterioration in cardiovascular status
2. Continued fall of core temperature by up to 3°C after initiation of rewarming and resuscitation probably due to reperfusion of cold extremities

Lab:
- Continuous EKG monitoring; check for Osborne J waves (wide upright slur in terminal QRS) at <80°F (27°C), may warn of impending vfib
- K^+ every 30 minutes
- Blood glucose
- CBC, coagulation profile due to incidence of cytopenia and DIC in this age group
- Toxicology screen
- Amylase/lipase
- ABG
- Digoxin levels

Rx:

- Gentle handling and moving essential, especially in profound hypothermia, to prevent vfib or asystole (Geriatrics 1999;54:51)
- Mild hypothermia: passive rewarming prevents further conduction, convection, radiation, and evaporation losses; warm sources such as radiant lights, forced warm air, electric blankets, warming mattress should be used at temperatures >31°C (87.8°F); warming will occur gradually 0.5–2.0°C/hr (Geriatrics 1999;54:51)
- Consider broad-spectrum antibiotic coverage for possibility of sepsis; thiamine (Conn Med 1995;59:515)
- Moderate to profound: do not do CPR as long as feel pulse, even if very slow, as CPR may cause vfib (Geriatrics 1999;54:51); CPR at half-nl rate; active core rewarming
- Heated, humidified O_2 mask (40–46°C/104–114.6°F) or endotracheal intubation; CO_2 retained in hypothermic state, therefore adjust vent for CO_2 level, not O_2
- Thoracic, pleural lavage with 40°F (104°F) saline rewarms at 2°C/hr
- Bypass rewarms at 4°C/hr
- Glucose if indicated (Conn Med 1995;59:515); avoid insulin for hyperglycemia; insulin action delayed until normothermic, causing hypoglycemia
- Try low-dose catecholamines for low BP if pt not responding to crystalloids and rewarming (Nejm 1994;331:1756)

2 Health Care Maintenance

2.1 ARTERIOSCLEROTIC CARDIOVASCULAR DISEASE

BLOOD PRESSURE

Arch Intern Med 1997;157:2413; U.S. Preventive Services Task Force. Guide to clinical preventive services. 2nd ed. Baltimore: Williams & Wilkins, 1996; Ann IM 1995;122:937; Jama 1995;274:570; Canadian Task Force on the Periodic Health Examination. The Canadian guide to clinical preventive health care. Ottawa, ON: Canada Communication Group, 1994; see Table 2-1

Issues: Systolic Hypertension in Elderly Persons (SHEP) study—systolic HT significantly decreased the incidence of stroke among the young-old (Canadian Task Force 1994:943; Jama 1991;265:3255)
Benefits may not be demonstrable among the old-old (Lancet 1995;345:825; Jama 1994;272:1932; J Hypertens Suppl 1986;4:S642); mortality inversely related to elevated systolic and diastolic BP in those patients aged 85 and older (BMJ 1988;296:887); however, higher rates of fatal MI in men w pharmacologically induced diastolic BP decrease from 90 to 86 mmHg (J Hypertens 1994;12:1183); 20% of elderly whose antihypertensive meds withdrawn while normotensive remained normotensive for 3 mo to 1 yr (J Intern Med 1994;235:581)
Intervention: Screen NH pts for HT, but use caution in treating those >80 yr; periodic trial off meds, particularly if become more sedentary (eg, pts w progressive disabilities, NH pts)

Table 2-1. Preventive Medicine and Screening in Older Adults: Summary of Recommendations

Maneuver Screening[a]	Recommendation (Frequency or Suggested Age)
Blood pressure	Every exam, at least q 1–2 yrs
Physician breast exam	Annually >40
Mammogram	Annually >40 or q 1–2 yrs 50–69 Continue q 1–3 yrs 70–85[b]
Pelvic exam/Pap smear	Every 2–3 yrs after 3 neg annual exams; can then decrease or discontinue after age 65–69[b]
Cholesterol	Adults q 5 years
Rectal exam, fecal occult blood test	Annually ≥50
Sigmoidoscopy	Every 5 years ≥50 or colonoscopy/BE q 10
Test/inquire for hearing impairment	Periodically in older adults
Mouth, nodes, testes, skin, heart, lung exams	Annually
Glucose	Periodic in high-risk groups; q 3 yrs starting at 45
Thyroid function (TSH)	TSH q 5 yrs for women ≥50
Electrocardiogram	Periodically >40–50
Vision/glaucoma screening	Periodically by eye specialist >65
Mental/functional status	As needed; be alert for decline
Osteoporosis (BMD)	If needed for treatment decision[b]
Prostate exam/PSA	Annually ≥50 if >10 yrs life expectancy NR esp. >70[b]
Chest x-ray	NR/as needed
Prophylaxis/Counseling	
Exercise	Encourage aerobic and resistance exercise as tolerated
Influenza vaccine	Annually >65 or chronically ill
Pneumococcal vaccine	23-valent at least once ≥65
Tetanus-diphtheria vaccine	Primary series then booster q 10 yrs
Calcium	800–1500 mg/d
Estrogen (or SERM)	Postmenopausal women
Aspirin	Middle aged to older men 80–325 mg qod
Vitamin E?, red wine?, NSAIDs?, Ginkgo?	May prevent/rx/slow progression of cardiovascular disease and dementia

NR = Not recommended for routine prevention/screening in asymptomatic individuals, though may be useful when clinically indicated.

[a] Screening recommendations for asymptomatic individuals; specific clinical circumstances may necessitate different testing and treatment schedules. Screening for occult disease may not be necessary/appropriate for the oldest old (approx. ≥85) and others with limited quality and quantity of life.

[b] Medicare will cover annual screenings for breast, cervical, prostate cancer, and osteoporosis (Balanced Budget Act of 1997).

Source: Adapted from Goldberg TH, Chavin SC. Preventive medicine and screening in older adults. J Am Geriatr Soc 1997;45(3):344–354. Update: J Am Geriatr Soc 1999;47(1):122–123.

PULSE

Canadian Task Force on the Periodic Health Examination. The Canadian guide to clinical preventive health care. Ottawa, ON: Canada Communication Group, 1994; Ann IM 1988;108:70

Issues: Risk of stroke for pts w afib w at least one other risk factor (HT, DM, TIA, h/o stroke) is 8% annually
Intervention: Check pulse in pts in whom aspirin or warfarin would be considered (Arch IM 1994;154:1443,1449)

PALPATION ABDOMINAL AORTA WIDTH

Canadian Task Force on the Periodic Health Examination. The Canadian guide to clinical preventive health care. Ottawa, ON: Canada Communication Group, 1994; Ann IM 1993;119:411

Issues: Palpation for abdominal aortic aneurysm 80–90% sens; elective nonemergent surgery risk for aneurysm >5 cm = 5% as opposed to emergent 50–70% mortality rate
Intervention: Palpate abdominal aorta in pt in whom surgery would be considered (Prim Care 1995;22:731)

CAROTID AUSCULTATION

Issues: 55–60+% reduction in relative risk results from endarterectomy in asx pts with >70% stenosis (Circ 1995;91:566; Jama 1995;273:1421); neither Canadian Task Force (1994) or European study (Lancet 1995;345:209) advocate endarterectomy for asx pts; carotid bruit auscultation has low specificity for carotid stenosis
Intervention: Where high-quality surgical services are available, auscultate carotids in high-risk pts <80 yr who are good surgical candidates (American Academy of Family Practice recommendations in Prim Care 1995;22:731) vs consensus against both endarterectomy and routine screening for asx carotid artery stenosis (Arch Neurol 1997;54:25)

CHOLESTEROL

Issues: High prevalence of hypercholesterolemia in asx elderly would require further lipid profiles in f/u, putting an enormous burden on the health care system (J Fam Pract 1992;34:320)

Low HDL cholesterol predicts coronary heart disease mortality in older persons (Jama 1995;274:539); total cholesterol levels relate directly to CAD in elderly (Ann IM 1997;126:753)

Computer simulation data suggest that treatment of those with established CAD is more cost-effective than primary prevention in the elderly (Ann IM 1995;122:539)

There have been no clinical trials to assess the risk or benefit of cholesterol-lowering meds in the elderly; inverse relationship between high cholesterol level and death from CAD by age 70–80 (Jama 1994;272:1335; Arch IM 1993;153:1065)

Intervention: Pts w >2 cardiac risk factors (Ann IM 1996;124:515); American Heart Association screen everyone into very old age; those pts with a life expectancy <3 yr should not be screened for hypercholesterolemia; lovastatin extremely well tolerated in older cohort (J Am Geriatr Soc 1997;45:8) and effective in preventing CAD, MI (Ann IM 1998;129:681; Jama 1998;279:1615; Nejm 1998;339:1349)

In NH setting, for LDL > 160 mg/dL or LDL > 130 mg/dL w established CAD (Nurs Hosp Med 1997(suppl D):1D); pts with decreased cholesterol may be at more risk than those with elevated cholesterol; low cholesterol indicates poor nutritional status and is associated with a high 6-mo mortality rate (J Am Geriatr Soc 1991;39:455)

ELECTROCARDIOGRAM

Issues: Screening EKGs have low specif and poorly predict future cardiac events; U.S. Preventive Services Task Force (1996) recommends EKGs in pts with 2 or more cardiac risk factors, but does not specifically address the elderly; discovery of silent ischemia on screening EKG could lead to treatment with significant side-effects (Ann IM 1989;111:489)

Intervention: Baseline EKG (comparison) for all NH pts and pts in continuity practices

COUNSELING (SMOKING, EXERCISE, ASPIRIN, ESTROGEN)

Issues: Cardiovascular benefits of smoking cessation do not diminish with age (Nejm 1988;319:1365); American College of Physicians, Canadian Task Force (1994), and U.S. Preventive Services Task Force (1996) recommend smoking cessation; difficult to achieve in the NH setting where pt's rights to freedom of choice are invoked

Increasing physical activity reduces the incidence of HTN, NIDDM, colon cancer, depression, anxiety, and coronary heart disease in F pts as old as 69 yrs (Jama 1997;277:1287); decreases cholesterol; may improve cognition and self-image (Nejm 1991;325:147; J Am Geriatr Soc 1990;38:123; Ann Rev Publ Hlth 1987;8:253; Nejm 1986;314:605; Jama 1984;252:544); moderate-intensity aerobic training improves glucose tolerance independent of adiposity (J Am Geriatr Soc 1998;46:875); decreased episodes of CHF in elderly who walked 4 h/wk at 75% of their maximum heart rate (Jama 1994;272:1442); older people who are already generally active start w increased volume of aerobic exercise or resistive training, eg, cycling, brisk walking, swimming (slow walking for 5 min and 5–10 min stretching before moderate exercise and after resistive training; free weights 70% of comfortable lift through a free range of motion one time increasing q mo; increase to 3 sets of 8–12 repetitions w 1–2 min rest between sets; exhale 2–4 sec w lift and inhale 4–6 sec w lowering weight (J Am Geriatr Soc 2000;48:318)

Estrogen cardioprotective via beneficial effects on lipid profile (PEPI trial in Jama 1995;273:199; American College Physicians in Ann IM 1992;117:1016,1038; Nejm 1992;326:1406; Nurses study in Nejm 1991;325:756); estrogen plus progesterone does not provide secondary prevention for CAD (Jama 1998;280:613)

Intervention: Strongly encourage even the very old pt to quit smoking unless life expectancy is <2 yr (J Fam Pract 1992;34:320); do not assume pts who have quit have done so forever, continue to counsel (Prim Care 1995;22:697)

Walking programs for appropriately selected ambulatory pts; weight-bearing exercises that avoid flexion of the spine for osteoporotic pts; Tai Chi (J Am Geriatr Soc 1996;44:489,498); encourage weight training

U.S. Preventive Services Task Force (1996) recommends aspirin for pts >40 yr with at least 2 risks for CAD (first-degree relative, smoking, HT, DM, h/o stroke or peripheral vascular disease, obesity, low levels of HDL) (J Am Geriatr Soc 1990;38:817,933); however, in the elderly the benefits may not outweigh the risks of aspirin, ie, GI bleeding (J Am Board Fam Pract 1992;5:127), does not prevent stroke (Arch Neurol 2000;57:326)

Estrogen Replacement: (See also 8.2 Coronary Artery Disease.) Avoid menstrual bleeding w daily estrogen 0.625 mg and progesterone 2.5 mg; use into very old age because not only cardioprotective but beneficial effects on osteoporosis (Byyny RL, Speroff L. A clinical guide for the care of older women: primary and preventive care. 2nd ed. Baltimore: Williams & Wilkins, 1996); not beneficial for secondary prevention of CAD

2.2 CANCER

Consider life-expectancy estimates that account for comorbidity, functional status, age; physical and psychological risks of false-negative tests (Jama 2001;285:2750)

BREAST CANCER

Issues: Breast cancer less aggressive than in premenopausal women; more poorly differentiated tumors with less organized cells (ie, no hormone receptors) selected out by aging, resulting in the more differentiated tumors lasting into old age; according to actuarial statistics healthy 80-yr-old women will live 9 more yr, but most NH pts have medical problems that will shorten their life expectancy; greater risk if >7 yrs of HRT (J Am Geriatr Soc 2000;48:842)

Morbidity: Fungating tumors, metastasis to bone, liver, lung, and 15% to brain; 50% of asx elderly women with breast cancer may have bony metastases (Ger Med Today 1989;8:27); local complications develop in nearly half of untreated 85-yr-old women with a breast lump; a demented 85-yr-old woman has a 75% chance of dying before these complications develop (J Am Geriatr Soc 1995;43:282)

Tamoxifen has been used in lieu of surgery in the frail elderly pt who develops breast cancer (J Am Geriatr Soc 2000;48:346; Br J Surg 1991;78:591); easily tolerated and may also protect against osteoporosis

Exercise ≥4-hr/wk decreases risk of breast cancer (Nejm 1997; 336:1269)

Intervention: In selected pts where the likelihood of developing morbidity from breast cancer will precede death from other causes, screen for breast cancer into late life w mammogram as well as breast exam (Lancet 1993;341:1973); annually or biennially until age 75, biennially or at least q 3 yrs after that w no upper limit of age as long as 4 yr life expectancy (NYFC III, IV CHF, DM w end organ damage, steroid or O_2-dependent COPD, severe dementia, malignancy) (J Am Geriatr Soc 2000;48:842); Medicare covers q 2 yr screening mammography

In the frail NH pt w average life expectancy limit screening to a breast exam (Ann IM 1995;122:539); low-risk rx, eg, tamoxifen, easily available for management

COLON CANCER

U.S. Preventive Services Task Force. Guide to clinical preventive services. 2nd ed. Baltimore: Williams & Wilkins, 1996; Lancet 1996;348:1467

Issues: Two-thirds of new cases of colon cancer diagnosed each yr are found in people older than 65; time for polyp to become malignant ranges from 5–12 yr (Ann IM 1991;115:807); dx and rx of colorectal cancer is curative or palliative and may improve quality of life, though perioperative mortality does increase with age

Digital Rectal Exam, Fecal Occult Blood Testing, and Sigmoidoscopy: 25% decrease in mortality associated with their use (Ann IM 1993;118:1; Nejm 1993;328:1365); well-designed case-control studies suggest protection remains unchanged for at least 10 yr after rigid sigmoidoscopy (U.S. Preventive Services Task Force, 1996); simple occult blood testing can lead to serial colonoscopies, expense, and discomfort without necessarily increasing longevity in debilitated elderly; controversial one-time screening with colonoscopy has been suggested for those >60 yr old (Jama 1994;271:1011; National Polyp Study in Am J Gastroenterol 1994;86:197; Nejm 1993;329:1977)

Intervention:
- General population of well elderly: screening with fecal occult blood tests yearly and sigmoidoscopies every 5 yr appropriate, q 10 yr colonoscopy (J Am Geriatr Soc 1999;47:122)
- Studies of colorectal screening targeting the growing NH population are needed to support more specific recommendations
  The Canadian Task Force (1994) finds insufficient evidence of benefit to include or exclude colon cancer screening of individuals >40 yr, asx or with family hx (Canadian Task Force, 1994)
- Take advantage of low cost of fecal occult blood screening and use repeat screening as valuable diagnostic tool when clinical suspicion is high; abstain from ASA >325 mg/d, substantial doses of NSAIDs, red meat, poultry, raw vegetables, fish, vit C for accurate study (J Am Geriatr Soc 2000;48:333)

CERVICAL CANCER

Issues: 40% of cervical cancer deaths occur in women >65 yr; 50% of women >65 yr have never had a pap smear, and an additional 25% have not had regular screening; women >65 who have never had pap smear have 2–3 times the risk of younger women for having abnormal pap (Am J Obgyn 1991;164:644); women >65 would benefit more than any age group from cancer screening with a 63% improvement in 5-yr mortality (Lancet 1990;335:97)
Canadian recommendations suggest that 2 neg pap smears are sufficient even in women never previously screened who are >65; cervical cancer screening, according to these guidelines, is about one-sixth the cost of mammography screening per yr of life saved
Women who have had any previous abnormal paps should be screened q 2–3 yr late into life (U.S. Preventive Services Task Force, 1996); w regularly documented neg pap smears, it is safe and cost-effective to stop screening at age 65 (Ann IM 1992; 117:529)

Pathophysiology of Cervix with Aging: As women age, the transformation zone migrates further into the cervix and is more difficult for the clinician to visualize; estrogen reverses this change; to obtain optimally reliable cytology in high-risk elderly women, use intravaginal estrogen for 3 wk prior to pap smear to avoid false-pos smears, because atrophic changes can be read as atypia on pap smear (Colposcopy course, Santa Fe, NM, 3/95)

Mechanical Barriers to Screening: Pelvic examination not only uncomfortable but also may lead to pain in severely arthritic, osteoporotic women; consider using "heels together, knees apart" position w assistant providing lateral knee support (rather than standard stirrups) for increased comfort; demented pts may be unable to cooperate with the procedure, so consider examination in left lateral decubitus position; decreased estrogen also makes vaginal introitus stenotic, shortened, narrowed

Natural History of Disease: Untreated cervical cancer usually involves local spread and subsequent ureteral and bowel obstruction causing death; rx options depend on the stage of the disease, progressing from cryosurgery, loop electrocautery excision procedure and laser, to surgery and radiation

Intervention: q 1–3 yr until age 70 (J. Am Ger Soc 2001;49:657) Cost-effective schedule of cervical cancer screening can be limited to previously unscreened women and women w previous abnormal pap smears who can tolerate the pap smear, colposcopy, and the various rx for dysplasia and cervical cancer

Other Gynecologic Cancers: Routine screening for ovarian cancer not yet proved to reduce morbidity or mortality (Jama 1995;273:491); a careful hx to elicit abnormal bleeding patterns requiring endometrial bx is the initial screening tool for endometrial cancer (J Fam Pract 1992;34:320)

PROSTATE CANCER

Issues: Most common cancer in men; second leading cause of cancer death in men >75 yr (after lung cancer; J Fam Pract 1992;34:320); >99% of men diagnosed with this disease die of other causes (Prog Clin Biol Res 1988;269:87); the American Cancer Society began recommending the PSA test along with digital rectal exam starting at 50 yr for men with a life expectancy of at least 10 yr (CA 1993;43:42); PSA may be more sens for aggressive cancers than non-aggressive cancers and may advance detection of early prostate cancer by 5.5 yr (Jama 1995;273:269)

Despite earlier detection of cancer and subsequent prostatectomy in the U.S., no change in the incidence of advanced disease or overall mortality; 1% incidence of death with prostatectomy, about the same as chance of dying of prostate cancer for older male (Lancet 1994;343:251); other risks of surgery include impotence and incontinence (often hidden by the pt); benefit of screening offset by morbidity of treatment (Jama 1994;272:773); long-term survival after conservative treatment of localized prostate cancer not changed with low-grade tumors (Jama 1995;274:626)

Intervention: Prostate cancer screening and rx are controversial even in otherwise well men and contraindicated in most NH pts whose average life expectancy is much less than 10 yr; rapidly developing literature demands attention by physicians and discussion w pts before screening; transrectal ultrasound not recommended (Ann IM 1997;126:480)

SKIN CANCER

Issues: Mortality from melanoma has increased by 50% in F >65 yr and by 100% in M >65 yr; high incidence of actinic keratoses combined w low incidence of conversion to squamous cell carcinoma; even basal cell carcinomas may rapidly disfigure, making early detection important to the pt

Intervention: U.S. Preventive Services Task Force (1996) recommends screening pts w yearly exam with increased sun exposure and with a family hx of dysplastic nevi; important for primary care provider to follow all abnormal lesions w serial exams for cost-effective management

ORAL CANCER

Issues: Tongue cancer most common (26%), then oropharynx (22%), then lip (19%), then gingiva (19%), then floor of the mouth (16%), then buccal mucosa (3%), then hard palate (2%); speckled leukoplakia, erythroplakia carry more risk than leukoplakia; <50% elderly survive oral cancer; 50% of elderly have undetected gum disease which can have a systemic impact on health; xerostomia common in NH elderly, especially those on anticholinergic drugs (Am J Nurs 1995;81:1135)

Intervention: Screen pts with a hx of tobacco or alcohol use for oral cancer, and other problems of the oral cavity as well; no well-designed controlled, cohort studies prove dental screening effective in the elderly, but easy to screen yearly with oral cavity exam (Gerodontics 1988;4:207)

2.3 INFECTION CONTROL

INFECTION SURVEILLANCE

Clin Ger Med 1995;11:467; Nurs Home Med 1995;3:207; Yoshikawa TT, Norman DC, eds. Antimicrobial therapy in the elderly patient. New York: Dekker, 1994; Clin Ger Med 1992;8:1821

Issues:

Nursing Home: Endemic (UTI, URI, skin) and epidemic (influenza, TB, gastroenteritis); approximately 1 infection/resident/yr; fever criterion should be lowered to rectal 37.2°C (99°F) or oral 37.7°C (100°F), and temperature rise of 2°F from baseline should be viewed as febrile response (J Am Geriatr Soc 1996;44:74); atypical clinical manifestations: anorexia, falling, incontinence, mental status change; MRSA infection: 10–25% of NH pts colonized, but only 3–5% infected

Intervention:

Nursing Home: Develop daily reporting system for nursing staff that includes criteria for infection from which infection rates in the NH can be determined

MRSA-colonized pts do not require isolation, but should not share room w pts w gastric feeding tubes, wounds, IV catheters, or immunosuppression (Am J Med 1993;94:313)

Vancomycin-resistant enterococci (VRE) (Nejm 1999;340:517,556; Inf Contr Hosp Epidem 1998;19:532; Nurs Home Med 1997;4:371): contact precautions for colonized or infected pts include grouping pts in same room, wearing gloves and gowns if pt or environmental surface contact anticipated, dedicating frequently used equipment, and barriers for shared equipment, eg, exercise machines; VRE infection control includes surveillance stool cultures or rectal swabs of roommates of newly discovered VRE-colonized pts; may remove contact precautions when 3 neg VRE cultures separated by wk intervals; antimicrobial rx associated w prolongation VRE carriage (J Am Geriatr Soc 1998;46:157); new medication for VRE and MRSA: Linezolid (Zyvox) 600 mg IV q 12 hr (Med Let 2000;42:45)

TUBERCULOSIS

Issues: Declining immune system leads to reactivation of quiescent infection; chronic cough, weight loss incorrectly attributed to COPD, or malnutrition could result in unrecognized TB epidemic

Intervention:

Nursing Home: Screen new admissions; screen staff yearly; screen pts yearly if high prevalence of TB in community and NH
- If PPD <10 mm after 48 h, PPD booster in 2 wk
- Use dermal controls for immunocompromised
- F/u pos PPD w chest x-ray and obtain 6 morning sputums for AFB; if pos PPD, and CXR negative and pt not a recent converter (2 yrs), check risk factors (see table from Am Fam Phys 2000;61:263); if pos risk factors, rx latent TB (chemoprophylaxis)

Chemoprophylaxis: Rx conversion of >15 mm within 2 yr with INH 300 mg, pyridoxine 50 mg 6 mo, check AST q 3 mo, discontinue rx if AST rises to 3 nl, re-challenge once AST nl, with 50 mg INH, increasing by 50 mg weekly to 300 mg/d; do not re-challenge if AST rises again

DECUBITUS ULCER

Issues: Prevalence in NH >20–30%; incurs 4 times risk of death
Intervention: Norton or Braden scales (see 12.19 Pressure Sores)
  Screen for risk of decubiti, taking physical and mental condition,
    activity level, mobility, and incontinence into account; for pts at
    high risk: ensure adequate repositioning schedules, check albumin
    and order high-protein diets (J Am Diet Assoc 1994;94:1301)
    (Table 2-2)

2.4 IMMUNIZATIONS

INFLUENZA

Issues: 4th leading cause of death pts >75 yr; 70% NH residents contact
  influenza during outbreak, 10–20% in non-epidemic years; fatality
  rate 30% (Jama 2000;1:S25), immunization rate 20–40% because
  physicians do not communicate to pts seriousness of illness
  (Clin Ger Med 1992;8:183); cost-effective, saving $117/person,
  $5 million in cumulative savings (Nejm 1994;331:778)
Intervention: Vaccinate all elderly (Jama 1997;278:1333); efficacy
  debated (Lancet 1998;357:399); drug-resistant pneumococci more
  common so liberalize use of vaccine (Nejm 1998;338:1861,1915)
  Aim to immunize 80% NH pts (Jama 1994;272:1133); during
    outbreaks begin prophylaxis regardless of vaccination status to
    both ill and non-ill pts; rimantadine has fewer CNS side effects,
    more expensive than amantadine (Geriatrics 1994;49:30); reduce
    side effects of amantadine by dosing according to calculated Cr
    clearance and decreasing other anticholinergic meds

PNEUMOCOCCAL PNEUMONIA

Issues: Increased incidence by 2–4 in pts >65 yr; 20% vaccination rate,
  partially due to low Medicaid/Medicare reimbursement through 1989
Intervention: Aim to vaccinate 60% NH pts; revaccinate q 6 yr in
  elderly w asplenia, nephrotic syndrome, or renal failure; revaccination
  w 23-valent vaccine should be considered for pts who were

Table 2-2. Jen Scale for Predicting Pressure Sore Risk

Patient's Name		Evaluator's Name		Date of Assessment
SENSORY PERCEPTION Ability to respond meaningfully to pressure-related discomfort	1. Completely Limited: Unresponsive (does not moan, flinch, or grasp) to painful stimuli, due to diminished level of consciousness or sedation. OR limited ability to feel pain over most of body surface.	2. Very Limited: Responds only to painful stimuli. Cannot communicate discomfort except by moaning or restlessness. OR has a sensory impairment which limits the ability to feel pain or discomfort over 1/2 of body.	3. Slightly Limited: Responds to verbal commands, but cannot always communicate discomfort or need to be turned. OR has some sensory impairment which limits ability to feel pain or discomfort in 1 or 2 extremities.	4. No Impairment: Responds to verbal commands. Has no sensory deficit which would limit ability to feel or voice pain or discomfort.
MOISTURE Degree to which skin is exposed to moisture	1. Constantly Moist: Skin is kept moist almost constantly by perspiration, urine, etc. Dampness is detected every time patient is moved or turned.	2. Very Moist: Skin is often, but not always moist. Linen must be changed at least once a shift.	3. Occasionally Moist: Skin is occasionally moist, requiring an extra linen change approximately once a day.	4. Rarely Moist: Skin is usually dry, linen only requires changing at routine intervals.
ACTIVITY Degree of physical activity	1. Bedfast: Confined to bed	2. Chairfast: Ability to walk severely limited or non-existent. Cannot bear own weight and/or must be assisted into chair or wheelchair.	3. Walks Occasionally: Walks occasionally during day, but for very short distances, with or without assistance. Spends majority of each shift in bed or chair.	4. Walks Frequently: Walks outside the room at least twice a day and inside room at least once every 2 hours during waking hours.
MOBILITY Ability to change and control body position	1. Completely Immobile: Does not make even slight changes in body or extremity position without assistance.	2. Very Limited: Makes occasional slight changes in body or extremity position but unable to make frequent or significant changes independently.	3. Slightly Limited: Makes frequent though slight changes in body or extremity position independently.	4. No Limitations: Makes major and frequent changes in position without assistance.

	1.	2.	3.	4.
NUTRITION *Usual* food intake pattern	**Very Poor:** Never eats a complete meal. Rarely eats more than 1/3 of any food offered. Eats 2 servings or less of protein (meat or dairy products) per day. Takes fluids poorly. Does not take a liquid dietary supplement. OR is NPO and/or maintained on clear liquids or IV's for more than 5 days.	**Probably Inadequate:** Rarely eats a complete meal and generally eats only about 1/2 of any food offered. Protein intake includes only 3 servings of meat or dairy products per day. Occasionally will take a dietary supplement. OR receives less than optimum amount of liquid diet or tube feeding.	**Adequate:** Eats over half of most meals. Eats a total of 4 servings of protein (meat, dairy products) each day. Occasionally will refuse a meal, but will usually take a supplement if offered. OR is on a tube feeding or TPN regimen which probably meets most of nutritional needs.	**Excellent:** Eats most of every meal. Never refuses a meal. Usually eats a total of 4 or more servings of meat and dairy products. Occasionally eats between meals. Does not require supplementation.
FRICTION AND SHEAR	**Problem:** Requires moderate to maximum assistance in moving. Complete lifting without sliding against sheets is impossible. Frequently slides down in bed or chair, requiring frequent repositioning with maximum assistance. Spasticity, contractures or agitation leads to almost constant friction.	**Potential Problem:** Moves feebly or requires minimum assistance. During a move skin probably slides to some extent against sheets, chair, restraints, or other devices. Maintains relatively good position in chair or bed most of the time but occasionally slides down.	**No Apparent Problem:** Moves in bed and in chair independently and has sufficient muscle strength to lift up completely during move. Maintains good position in bed or chair at all times.	

For additional information on administration and scoring: Braden BJ, Bergstrom N. Clinical utility of the Braden Scale for Predicting Pressure Sore Risk. Decubitus 1989;2:44–6,50–1.

HEALTH CARE MAINTENANCE

vaccinated w 14-valent vaccine (Am Fam Phys 1995;51:859); U.S. Preventive Services Task Force (1996) revaccinate q 6 yr (Jama 2000;1:S25)

TETANUS

Mmwr 1998;47(SS-2):1

Issues: Increased incidence with age because protective antitoxin levels decline; 28% have protective levels over the age of 70 (Nejm 1995;332:761); 10% pts are fecal carriers of *Clostridium tetani*, leaving pressure ulcers at high risk for contamination; case fatality rate 50%

Intervention: Give tetanus immune globulin to pts with contaminated ulcers who have completed primary series but have not had re-immunization within 10 yr; give primary series to pts with unknown immunization status (J Am Geriatr Soc 2000;48:949); pts in the military after 1941 have received at least one tetanus toxoid dose (Inf Contr Hosp Epidem 1993;14:591); primary immunization series consists of second dose 4–6 wk after the first and third dose 6–12 mo later (Sci Am 2000; "Clinical essentials" in Adult Snow C. Preventive Health Care)

2.5 FUNCTION

FUNCTIONAL ASSESSMENT

Issues: Emphasize quality of life issues over extension of life; screening emphasizes preservation of function; the Canadian Task Force (1994) and the U.S. Preventive Services Task Force (1996) recommend screening for functional assessment in the elderly

INTERVENTION

In Office and NH: Nurses perform a yearly functional assessment (Kane RL, Ouslander JG, Abrass IB. Essentials of clinical geriatrics. 3rd ed. New York: McGraw-Hill, 1994)

Katz functional assessment is one of the most common; assesses actual capacity and not performance and records loss of independence in 6 skills in the order in which they are lost; bathing, dressing, toileting, transferring, continence and feeding; skills usually regained in reverse order

SENSORY—HEARING AND VISION

HEARING

Issues: The Canadian Task Force (1994) and U.S. Preventive Services Task Force (1996) recommend screening for hearing loss in the elderly; particularly effective screen in the old-old pt (J Fam Pract 1992;34:320); 41% of pts >65 yr are hearing impaired (Ear Hear 1990;11:247)

Intervention: (Am Fam Phys 1997;56:2057) Whispered voice and otoscopy most sens and specif screens (86–96%) (Canadian Task Force, 1994; Ann IM 1990;113:138); observation of listening behavior helpful; obtain a continued hx of hearing loss, perform otoscopy for cerumen impaction and f/u w portable audiometry for presbycusis where indicated; pts sometimes refuse to wear hearing aids; ascertain the cause of their noncompliance, eg, poor fit, difficult to manipulate, change in hearing deficit, depression, dementia, rather than assuming indifference or stubbornness

VISION

Issues:

Community: 9% >65 yr, 50% >75 yr have visual impairment, optical changes in aging (Mangione CM, Intensive Course in Geriatric Medicine and Board Review, 1/96)

- Increased light absorption by crystalline lens reducing intensity reaching photoreceptors
- Senile miosis: older pupils smaller, leading to less light getting to retina in low-light conditions

- Increased intraocular light scatter, leading to heightened sensitivity to glare
- Decreased amplitude of accommodation of the lens (presbyopia) so by 60–70 yr most need glasses for near vision
- Axis of astigmatism changes, requiring refraction
- Neural change w loss of blue-yellow discrimination; no prospective studies show that screening elderly for visual acuity worthwhile

Nursing Home: 17% of pts in NHs blind and another 19% have <20/40 vision; 20% of blindness and 37% of impairment remediable with adequate refraction (Nejm 1995;332:1205); Baltimore eye study: un-operated cataracts accounted for 27% of all blindness in blacks, suggesting that elderly with less access to eye care would benefit from screening for cataracts (Mangione 1996; Nejm 1991;325:1412)

Macular degeneration leading cause of blindness among whites (3% of all whites >80 yr); early treatment w laser effective in slowing progression in minority of patients who have neovascularization (see 1.7 Vision, Macular Degeneration); referral to low-vision services may help pt to maximize peripheral vision

Diabetic retinopathy most treatable in presymptomatic phase when neovascular changes have just begun

Impaired visual acuity linked to falls and hip fx; thus screening elderly may be beneficial (Nejm 1991;324:1326)

Screen using combination of visual field exam, tonometry, and direct ophthalmoscopy by ophthalmologist w pt's eyes completely dilated (2.5% phenylephrine w tear duct occlusion to decrease systemic absorption); long asx and potentially treatable phase before irreversible vision loss (UCLA intensive board review, 1/96). However, reliable screening tests for glaucoma are not available and early treatment does not improve pt outcome (Surv Ophthalmol 1983;28:194)

Intervention: Screen for visual acuity yearly; visual acuity screening criteria for referral to specialist: best eye <20/40 (wearing correction), >2 Snellen lines difference between two eyes; hx of night driving problems helpful for accident prevention; vs vision screening no apparent benefit—many causes untreatable (BMJ 1998;28:316)

DEMENTIA

Nejm 1990;322:1212

Issues: Screening recommended by the American College of Physicians, Canadian Task Force (1994), and U.S. Preventive Services Task Force (1996); Mini Mental State Exam (MMSE) has a broad range; moderate but not mild deficits can be picked up; Wechsler identifies subtle deficit, but lengthy to administer; 4–7-yr delay in presentation to health care provider; EXIT interview screens for subcortical dementias by testing executive function (see 5.5 Dementias)

Intervention: Use MMSE to pick up attention-span deficit associated with the reversible dementias (and delirium), ie, thyroid disorders, other metabolic abnormalities, and acute infections; MMSE helps identify the type and stage of dementia; prevent unnecessary agitation in demented pts by providing stage-appropriate challenges without overstimulating them with activities that are too difficult for them; careful spouse and family hx probably undervalued as dx tool

DEPRESSION

Issues: 10–15% of general geriatric population depressed; 60% of NH elderly may be depressed; masked depression more common among the elderly presenting w agitation, jealousy, or somatization

Intervention: Asking single question "Have you been feeling depressed?" may be just as effective as Geriatric Depression Scale (GDS) (J Am Geriatr Soc 1994;42:1006); anhedonia (failure to find usual pleasures) can be sensitive sx; GDS only requires yes/no answers, has a shortened form, but may lack specif among medically ill pts; Beck, Zung, and Hamilton depression inventories rely heavily on somatic complaints and so are less useful in the elderly; nonverbal depression scale developed by Hayes and Losche useful in more debilitated NH pts (Clin Gerontol 1991;10:3)

HEALTH CARE MAINTENANCE

ALCOHOL PROBLEMS

J Am Geriatr Soc 1995;43:415

Issues: Prevalence of alcohol problems = 10% in community; in the NH ranges from 2.8–15%; 33% of the pts who enter NH will return to their community, making alcohol rehabilitation more relevant (Ger Rev Syllabus 1996). Knowledge of ETOH hx may add to the understanding of family-pt interactions; behaviors exhibited with the staff such as "dry drunk" spells will take on new meaning as well; move to retirement communities associated w increased ETOH use

Intervention: Screening with either a CAGE or MAST-G (see 5.3 Alcohol Misuse) yields 82/90% and 93/65% sens/specif, respectively (Ger Rev Syllabus 1996); CAGE not reliable as only screening tool in outpts >60 yr; directly ask about number of drinks/wk (Jama 1996;276:1964); watch for reluctance to appropriately modify ETOH use w illness, new meds; pointing out percentage of daily calories provided by 1, 2, 3, etc. drinks may help to improve nutrition

FALLS

Issues:

Community: Lower extremity dysfunction predicts subsequent disability (Nejm 1995;332:556); one-leg balance important indicator of injurious falls (J Am Geriatr Soc 1997;45:735); slowed, timed chair stands, decreased arm strength, decreased vision and hearing, high anxiety or depression score also predictors for falls (Jama 1995; 273:1348)

Nursing Home: Increased fall rates in NH residents after relocation in a new facility (J Am Geriatr Soc 1995;43:1237); pts who fall infrequently are at most risk for injury; they tend to be going at faster speeds at point of impact; these pts as well as those who fall frequently can be helped by intervention that determines etiology of falls; fear of falling leads to functional decline (Gerontol 1994;40:38) and should be considered important part of all fall management

Intervention: (See 10.1 Osteoporosis, 10.2 Hip Fracture.) Screen all outpts and ambulatory NH pts with an assessment of balance and gait; Tinetti assessment tool (J Am Geriatr Soc 1986;34:119) evaluates nl and adaptive ability to maintain balance when arising from chair, standing with eyes closed, turning, and receiving sternal nudge; also evaluates several components of gait (step height, postural sway, path deviation); abnormalities in particular parts of the exam point to specific intrinsic etiologies of falling, eg, "uses arms to assist in standing—may have proximal muscle weakness and might be helped by strength training for hip and quad muscles"; foot scuff during swing phase—anterior tibial muscle weakness that might be aided by an ankle/foot orthosis or reconditioning; observational gait analysis (Table 2-3)

Prevent falls by using both intrinsic and extrinsic approaches; increased muscle strength associated with decreased falling (J Am Geriatr Soc 1994;42:953); exercise training decreases falls (Jama 1995;273:1341); work with physical therapist to develop care plan; use antigravity exercises that do not flex the spine to avoid vertebral compression fractures in severely osteoporotic pts

Osteoporosis likely in pts whose height has decreased on yearly screening; high risk: white, Asian, thin, nulliparous, sedentary, kyphotic women with past or family hx of fx, both M/F who smoke, have COPD, or take steroids chronically; post-menopausal estrogen therapy at any age prevents further bone loss and serious injury from falls; if no preexisting breast cancer, prescribe estrogen (several different regimens see 1.3 Geriatric Pharmacology), vs estrogen begun 5 yr after menopause no fx prevention benefit at any site (Ann IM 1995;122:9); calcitonin via intranasal route a costly option for pts with fx pain in whom estrogen is contraindicated (Ann IM 1992;117:1038); alendronate (see 10.1 Osteoporosis)

Hip fx <23% when adequate calcium supplementation prescribed (1.2 gm/d) with 800 IU of vit D (Osteoporos Int 1994;4(suppl 1):7); adequate levels of vit D found in most OTC vit supplements (J Endocrinol Metab 1995;80:1052); unless elderly F have hx of renal stones, should have total calcium intake = 1.2 gm/d and add vit D if they are not exposed to direct sunlight for at least one-half h/d; serving of broccoli or dairy product equivalent to 1 Tums tab (0.2 gm elemental calcium); use as guide to decide calcium tab supplementation

Extrinsic approaches: hip pads and chariot ambulators maintain independent walking, prevent serious injury (Lancet 1993;341:11); restraint reduction does not increase serious falls (J Am Geriatr Soc 1994;42:321,960; Arch IM 1992;116:368); evaluate meds: sedatives, narcotics, neuroleptics, and antihypertensives

Table 2-3. Observational Gait Analysis

3 × 3 × 3 MODEL	
Ask:	Which of the three essential components is involved? **1. FOOT CLEARANCE IN SWING** **2. UPRIGHT SUPPORT IN STANCE** **3. CONTROLLED FORWARD MOVEMENT**
Then Ask:	Where does the problem occur? **1. GATHERING INFORMATION** **2. PROCESSING INFORMATION** **3. PRODUCING MOVEMENT**
Finally:	What can be done? **1. PREVENTION** **2. CORRECTION** **3. COMPENSATION**

FOOT CLEARANCE IN SWING PHASE	UPRIGHT SUPPORT IN STANCE PHASE	CONTROLLED FORWARD MOVEMENT
	Gathering Information	
Proprioceptive loss	Paresthesias	Vestibular disturbance
Compensatory strategy: orthotics hard-soled shoes	*Preventative strategy: foot care*	*Corrective strategy: desensitization exercises*
	Processing Information	
Poor coordination	Polypharmacy	Difficulty initiating or terminating movement, eg, Parkinson's disease
Compensatory strategy: enhance safety with architectural redesign	*Corrective strategy: streamline medication*	*Preventative strategy: prevent secondary problems of weakness, inflexibility, and poor joint mobility*
	Producing Movement	
Tight gastroc-soleus, eg, 15° of ankle dorsiflexion necessary for normal gait	Weak hip abductors, eg, Trendelenburg	Arthritis pain
Corrective strategy: stretching	*Corrective strategy: strengthening*	*Preventative strategy: shock-absorbing inserts, prevent deconditioning*

Data from C Rosemond, PT, GCS, University of North Carolina, Chapel Hill.

INCONTINENCE

Urinary Incontinence Guideline Panel. Urinary incontinence in adults: clinical practice guideline. AHCPR Pub. No. 92–0038 (1992)

Issues: 50% of NH pts incontinent of urine resulting in social embarrassment and medical complications such as skin infections; high hidden prevalence in both M/F in community

Intervention: (See 1.9 Incontinence.) Screen for reversible causes of incontinence, ie, local causes: bladder infection, atrophic vaginitis, stool impaction; functional causes: delirium, depression, immobility; systemic illnesses: CHF, hyperglycemia; meds: anticholinergic and adrenergic agents; diet: excess caffeine, soda, alcohol (all "bladder irritants")

Collaborate with nurses to determine cause of incontinence, obtaining signif pos hx for urge, stress, overflow, or functional incontinence; fluid intake, voiding pattern, PVR volume, and UA are w/u necessary for empiric rx; screening in this way allows for identification of select number of pts likely to respond to bladder retraining, an intervention requiring significant staff time and commitment; careful management of early dx and management (change of habits, exercise, meds) of community elderly can be rewarding

SEXUAL FUNCTION

Nurs Home Med 1995;3:56

Issues: Among NH residents 70% (M) and 50% (F) have thought about being close or intimate (Arch Sex Behav 1988;17:109); sexual contacts often casual and involve manual or oral genital stimulation, rather then coitus; privacy rooms often lacking or ill equipped for a couple engaging in a mutual sexual act, even for an able-bodied couple; private space infrequently made for heterosexually wedded couples, almost never made available for gay, lesbian, or bisexual couples; public masturbation may occur when pts seek out stairwells or alcoves, attempting to avoid the scrutiny of the staff

67% of men >80 yr have sex 1/wk; primary reason older women do not have sex is unavailability of partner (Arch Sex Behav 1994; 23:231; 1993;22:543) (see 1.10 Female Sexual Dysfunction)

Intervention: Remove barriers to sexual expression by encouraging privacy (do-not-disturb signs, closed doors), allowing conjugal or home visits, evaluating complaints of sexual function and changing meds that may affect sexual function; counsel interested pts about sexuality, assess decision-making capacity of impaired elderly, provide staff education (Am Fam Phys 1995;51:121); situation capacity: voluntariness, avoidance of harm, avoidance of exploitation, avoidance of abuse, ability to stop and start an interactive behavior when desired, appropriateness of time and place (Assessing Capacity to Give Sexual Consent, Kelly, AMDA meeting Mar 5 1998, San Antonio, TX)

Outpatient: Educational counseling to increase pt comfort in addressing sexual issues and enlarge views of sexuality to link w larger intimacy issues and wide variation for "healthy" sexual adaptation

2.6 OTHER ANTICIPATORY MEASURES

ADVANCED DIRECTIVES

Ouslander JG, Osterweil D, Morley JE. Ethical and legal issues. In: Medical care in the nursing home. New York: McGraw-Hill, 1991:358

Issues: Definition of medical futility nebulous; pts >69 have a 5% chance of surviving CPR, but physicians underestimate what pts consider futile; some pts would consider these odds encouraging and preferable to death (Jama 1995;273:156; Ann IM 1989;111:199); demented pts may be capable of making *some* decisions about their health care (Jama 1988;260:797; 1995;273:124), eg, options regarding a gangrenous leg may be more difficult to comprehend than whether to do CPR (J Am Board Fam Pract 1992;5:127)

Pts and families may fear that advanced directives are not readily carried out in many hospitals; failure of pts to review advanced directives w adult children may lead to conflicts within the family at the time of health crisis; strength of documents can depend on regular reiterations of values and wishes to personal physician recorded in medical record

Intervention: End-of-life decisions should be discussed with the pt or their guardian and family members; include discussion of the following: CPR, ventilator support, hospital or ICU admission, blood transfusion, IV therapy, tube feeding, antibiotics; values questionnaires may be useful to help facilitate discussions (Arch Fam Med 1994;3:1057); early discussions (time of dx of terminal illnesses, including dementia) helpful

MEDICATIONS

Nurs Home Med 1995;3:6

Issues: Risk of adverse drug reaction directly proportional to number of meds pt is on (Ger Rev Syllabus, 1996:31); The Omnibus Budget Reconciliation Act of 1987 (OBRA) mandates strict review of psychotropic meds; psychotropic usage has decreased by 50% since OBRA implementation; use same principles for nonpsychiatric drugs

Intervention:

Community: If pt has multiple physicians, use "brown bag" strategy to determine complete med list (Prim Care 1995;22:697)

Nursing Home: Avoid excessive dosing frequency, prolonged duration of med, duplicate therapy, and side effects that outweigh benefits of drug; do not add med to relieve the side effects of another medicine except perhaps when using anticholinergics to treat extrapyramidal side effects, progesterone to oppose estrogen replacement, or misoprostol to prevent NSAID gastritis; consider cost; interdisciplinary teams including consultant pharmacists can review drug–drug and disease–drug interactions regularly; consider all drugs candidates for regular reevaluation (Table 2-4)

Table 2-4. Lab Work to Follow Effects of Medications for Nursing Home Patients

Practice	Frequency
Pts on NSAIDs: check BUN, Cr, hct	q 2 mo
Pts on iron replacement: hct	q mo until stable, then q 3 mo
Pts on diuretics: BUN, Cr	q 4 mo
Pts on digoxin, phenytoin, quinidine, procaine amide, theophylline, nortriptyline	Levels q 6 mo
CBC, FBS, lytes, BUN, albumin	Yearly
EKG	On admission

Modified from Ann IM 1994;121:584.

ELDER ABUSE

J Am Geriatr Soc 1996;44:65; Nejm 1995;332:437; J Am Geriatr Soc 1994;42:169; Prim Care 1993;20:375

Issues: Prevalence not well documented; family, caregivers, and other neighbors (J Am Geriatr Soc 1998;46:885) of community-dwelling elderly, other NH residents, NH staff, or visitors may be implicated in acts of abuse; stressed caregiver, especially of pts w significant functional disabilities, represent the overwhelming majority (Canadian Task Force, 1994); also associated w child abuse and low income (J Am Geriatr Soc 2000;48:513)

Nursing Home: Inadequate and inconsistent training of caregivers may contribute to abuse; in one study 10% of nursing assistants admitted to at least one act of physical abuse and 40% admitted to at least one act of psychological abuse in the preceding year

Poor hygiene, signs of dehydration, multiple skin lesions with various degrees of healing, wrist or ankle restraint bruises, and pain with occult fx; may be subtle: unjustified chemical restraint, verbal and emotional attack, or failure to follow an appropriate care plan; pts with cognitive and physical impairment and violent, disruptive, or annoying behavior at particular risk for abuse

Assess environment early

Baseline physical exam and long-term perspective may allow the physician to perceive changes in demeanor such as withdrawal, depression, or injuries that suggest abuse

Question capable residents directly to clarify any concerns of abuse or neglect: Has anyone ever tried to hurt you? Has anyone ever made you do things you didn't want to do? Has anyone ever taken anything away from you without your consent?

Evaluate mental status to validate the hx, check driving status

Address spiritual concerns

Interview family members, close friends, and staff to determine general social, psychological status and support; differences in details of unlikely explanations of events from various parties may heighten suspicions of abuse; document physical abuse with photographs where possible (AHCPR Pub. No. 92–0038, 1992)

In most states it is mandatory to report suspected abuse to the ombudsmen (U.S. Preventive Services Task Force, 1996)

Intervention:

Community: Home care agencies, volunteer organizations, adult daycare, other forms of respite

Nursing Home: Weekly decompression groups for staff to discuss their feelings of frustration in caring for challenging pts provide a forum for creative and constructive changes in care plans; behavioral modification techniques

3 Endocrinology

3.1 DIABETES MELLITUS

Ger Rev Syllabus 2000:49; Clin Ger Med, Advances in the Care of
Older People w Diabetes 1999;15:211; Am Fam Phys Monograph
1995;1:1; Sci Am Med 1995;9:vi

Cause: Resistance to effects of insulin peripherally as well as impaired
insulin release w aging (Diabetes Care 2000;23:S1); secondary
causes: glucocorticoids, hydrochlorothiazide, β-blockers, estrogen,
hemochromatosis, Cushing, acromegaly, pheochromocytoma

Epidem: Frank diabetes in 10% patients >65 yr, 20–40% of patients
>80 yr old; half the cases of type 2 not diagnosed (Diabetes Care
1993;16:642); 18% prevalence, non-whites at risk (Nejm 1989;321:
1074; Diabetes 1988;37:878; Diabetes 1987;36:523)

Pathophys: Insulin resistance and decreased insulin production (Diabetes
Care 2000;43:S1); genetic peripheral insulin resistance in the obese
pt; increased levels cause eventual β-cell exhaustion (Ann IM
1990;113:9050); impaired/delayed insulin release and action in
response to glucose load also allows hepatic gluconeogenesis to
persist 1–2 h, then insulin overshoot occurs (Nejm 1992;326:22);
DM like aging 10 yrs, causing increased collagen cross-linking
wrinkles, increased capillary basement membrane thickening,
increased cataracts, atherosclerosis, decreased cognitive function,
decreased bone density; Amylin increased in aging leading to
increased glucose; Lysin decreased w aging leading to increased
adiposity (Morley, Diabetes at AMDA Annual Conference 3/5/99
Orlando, FL); more commonly elderly w type 2 at risk for
hyperglycemic hyperosmolar nonketotic coma (HHNC), secondary
to stress, steroids, tube feeding; failure to replace water because of
impaired thirst and mental status increases osmolarity

Cardiovascular Dysmetabolic Syndrome (Syndrome X): hyperinsulinemia, hyperglycemia, hypertriglyceridemia, HT caused by nitric oxide synthetase, which is inhibited by metformin (Clin Ger Med 1999;15:211)

Sx: Usually atypical presentation, eg, slowly resolving infection, weight loss, fatigue, weakness, acute confusional states, depression

Si: Necrobiosis lipoidica (95%) = pigmented skin plaques with white lipid center, irregular, atrophic; fatty hepatomegaly; retinopathy w hard exudates, microaneurysms, and hemorrhages (photos in Nejm 1993;329:320); neuropathy w decreased sensation, vibratory sense, position sense

Crs: Years before onset of type 2 diabetes, pts have hypertriglyceridemia, low HDL, and HT; factors affecting diabetes control in the elderly: decreased vision, altered taste, poor dentition, arthritis, tremor; living alone impairs food preparation and consumption, as well as med administration

Cmplc:
- Glucotoxicity leads to increased infections and increased pain perception
- HHNC: hyperglycemia >600 mg/dL without ketosis or ketoacidosis, w severe volume depletion (25% body weight); serum osmolality >350 mOsm/kg usually compounding an illness; steroid therapy or tube feeding w concentrated carbohydrate solutions
- Cardiovascular disease 2–3 times greater in type 2 DM than general population; MI and peripheral vascular disease cause 60% of deaths from type II DM, HbA_{1C} <6 decreases risk of MI; half of nontraumatic amputations due to type 2 DM (Lebovitz HE, ed. Therapy for diabetes mellitus and related disorders. 3rd ed. Alexandria, VA: American Diabetes Association, 1998)
- Retinopathy: after 15-yr duration, HbA_{1C} <7 decreases risk of retinopathy (Lancet 1998;352:854; J Am Geriatr Soc 1994;42:142); proliferative in 25% of type 2 on insulin and 5% of those on diet and oral agents (Diabetes Metab Rev 1989;5:559); nonproliferative most common; loss of supporting cells of the retina vasculature leads to microaneurysms, especially at the macula, affecting central vision and visual acuity; when microaneurysms leak, they form punctate "dot-and-blot" hemorrhages that then form hard exudates which can cause macular edema if they accumulate near the macula
- Nephropathy: highest mortality of all the complications; >20% of pts w NIDDM develop nephropathy (Arch IM 1989;111:788);

begins w microalbuminuria 30–300 mg/24 h; risk factors for nephropathy include duration of DM and HT (Nejm 1988; 318:140), inherited tendencies toward ASHD (Nejm 1992; 326:673) and w higher infection rates; symmetric sensorimotor peripheral neuropathy most common ("stocking-glove"); dysesthesias progress to more severe anesthesia and neuropathic foot ulcers; asymmetric mononeuropathies affecting both peripheral and cranial nerves secondary to nerve infarcts; entrapment syndromes such as carpal tunnel syndrome; autonomic neuropathy leading to gastroparesis (delayed gastric emptying, early satiety, fullness, nausea and vomiting), postural hypotension, atonic bladder; polyneuropathy more common in pts w NIDDM and hypoinsulinemia (Nejm 1995;333:89)

- Associated w cognitive decline (Arch IM 2000;160:174; Neurology 1999;52:97; Lancet 1998;352:837)
- Decreased visceral pain perception, eg, silent angina and MIs (Ann IM 1988;108:170), vs silent MIs not any more common in diabetics (Circ 1996;93:2097)

Lab:
- American Diabetic Association (ADA) criteria: 2 FBS >126 mg/dL, or any 2 random >200
- Serum fructosamine, marker for short-term diabetic control (J Am Geriatr Soc 1993;41:1090)
- Monitor HbA$_{1C}$ q 3–6 mo, keep under 8% to avoid microvascular complications

Rx:

Preventive: Annual exams to detect early retinopathy; foot care; detect neuropathy early (10 gm monofilament sensory exam q yr), screen for microalbuminuria; w tight control of blood sugars there is less progression (J Am Geriatr Soc 1994;42:142)

Therapeutic: See Table 3-1
- Any lowering of blood glucose reduces rate of complications (BMJ 2000;321:405)
- Minimally impaired (8 + yr life expectancy): euglycemia the goal; dementia, complex medical problems: control DM w pharmacologic management, minimize hypoglycemia; terminal (<1 yr life expectancy) goal postprandial <200 mg/dL unrestricted diet (table of NH standing orders in Ann LT Care 6:100:109)
- Diabetic pts have more difficulty losing weight than those without; 20% of pts initially control their diabetes by diet alone (Diabetes

Table 3-1. Special Considerations for Diabetes Management in the Elderly

Diagnosis

Recognition of worsening glucose tolerance with aging that contributes to the
  increasing incidence of type 2 diabetes in the elderly population

Use of screening guidelines to help uncover diabetes at its earliest, asymptomatic
  stages

Treatment

Use of diet and exercise to help improve insulin resistance and maintain lean body
  mass

Avoidance of hypoglycemia when choosing drug therapy

Prevent mental status change and adrenergic discharge during low blood glucose

Thiazolidinediones are safe and well-tolerated in the elderly (best studied with
  rosiglitazone).

α-glucosidase inhibitors are safe but limited by potential gastrointestinal side effects.

Use of metformin will also avoid hypoglycemia; however, loss of glomerular
  filtration with aging and decline in renal function needs to be considered.

If employed, short-acting insulin secretagogues and newer agents (repaglinide,
  glimepiride) are safest; avoid chlorpropamide and other insulin secretagogues
  with long half-lives.

1995;44:1249); avoid diabetic diets in NHs where patients at risk
for malnutrition because not eating unappetizing diets
- 20-min exercise 3/wk decreases risk type 2 diabetes (Nejm
  1991;325:147); exercise 1/wk decreases risk developing DM
  by 40%, 60% for overweight men
- Stop hyperglycemic-producing meds, eg, thiazides; try low dose
  12.5 mg, glucocorticoids, sympathomimetics (see list in Ann IM
  1993;118:536)
- Conditions requiring drug therapy: sx secondary to hyperglycemia
  not controlled by diet alone, hyperglycemia leading to risk of
  dehydration, ketones are present; weight loss is rapid and
  uncontrolled; hyperlipidemia–hypertriglyceridemia; in elderly, main
  goal to prevent sx of hyperglycemia, these sx usually begin to occur
  at glucose concentrations 200–250 mg/dL (Nejm 1996;334:574)

First Choice for Drug Therapy:
- Antihyperglycemic meds: for overweight on <40 U/d insulin;
  stimulate endogenous insulin; 2nd-generation hypoglycemics have
  fewer interactions with other meds than the 1st generations but
  more frequently cause hypoglycemia, especially the longer-acting
  ones; glyburide more hypoglycemia than glipizide (J Am Geriatr Soc
  1996;44:751), so start w low doses and increase every 4–7 d;

sustained-release glipizide qd; 20% primary failures and 10–15%; autonomic warning of hypoglycemia (sweating, palpitations) decreased in elderly

- Insulin + oral hypoglycemic: increase bedtime insulin by 2 units q hs until fasting glucose approaching normal giving oral agent opportunity to work
- Rx glucose-induced insulin release in lean elderly w sulfonylurea to stimulate insulin secretion, or give insulin
- Consider rx resistance to insulin-induced glucose disposal in overweight elderly w thiazolidinediones which enhance insulin action (Clin Ger Med 1999;15:239)

Second Choice for Drug Therapy:

- Biguanides (metformin, Glucophage) inhibit gluconeogenesis and increase insulin-mediated glucose uptake, do not cause weight gain (Nejm 1995;333:550); metformin decreases mortality (Lancet 1998;352:854); 500–850 mg po bid; increase by 500 mg q 1–2 wk not exceeding 2500 mg; give w meals; will not cause hypoglycemia as monotherapy; give after failure of diet therapy or add after sulfonylurea fails; moderate decrease in triglycerides, LDL-C, moderate increase HDL-C; side effects: GI (diarrhea, nausea, anorexia, abdominal discomfort, metallic taste, decreased absorption of vit B_{12}, folate); lactic acidosis, especially w liver and renal impairment (abnormal LFTs, Cr >1.5); no Metformin in patients older than 80 yrs old unless Cr clearance nl; contraindications; cardiac or respiratory problems that would lead to hypoxia, severe infection, alcohol abuse, radiographic contrast agents (Nejm 1996;334:577); $47.00/mo (Med Let Drugs Ther 1995;37:41)

Third Choice for Drug Therapy:

- Acarbose and glucose inhibitors: delays digestion and absorption of disaccharides 25–100 mg po ac tid (Ann IM 1994;121:928); GI side effects may be troublesome (diarrhea, abdominal pain, flatulence); may not want to use w metformin because of additive effects; treat hypoglycemia w glucose not sucrose because sucrose may not be adequately hydrolyzed or absorbed (Med Let Drugs Ther 1996;38:9); w Miglitol (Glyset) do not have to monitor liver function
- Thiazolidinediones: Pioglitazone (Actos) 15–45 mg max qd monotherapy and max 30 mg qd for combination therapy, Rosiglitazone (Avandia) 4–8 mg qd-bid improve insulin resistance

without stimulating insulin secretion; give before pancreas fails; may also help w HT, dyslipidemia, atherosclerosis (Am Fam Phys 1997;56:1835; Clin Diabetes 1997;15:60); ALT increased 3 times (Nejm 1998;338:861); ALT q 2 mo × 1 yr and periodically thereafter, stop w abnormal liver function × 2.5; Rosiglitazone plus metformin improve glycemic control in type 2 DM within 2 mo (Jama 2000;283:1695)

• Meglitinides
• Benzoic acid derivatives or meglitinides: repaglinide (non-sulfonylurea insulin secretagogue) stimulating insulin secretion, more rapidly acting, decreased frequency of hypoglycemia (Ger Rev Syllabus 2001:260); short half-life so do not use in NH where meals can be delayed

Insulin has more beneficial effect on lipids (Ann IM 1988;108:134); HbA_{1C} <8.1% reduces renal failure (Nejm 1995;332:1267); hypoglycemia from insulin less prolonged than with oral agents

Types of Insulin: Regular—onset 15 min, peak at 3–4 h, duration 6–8 h; NPH—onset in 3 h, peak at 4–8 h, duration 12–16 h; first-choice regimen (Med Let Drugs Ther 1989;31:363): hs NPH and regular plus NPH in morning; or hs NPH and regular before each meal (Nejm 1993;329:977); start at 5–10 units and increase by 2–3 units every 3–4 d; once stabilized only need to monitor 2 fasting and 2 bedtime measurements a week; ultrafast peak 1 h (Table 3-2)

• Metabolic control of diabetes decreased risk of coronary heart disease (Diabetes 1994;43:960), but associated with more driving accidents (J Am Geriatr Soc 1994;42:695)
• HHNC: look for precipitating infections; replete volume deficit w one-half normal saline; low-dose insulin infusion, 50% mortality; usually insulin rx not required in long-term if pt recovers
• Retinopathy: proliferative retinopathy and macular edema respond to laser rx (Ophthalm 1991;98:766); vitrectomy for vitreous scarring may restore sight (Arch Ophthalm 1985;103:1644)
• Nephropathy: control HT (BMJ 2000;321:394,412; BMJ 1998;317:713; Nejm 1998;338:645), restriction PO_4 (Nejm 1991;324:78), intensive diabetes rx (Nejm 1993;329:977), ACE inhibitors prevent proteinuria (Arch IM 1994;154:625; Jama 1994;271:275; Med Let Drugs Ther 1994;36:46; Nejm 1993;329:1456); β-blocker same improved mortality; do not use ACE inhibitor in patients >80 yrs because K^+ and Cr clearance

Table 3-2. Insulin Types and Blood Glucose Monitoring

Insulin Types and Actions

Insulin Type	Action	Onset (hours)	~Peak	~Clinical Duration
Lispro	Ultrafast	$1/4$	1 hour	3–4 hours
Regular	Fast	$1/2$–1	3 hours	6–8 hours
NPH & Lente	Intermediate	2–3	6–8 hours	14–16 hours
Ultralente (human)	Long	4–8	6–16	18–24 hours
Glarginc	Basal/Very Long	?	None	>24 hours

Time of Blood Glucose Monitoring

	Before Breakfast	Before Lunch	Before Dinner	Bedtime
Insulin dose affecting blood sugar level	Bedtime NPH OR Evening NPH	Breakfast Reg OR Breakfast Lispro	Morning NPH OR Lunch Regular/Lispro	Dinner Regular OR Dinner Lispro
Meal affecting blood sugar level	N/A	Breakfast	Lunch	Dinner

Tom Bartol, RN-C, MN, CDE, 2000.

likely to be abnormal (BMJ 1998;317:720); end-stage renal disease: peritoneal rather than hemodialysis because increased risk of cardiovascular event and retinal bleed w BP fluctuations and anticoagulation; if renal failure occurs in the absence of proteinuria or retinopathy, search for other causes, eg, NSAIDs or UTI

- Neuropathy: rx peripheral neuropathy w Neurontin, tricyclic antidepressants; paroxetine plus imipramine may be more effective than a placebo (Pain 1990;42:135); phenytoin, carbamazepine, capsaicin (Arch IM 1991;151:2225)—questionable benefit, $27.00/oz (Med Let Drugs Ther 1992;34:61); rx diarrhea w clonidine (Ann IM 1985;102:97); rx impotence with Viagra

Team Management:
- Antioxidants, vit C and E, enhance glucose-induced insulin release (Clin Ger Med 1999;15:239)
- Exercise (Jama 1999;282:1433)

- Occupational therapy: magnifiers to wrap around syringes, spring-filling devices that click, "talking glucose meters"; family or nurse may need to do supply setup weekly
- Foot ulcers/infections (Nejm 1994;331:854) w anaerobes and *Pseudomonas*; rx w parenteral imipenem or clavulanate potassium-ticarcillin disodium (Timentin), or oral fluoroquinolone plus clindamycin po 10–14 d; r/o osteomyelitis (Jama 1995;273:712); avoid barefoot walking, rx calluses, check water temperature when bathing feet, toenails clipped straight across; zinc 220 mg tid (70 mg elemental zinc) (Morley 1999 AMDA Annual Meeting Orlando, FL) can irritate stomach (Ger Rev Syllabus 1999–2001: 132)
- Footwear: one pair of shoes and two inserts covered by Medicare per yr (Clin Ger Med 1999;15:351)

3.2 THYROID

HYPOTHYROIDISM

J Am Geriatr Soc 1995;43:592; Clin Ger Med 1995;11:231, 239; Jama 1995;273:808; J Am Geriatr Soc 1994;42:984; J Am Geriatr Soc 1993;41:1361

Cause: Autoimmune thyroiditis; iodine-containing drugs decrease thyroid hormone secretion (Nejm 1995;333:1688), eg, radiographic contrast agents; amiodarone (Br J Clin Pract 1993;47:123); cough medicines, eg, codeine phosphate-dextromethorphan hydrobromide (Tussi-Organidin); antiseptic solutions, eg, povidone-iodine (Betadine); long-term lithium (South Med J 1993;86:1182); cholestyramine; aluminum hydroxide; sucralfate (Carafate) decreases T_4 absorption; rarely tumors of pituitary, hypothalamus

Epidem: 2–5% prevalence; F/M = 5:1; risk factors for thyroid failure: family hx of any thyroid disease, hx of hyperthyroidism, subacute thyroiditis, postpartum thyroid disease, radiation (head, neck, chest), other autoimmune disease, eg, Addison, pernicious anemia; 50% pts with PMR developed hypothyroidism (BMJ 1989;298:647)

Sx: Neither pt nor family aware of changes over number of yrs; debilitation and apathy (66%); falls (17%); frequently subclinical (14%)

Si:

- Skin: myxedematous infiltration of dermis loosening interface dermal-epidermal layers causing shiny tissue paper appearance; hair loss in scalp
- Head/neck: goiter rare, hoarse voice (0.8%), hypothyroid facies (3.3%) (J Am Geriatr Soc 1995;43:59); ophthalmologic—primary open-angle glaucoma (Ophthalm 1993;100:1580; Can J Ophthalm 1992;27:341)
- Neurologic: decreased hearing, carpal tunnel syndrome, paresthesias, positional vertigo, myopathy (1.7%)
- Mental status: withdrawn, confused (3.3%), psychotic (Int J Psychiatr Med 1990;20:193), cognitive deficit (J Am Geriatr Soc 1992;40:325), treatable dementia (Am J Phys Med Rehab 1992; 71:28)
- Cardiovascular: pleural effusions (11%), angina (8%), CHF (5.2%), pleural CVA (3.3%), CPK-MB elevated, bradycardia, infrequent HT
- Respiratory: airway obstruction secondary to swollen tongue, pharynx
- Metabolic: SIADH, hypothermia (1.7%)
- Anemia may be only manifestation; screen for hypothyroidism in pernicious anemia (Arch IM 1982;142:1465)

Cmplc: Myxedema coma (lethargy, confusion, psychosis, sometimes frontal/occipital headache) associated with severe infection, cold exposure, psychoactive meds (Ger Clin N Am 1993;222:279)

Lab:

- TSH >10 mU/L; TSH may be increased by dopamine blocker; there may be an acute elevation of TSH in non-thyroidal illness, recheck 4–6 wk after illness resolves; associated w elevated cholesterol
- R/o hypothalamic-pituitary axis damage: look for DI, acromegaly, hypogonadism, adrenal insufficiency
- If no sx, check antimicrosomal antibody; if increased, likely that subclinical hypothyroidism will convert within 5-yr period to clinical hypothyroidism

EKG: Sinus bradycardia, low-voltage, prolonged QT, AV block, intraventricular conduction delay

Xray: Pleural effusion

Rx:

Preventive: Screen women (U.S. Preventive Services Task Force. Guide to clinical preventive services. 2nd ed. Baltimore: Williams & Wilkins, 1996) and men (= 2.5% subclinical; Arch IM 1990;150:785); low threshold for ordering in pts w nonspecific complaints (J Am Geriatr Soc 1996;44:50)

Therapeutic: L-thyroxine (Synthroid) 0.05 mg/d unless cardiac concerns; increase by 0.025 mg/d q 4–6 wk; in exceptional cases, eg, pts w heart disease may start as low as 0.0125 mg/d

Switching from desiccated thyroid preparation, which has variable bioavailability, to L-thyroxine may lead to iatrogenic hyperthyroidism

Hypothyroid pts with angina can undergo surgery without replacement; do not delay emergent CABG in hypothyroid patients with unstable angina; be careful of CNS-active meds that are cleared more slowly in hypothyroidism (Am J Med 1984;77:261; Ann IM 1981;95:456)

Thyroid replacement does not effect bone density

Myxedema coma: initial T_4 IV 100–500 μg; subsequent dose 100 μg IV qd 1 through 10 d, then po

Pts w profound hypothyroidism requiring emergency general surgery should receive preoperative L-thyroxine 300–500 μg slow IV infusion + hydrocortisone 300 mg IV; Swan-Ganz monitoring; watch for prolonged ileus and infection (altered febrile response) (Clin Ger Med 95;11:251)

Some argue if TSH mildly elevated and T_4 nl, treat to slow atherosclerosis and lower cholesterol (Solomon D, Intensive geriatric review course, UCLA, 1996)

HYPERTHYROIDISM

Clin Ger Med 1995;11:181; Jama 1995;273:808

Cause: Most common cause is toxic nodular goiter; Graves or diffuse nodular goiter less common in late life; iatrogenic: takes T_4 5–6 half-lives to reach steady state in the elderly, or 6–7 wk in pts 80–90 yr old; thus may induce hyperthyroidism if do not wait appropriate amount of time before increasing dose; T_4 may be suppressed in T_3 toxicosis (almost exclusively seen in the elderly);

due to paucity of complaints, important to screen q 2 yr w TSH (J Am Geriatr Soc 1996;44:50)

Epidem: 15–25% of cases occur in the elderly; 0.47% prevalence in community-based elderly

Pathophys: Apathetic thyrotoxicosis diminished postreceptor responsiveness to thyroid hormone w age

Sx: Rarely report loose stools but may note a correction of constipation; reduction in appetite, consume fewer calories, weight loss; inability to rise from chair due to proximal muscle weakness; apathetic hyperthyroidism

Si: Coarse tremor; less common in elderly; most frequent cardiac manifestation is sinus tachycardia; afib

Cmplc: Accelerates bone turnover, leading to osteoporosis; causes insulin resistance (2–3% of thyrotoxic pts develop clinically significant diabetes); CHF (60% of elderly persons w hyperthyroidism develop CHF); high-output failure leads to widened pulse pressure; 50% have afib; 20% have angina (Nejm 1992;327:94); thyroid often largely substernal

Lab: TSH lowered by dopamine agonists and corticosteroids (Drinka P 1997 AMDA Annual Meeting, Phoenix, AZ)

Xray: Diagnosis confirmed by increased uptake of radioactive iodine

Rx:

Preventive: If asx but TSH low w normal T_3, T_4, monitor more frequently for sx and increase in T_3, T_4 and treat

Therapeutic:

- I^{131} for toxic multinodular goiter requires 2–3 times the radioisotope dose for diffuse toxic goiter; for Graves: irradiation (Table 3-3), propylthiouracil (PTU) for 3 wk before radioactive iodine therapy to eliminate the possibility of radiation-induced thyroiditis; major complication of radiation is hypothyroidism: 50% develop hypothyroidism within 20 yr
- Methimazole (Tapazole) when TSH low, T_3, T_4 normal but patient is sx (J Am Geriatr Soc 1996;44:573)
- Graves: β-blockers: for heat intolerance, anxiety, myopathy; adverse effects: cardiac, pulmonary, memory, mood, sleep disorders, fatigue
- PTU 100 mg or methimazole (Tapazole) 10 mg q 6–8 h blocks hormone synthesis; large goiters may require twice as much, rarely up to 1000 mg/d of PTU; euthyroid in 6 wk, then can begin maintenance 50–300/d × 1 yr; > one-third respond permanently; adverse effects include hypothyroidism, agranulocytosis (0.5%)

Table 3-3. Radioisotope Use in Thyroid Disease

Iodine 131	Iodine 123	Technetium 99m
$t_{1/2}$ = 8 d, 30% detection hyperactive thyroid, readily available, low cost, use to rx hyperthyroidism, thyroid cancer	$t_{1/2}$ = 13 h, 80% detection, not easily available, high cost	$t_{1/2}$ = 6 h, 90% detection, readily available, low cost, use to image thyroid when pt has had thyroid-blocking agents

Drugs that interfere w thyroid iodine absorption: adrenocorticosteroids, nitrates, PTU, ASA, sulfonamides, methimazole for 2 mo, myelogram contrast agent for 2 yr.

(early in treatment, w large doses, reversible w withdrawal, baseline WBC, and repeat w signs of infection—fever), skin rash, arthralgia, myalgia, neuritis, SLE, psychosis

- Prior to surgery on those with untreated hyperthyroidism: IV loading dose of PTU 1000 mg or ipodate sodium 500 mg po × 5 d prior to surgery, or propranolol IV 1 mg/min during surgery

Epidem: More common in elderly and more frequently malignant, and when malignant more aggressive than in younger patients; more common among women; differentiated tumors more aggressive at age >45 yr; anaplastic exclusively at age >65 yr

Sx: Dysphagia, pain suggest cancer

Si: Hard nodules, enlarged lymph nodes, rapid growth should raise suspicion of cancer

Crs: Variable and dependent on pathologic grade

Cmplc: Of multinodular goiter: thyrotoxicosis, subclinical thyrotoxicosis (Clin Endocrinol 1992;36:25), vocal cord paralysis, tracheal compression (Am J Med 1988;84:19)

R/o benign: colloid (60%), adenomas (30%); carcinoma (Table 3-4), lymphoma frequently in persons w underlying Hashimoto thyroiditis

Lab:

Pathologic: Fine-needle aspiration (FNA) bx—malignant reports in 5% of specimens, and an indication for surgery (except w lymphoma or anaplastic carcinoma); false-pos rate of 5–7%; bx several areas of multinodular goiter (larger, harder ones, those that are cold on scan)

Xray: Both US and radionuclide scan more sens than palpation; nodules frequently cold and solid

Rx:

Table 3-4. Thyroid Carcinoma

	Papillary	Follicular	Medullary	Anaplastic
Cause	Graves: LATS	—	—	—
Epidem	75% of thyroid cancers	15%	5%	3%
Pathophys	—	—	Associated w MEN IIA, hyperparathyroidism, pheochromocytoma	—
Sx	30% present as occult tumors; lymph node enlargement; hoarseness, dysphagia, neck pain	Slow-growing goiter; lymph node not as common as papillary; 50% metastatic at presentation; occasionally thyrotoxicosis	—	Sudden increase in size of goiter; difficulty breathing
Si	Bilateral	—	Mostly bilateral	Firm, tender w soft areas of hemorrhage, necrosis
Crs	Good prognosis if <1.5 cm despite lymph node involvement; 55% 10-yr survival; enters more malignant phase after 10 yr w metastases to lung, bone (lytic), brain, and soft tissue	High mortality w vascular invasion	To lymph node liver, bone, adrenal	Mortality 6 mo to 1 yr
Lab	Psammoma bodies pathognomonic on histology	—	Calcitonin >250 pg/mL indicates cancer	—
Rx	Surgery: total thyroidectomy w excision suspicious lymph nodes, ablate postoperatively w ^{131}I; watch calcium levels postoperatively; f/u T4 q 6 mo, if elevated, check radioiodine scan and rx recurrent disease w [131]I	Radioactive iodine; replace w T3 because shorter-acting and can discontinue for only 2 wk when checking radioactive scan yearly	Not responsive to radioiodine; rx w surgery	Radiation shrinks tumor (4–5000 rads); may cause tracheal obstruction; undifferentiated cancer fatal in 1 yr; rx doxorubicin (De Vita VT, Cancer principles and practice of oncology, 4th ed, Lippincott, 1993: 1333)

LATS = long-acting thyroid stimulator; MEN = multiple endocrine neoplasia.
Source: Gupta KL. Neoplasm of the thyroid gland. Clin Geriatr Med 1995;11:271–90.

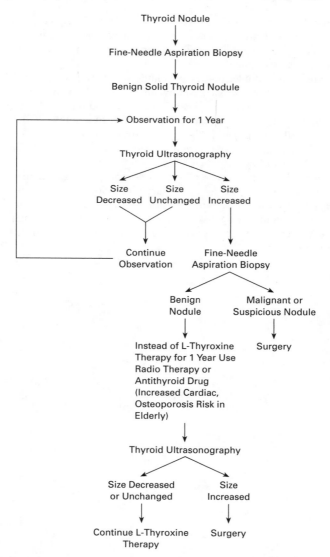

Figure 3-1. Decision making for treatment of patients with benign thyroid nodules. (Reproduced by permission from Mehta V, Savino JA. Surgical management of the patient with a thyroid disorder. Clin Geriatr Med 1995;11:291–309.)

Therapeutic: See Figure 3-1; thyroid replacement: if TSH elevated, reassess nodule after 2 mo of thyroid replacement; multinodular goiters do not respond as well to suppressive therapy as Hashimoto thyroiditis or simple diffuse goiters

Of hot nodules: older pts w hot nodules, nl T_4, but suppressed TSH (subclinical thyrotoxicosis) have increased risk for osteoporosis and possible underlying heart disease; should have lower threshold for radioactive rx, solitary autonomously functioning nodule 200–400 µCi/gm and 80–100 µCi/gm for toxic multinodular goiter, surgery if rapid decompression vital structures (Nejm 1998;338:1438)

If benign FNA and nodule <2 cm, use suppression rx; if benign FNA and >2 cm, surgery indicated (larger nodules not as responsive)

Preoperative cardiac screening indicated for pts undergoing thyroid surgery w following risk factors: Q wave MI on EKG, angina, DM, ventricular ectopy requiring rx, advanced age (Ann IM 1989;110:859)

4 Neurology

4.1 STROKE

Am J Med 1996;100:465; Circ 1996;94:1167; Arch Neurol 1995;52:347; Am Fam Phys 1994;49:1777; Clin Ger Med 1993;9:705; Reuben DB, Ger Rev Syllabus Suppl 1993:126S; Ger Rev Syllabus; 2001:224; Circulation 2000;102:11; Stroke 2001;32:803

Cause: Carotid or aortic arch (Nejm 1992;326:221), basilar system plaque and/or platelet emboli, cardiac emboli, vascular spasm, hypercoagulable states, idiopathic

Risk Factors: HT, DM, CAD, MI, afib (14% risk embolic stroke at onset and 5%/yr), peripheral vascular disease (PVD), smoking, lipids, homocystinemia (Jama 1997;227:1775; Ann IM 1995;123:747; Jama 1995;274:1526; Nejm 1995;372:286,328); cholesterol associated positively with ischemic stroke risk and negatively with hemorrhagic stroke (Jama 1997;278:316)

Hemorrhagic Stroke: 50% are due to HT, 17% from amyloid angiopathy, 10% from anticoagulation rx, 5–10% from brain tumors, 5% from smoking (Nejm 1992;326:1672; Curr Concepts Cerebro Dis 1991;26:1; 1990;25:31)

Epidem: 75% of pts w CVA are >75 yr; 2% incidence/yr for elderly; 35,000 pts/yr in NH; 100,000 pts/yr at home

Pathophys: Occasionally is vasospastic and can rx w calcium channel blocker (Nejm 1993;329:396) (Table 4-1)

Sx:
- TIA: most resolve <24 h, 70% <1 h
- Infarct: h/o TIA (80%); 60% onset in early morning hours awakens w stroke

   Anterior circulation sx: amaurosis fugax (Stroke 1990;21:201); weakness of arm > face > leg paresis (middle cerebral artery

NEUROLOGY

Table 4-1. Stroke Types and Mortality

Cerebral Infarct (75%)	Intracerebral Hemorrhage (15%)	Subarachnoid Hemorrhage (10%)
40%	80%	50%

    affected pattern); leg > arm > face paresis (anterior cerebral artery pattern); depression; abulia; delusions; aphasia if dominant hemisphere

    Posterior circulation sx: diplopia, numbness in face and mouth; slurred speech; loss of consciousness; crossed signs CN vs body; headache (HA); vomiting; dizziness; ataxia

    Lacunar: pure motor w internal capsule; pure sensory w thalamus; dysarthria and clumsy hand w pons; ataxia and hemiparesis w base pons, genu and internal capsule

- Embolism: 75% middle cerebral, 90% maximum loss at onset, loss of consciousness (LOC) common, seizure
- Hemorrhagic infarct: during physical activity, most commonly from Berry aneurysm or microaneurysm from HT; decreased alertness, vomiting; hemiparesis w putamen or thalamus bleed; bilateral signs and coma w brainstem; HA, vertigo, ataxia, gaze, and facial palsy w cerebellar

Si:

- TIAs: in elderly, asx bruit present in 10% and does not correlate with CVA rate in or out of affected carotid distribution
- Infarct: specific occlusion patterns

    Middle cerebral: face and arm motor; expressive aphasia (Broca)

    Carotid watershed: parietal aphasias, weakness arm > face > leg

    Posterior cerebral: homonymous hemianopsia, hemisensory loss, memory loss (Curr Concepts Cerebro Dis 1986;21:25)

    Lateral medullary plate syndrome (PICA: posterior inferior cerebellar artery; Curr Concepts Cerebro Dis 1981;16:17): ipsilateral pain and temperature loss on face, contralateral for rest of body, hoarseness, swallowing dysfunction, Horner, hiccoughs, ipsilateral cerebellar si

- Subarachnoid hemorrhage: HT, stiff neck
- Cerebellar hemorrhage: awake, alert even with ophthalmoplegias; acute hypotonia; conjugate gaze paresis; skew deviation
- Cerebral hemorrhage: seizure (13%) w onset or within 48 h

- Brainstem hemorrhage: early loss of consciousness, brainstem si, quadriplegia

Crs:

- 20% of pts w TIAs will have CVA within 1 mo; 50% in 1 yr; 50% of pts w TIAs die of CAD while 36% die of CVA; association of TIA w MI as strong as MI and 3-vessel CAD (Am Fam Pract Series III Home study monograph 1995:195)
- Infarct: if there is even slightest voluntary twitch within 7 d of stroke onset, full upper extremity recovery may be expected; voluntary hip flexion predictor of ambulation, spasticity resolves, hyperreflexia persists
- Embolic stroke: 15% 30-d mortality; 12% of cardiac embolic stroke have second embolus within 2 wk of first event
- Hemorrhagic stroke: over 1 mo 33% die, 33% are impaired, and 33% are OK (Nejm 1993;311:1547)

Cmplc:

- TIA: r/o migraine, subdural, hematoma, seizures, hypoglycemia, tumor, MS
- Stroke: r/o MI w EKG
- CVA: seizures, 33% of which occur within 2 wk after infarction; depression occurs in 40% of L-hemisphere infarction; probably physiologic not psychological phenomenon (Stroke 1994;25:1099); arthritis of shoulder after hemiplegia despite passive range of motion exercises; pulmonary emboli; pneumonias; UTIs
- Reflex sympathetic dystrophy: burning pain, vasomotor instability, trophic changes skin, bony demineralization of hand or foot secondary to abnormal stimulation of sympathetic nervous system; rx is short course high-dose steroids, physical therapy, sympathetic nerve block (Lancet 1993;342:1012)

Lab:

Noninvasive: Carotid duplex US, carotid Doppler US, MRA all about 85% sens and 90% specif (Ann IM 1988;109:805,835; 1995;122:360); CBC w platelets, PT/PTT; VDRL; EKG (r/o MI, arrhythmia), which often shows abnormal "anterior MI" patterns (Nejm 1974;291:1122; J Neur Surg 1969;30:521)

Hemorrhagic Stroke: LP preferably only after CT to r/o mass lesion; CSF: some intracerebral bleeds and all subarachnoid bleeds show grossly bloody tap w >1000 rbc/dL (100% sens, 80% specif), protein >1 gm/dL; xanthochromia present in 90% (centrifuge immediately to avoid false-pos); rbc decrease 10-fold from first to third tube (Ann IM 1986;104:880)

Xray: W/u TIA w US Doppler; CT best for acute bleed; MRI for lacunar—not good for acute bleed; old strokes often found during acute CT in elderly; MRI-A as good as angiography; videofluoroscopy to determine aspiration and subsequent pneumonia risk (Arch Phys Med Rehabil 1996;77:707)

Hemorrhagic Stroke: 25% of subarachnoid bleeds will not show blood on CT

Rx:

Preventive: Decrease systolic BP to 140 even in pts >80 yr; decreases long-term incidence of CVA by 3% and MI by 5.5%; prefer thiazides and β-blockers, ACE inhibitors (for acute BP management, see treatment section)

Control blood sugar in diabetic pts

If smoke >20 cigarettes/d, have 6 times increased risk for CVA (Cullison S, Cerebral vascular disease, strokes and TIAs, at Family Practice review course, Seattle, WA, 3/95); incidence falls significantly after 2 yr of not smoking and falls to risk of nonsmokers after 5 yr of not smoking

ASA after TIA reduces recurrence of nonfatal stroke, MI, and vascular death by 20–25% (BMJ 1994;308:81,1540; Curr Opin Neurol 1994;7:48)

Warfarin for all afib unless contraindications (Jama 1995;274:1839; Nejm 1995;332:238; 1995;333:5; Ann IM 1994;121:41,54)

Versus ASA for pts w nonvalvular afib <60 yr; warfarin (Coumadin) for pts w nonvalvular afib 65–75 yr; ASA for pts w nonvalvular afib >75 yr (Lancet 1994;343:687); pts w nonvalvular afib can be rx w ASA if low risk, eg, do not have CHF or EF <25, previous thromboembolism, systolic BP >160 mmHg, W >75 yrs (Jama 1998;279:1273)

Warfarin for pts w 60% carotid stenosis (Jama 1995;243:1421; Nejm 1995;332:238)

Statins to reduce risk of nonhemorrhagic stroke (Nejm 2000;343:317; Ann IM 1998;128:89)

Folic acid 1 mg po qd to reduce risk of ASCVD (Jama 1998;279:359; Nejm 1998;338:1009)

Therapeutic:

- TIA: endarterectomy if >70–80% stenosis (Lancet 1998;351: 1373,1379; Jama 1995;273:1421; Nejm 1991;325:445); consider if combined cmplc rate of angiography and surgery at your hospital is <3%, since often morbidity is 14% in community hospitals, but only 1% in big centers; more risk of MI s/p endarterectomy in pts >70 yr old (Cardiovasc Surg 1993;1:30); ETT if any cardiac risk factors; warfarin 3-mo course; if risk of bleeding, ASA 300 mg; if risk of bleeding ticlopidine (Ticlid) better (Med Let Drugs Ther 1992;34:65); adverse effects of ticlopidine: diarrhea, abdominal cramps, rarely neutropenia (monitor blood counts q 1 mo for 3–4 mo) (Ann IM 1994;121:45)

- Stroke in evolution: IV TPA within 3 h of onset of stroke results in 30% improvement in clinical outcome but increased incidence of intracranial hemorrhage within 36 h (6.45% vs 0.6%) (Jama 1996;276:961; Nejm 1995;333:1581) in pts up to 85 yr (Circ 1996;94:1826); alteplase (Activase) (Med Let Drugs Ther 1996;38:99)

- Nonhemorrhagic infarct: use anticoagulant only w CVA in evolution, TIA in pt on ASA or ticlopidine; otherwise risk of bleeding too great (American Heart Association, Stroke 1994;25:1901)

Acute Care (Curr Concepts Cerebro Dis 1989;24:1): Rx diastolic BP >140 or systolic >230 acutely with IV nitroprusside; if diastolic persists >105 or systolic >180 for 1–2 h, then rx with labetalol IV or po, mannitol 25–50 gm as 20% soln over 30 min q 3–12 h and/or furosemide IV, and/or nifedipine sl or po (sl nifedipine may lower BP too abruptly) (American Heart Association, Stroke 1994;25:1901); keep Pco_2 at 25–30 mmHg if on respirator; monitor; give 100–125 mL/h of Ringer's or D5S

Supportive Care: Heparin sc to prevent DVT, which occurs in 70% (Ann IM 1992;117:353); pneumatic compression further prevents DVT in stroke pts (Neurology 1998;50:1683); post-stroke depression: SSRIs (Stroke 1994;25:1099) or nortriptyline (Lancet 1984;1:297)

Follow-up Care:

- Embolic stroke: decreased by 86% if anticoagulate 2 yr; annual bleeding rate 2.5% (Ann IM 1992;320:352,392); maintain INR 2–3; warfarin if abnormal echocardiogram; anticoagulate >60% occluded asx carotid stenosis w intermittent or chronic afib to decrease embolic stroke, NNT = 16 (Jama 1995;273:1421); surgically fix >70% carotid stenosis (Nejm 1995;332:238)

- Hemorrhagic infarct: prevent aspiration; hydration control; do not lower BP; supratentorial >5 cm size bad prognosis; pontine >3 cm bad prognosis

Rehab (Clin Ger Med 1999;15:819,833):

- Prognosis for pts w CVAs >65 yr: 10% no dysfunction, 40% moderate dysfunction, 40% severe dysfunction, 10% institutionalized; begin physical therapy right away after stroke w progression to full program as able; good prognostic signs: motivated to participate in rehab, follows one-step commands, memory to learn, bowel and bladder control, feeding and grooming skills, strong social support; successful rehab not associated w size or site of infarction (Arch Phys Med Rehab 1989;7:100) or age alone

- 6 mo to regain motor function w continuous gains for 2–3 yr; 2–3 yr to regain language function

- Upper extremity motor skills can improve despite residual spasticity (Stroke 1998;29:75); whole-task and meaningful-task better than part-task practice (Am J Occup Ther 1997;51:508)

- Reimbursement from Medicare for rehab requires multidisciplinary approach, documentation of goals, documentation of improvement; goal cannot be maintenance

- Criteria for admission to acute rehab facility: expected rapid rate of improvement, eg, 3–4 wk; tolerate 3 h/d of combined therapy 6–7 d/wk; minimal dementia; may want to use methylphenidate HCl (Ritalin) for severely depressed pts to ensure their candidacy for rehab but would try SSRIs first; Ritalin good prior to SSRI b/c of rapid onset of action

- To obtain rehab in the home, must need two therapies daily, as well as daily nursing and 24-h physician availability; location of rehab program may vary w managed-care programs

Team Management: (post-stroke rehab in AHCPR Pub No. 95–0663, 1995; Clinical Practice Guidelines in Jama 1997;45:881)

Physical Therapy: Return of function 3–12 mo: start brace when have "en masse" flexor or extensor synergism of all joints and 4/5 strength and can balance on good leg; then work on selective flexion and bed access; metal brace for spasticity

Shoulder pain common and has many possible causes: adhesive capsulitis, shoulder subluxation, rotator cuff injury, tenosynovitis, rarely reflex sympathetic dystrophy (cutaneous sensitivity and swelling of hand and arm); rx w ROM exercises, hot and cold contrast baths; if unresponsive, can try high-dose corticosteroids, stellate block; rx spasticity w baclofen, dantrolene or tizanidine (D_2-adrenergic agonist not yet released on U.S. market), all of which cause sedation

Occupational Therapy: Diagnose and rx perceptual, cognitive losses and ADL deficit, and help pt begin to engage in social activity again

Swallowing Evaluation: (See Table 4-2) 6 nerves and 25 facial and oral muscles involved; 40–50% of stroke pts have some degree of dysphagia, which can carry up to a 40% risk of aspiration; transit time is measured by placement of examiner's index and third fingers at the top and bottom of the thyroid cartilage while pt swallows; delay >10 sec is associated w a significant risk of aspiration (Am Fam Phys 1994;49:1777); methylene blue dye test useful for pts w tracheostomy, dye in tracheal secretions after oral intake of dye in foods indicates aspiration (Am J Nurs 1995;95:34)

Feeding Recommendations:
1. 30-min rest before eating
2. Observation of eating essential until degree of risk established
3. Call button if eating without assistance
4. Allow 30–40 min for pt to eat meal
5. Juice better than water because taste helps locate food in mouth; the pulp in citrus juices may pose a problem
6. Avoid sticky, dry foods and mucus-producing foods such as milk products; just because pt has gag reflex does not mean will not aspirate; small amounts of food may not stimulate a gag reflex; may need to thicken fluids; chopped better than puree
7. Have pts clear their throat before swallowing, say "ah," and if sound is gurgly, may have aspirated; pt can perform finger sweep between swallows
8. Straws deposit food too far back in the throat; if pt has a weak swallow reflex, keep drinking glass three-fourths full so pt does not have to tilt head too far back
9. Keep pt upright 45–60 min after eating
10. Pt education about risk factors (Jama 1998;278:1324)

NEUROLOGY

Table 4-2. Four Phases of Swallowing

Phase	Description	CN	Dysfunction	Assess
Oral preparatory	Lips closed, lubrication, chewing, tongue places bolus of food between tongue and palate	V, VII, XII, voluntary, cortical	Drooling, food pocketed on affected side, because no sensation	"Mi, mi, mi"
Oral	Food received into the pharynx beginning the reflex of swallowing	XII, voluntary, cortical	Coughing, choking	"La, la, la"
Pharyngeal	Tongue and pharynx walls push food into the esophagus, laryngeal elevation triggers closure of the epiglottis and vocal cords	IX, X, XI, involuntary, brainstem	Food stuck in throat, nasal regurgitation, coughing, choking, hoarseness	"Ga, ga, ga"
Esophageal	Upper esophageal sphincter closes, peristalsis moves food from esophagus to stomach	X, involuntary, brainstem		

Reproduced by permission from Gauwitz DF. How to protect the dysphagic stroke patient. Am J Nurs 1995;95:34–8.

4.2 PARKINSON DISEASE

Robbins L, UCLA, geriatrics review course lecture on Parkinson's disease, 1/96; Neurol 1994;44(suppl 10)

Cause: Environmental factors (blacks in America have 5 times risk of blacks in Nigeria); genetic cause chromosome 4 (Science 1996;274:1197); parkin enzyme deficiency leads to build-up of toxic synuclein in nigostriatal neurons (Science 2001;293:263); drugs w antidopaminergic properties: some calcium channel blockers, haloperidol (Haldol), metoclopramide (Reglan), prochlorperazine (Compazine), reserpine, amoxapine (Asendin), lithium, methyldopa (Aldomet); drug-induced Parkinson in first 3 mo of therapy (Table 4-3), and reversible when discontinued usually within weeks to months

Epidem: 50,000 new cases annually; 1/100 elderly vs 1/1000 general population; prevalence second only to Alzheimer among degenerative neurologic diseases; cigarette smoking associated w decreased risk of Parkinson (Neurology 1995;43:1041); high intake of caffeine associated w decreased incidence of Parkinson (Jama 2000;283:2674); NH pts w Parkinson undertreated: lacking in physical therapy, rx of depression, adequate social interaction (J Am Geriatr Soc 1996;44:300; Nejm 1996;334:71)

Pathophys: Loss of pigmented neurons in substantia nigra and brainstem, Lewy bodies (concentric hyaline cytoplasmic inclusions); dopamine reduced in substantia nigra and corpus striatum; clinical symptoms when 80% depletion of striatal dopamine; neurotoxins: manganese toxicity, copper in Wilson disease destroys dopaminergic neurons (Onion DK. The little black book of primary care. Malden, MA: Blackwell Science, 1996)

Si: (See Table 4-4, Table 4-5) Bradykinesia, rigidity (no loss of muscle strength), tremor (3–7 Hz), pill-rolling tremor (not as common in drug-induced Parkinson or atherosclerotic Parkinson) (Lancet 1984;2:1092; UCLA intensive review course, 1996), hypophonia, micrographia, depression 15–40% (serotonin pathway may be affected too), drooling, constipation, seborrheic dermatitis

Crs: Average life expectancy = 12.3 yr, some live 20+ yr, more rapid course in elderly, declining 5 yr after diagnosis

Cmplc: R/o vascular parkinsons: gait, balance problems out of proportion to rigidity, tremor doesn't respond to meds

NEUROLOGY

Table 4-3. Parkinson Disease and Other Disorders

	Bradykinesia	Tremor	Automatic Dysfunction	Dementia	Depression	Vertical Gaze Paralysis/PDD	Other Neurologic Signs
Parkinson's 130/100 000	Facial Psychomotor slowing (cog wheeling) Slowed gait, decreased arm swing, forward flexion of neck and trunk Decrease turning (truncal rigidity) Decrease stride, step height (festonating gait) Drooling Hypophonic speech Micrographia	Alt. flexion ext fingers; resting; disappears with action; 4–8 c/sec; 70%	Hypotension Constipation (Shy-Drager) Increased salivation Increased sebum Dysphasia	40%; increased SE with meds	60%	Absent/absent	Absent
Supranuclear palsy	Axial rigidity Neck extension posture	Absent	Absent	Decreased cognition Decreased memory Decreased abstract thought	Present	Present/present	Absent

					Emotional lability		
Lacunar infarct	Present	Absent	Present	—		Absent/present	Present
Hypothyroid	Delayed response Slowed movement	Absent	Absent	Present	Present	Absent/absent	Present
Hypoparathyroid	Present	Absent	Absent	Absent	Absent	Absent/absent	Present, cerebral dysfunction
Drugs Methyldopa Diazepam Lithium Reserpine Cholinergics Phenothiazines Excess vit B₆	Present	May be present	Absent	Delirium	May be present	Absent/absent	Absent
Other AIDS Neoplasia Trauma Creutzfeldt-Jakob Viral postencephalitis Hydrocephalus	Present	—	—	—	—	Absent/absent	—

Alt = alternating; ext = extension; SE = side effects; PPD = pseudobulbar dysarthria, dysphagia.

Table 4-4. Clinical Classification of Tremors

Feature	Parkinsonian	Exaggerated Physiologic	Essential	Cerebellar
Frequency (Hz)	4–7	6–12	6–12	3–5
Amplitude	Coarse	Fine	Variable	Variable
Tremor at rest	++++	+	+	+
Tremor with action				
Postural	++	++++	+++	+++
Intention	++	++	++	++++
Distribution	Limbs, jaw, tongue	Limbs	Hands, head	Limbs, head

Table 4-5. Parkinson Disease Age-related Characteristics

Older Pts (>65)	Younger Pts (<65)
Tremor (63%)	—
Bilateral (50%)	Unilateral (90%)
Difficulty walking (33%)	Stiff muscles (43%)

Reproduced by permission from Blin J, Bonnet AM, Agid Y. Does levodopa aggravate Parkinson's disease? Neurology 1988;38:1410–6.

- R/o essential tremor, which is sporadic or hereditary w onset at early age; interferes w volitional movements, eg, writing, eating, highly skilled occupations; alcohol helps; β-blockers (propranolol 40–320 mg/d) significant improvement in one-half pts; primidone (Mysoline) (125–750 mg/d) also effective; clonazepam third choice
- R/o Lewy body disease: sx of dementia preceded by depression/sleep disorder, drug-induced hallucinations and may respond to Levodopa in early stages
- R/o progressive supranuclear palsy (axial rigidity, vertical and later horizontal gaze paralysis, very little in the way of tremor); nortriptyline 100 mg/d to rx depression of supranuclear palsy (J Am Geriatr Soc 1997;45:1034), progresses to death 5–10 yrs. Sleep disturbance common problem (J Am Geriatr Soc 1997;45:194); drugs causing tremor: xanthines, β-agonists, valproate, heavy metals (Hg, Pb, As), thyroid, corticosteroids, multiple environmental toxins, methylphenyltetrahydropyridine (MPTP)
- Shy-Drager seen w bradykinesia, autonomic dysfunction, and cerebellar ataxia due to degeneration of sympathetic preganglionic

nerves of thoracic and upper lumbar spinal cord, and not responsive to L-dopa; hypotension resulting from rx of Parkinson can be treated w high-salt diet or fludrocortisone or midodrine (Geriatrics 1999;54:44)

Hallucinations associated w Parkinson dementia (see subcortical dementia in 5.5 Dementias) chief reason for admission to NH for Parkinson pts (J Am Geriatr Soc 2000;48:938)

Lab: CBC, chem profile, albumin (nutritional assessment), thyroid profile, VDRL, Pb level

Xray: Chest xray—baseline for aspiration changes

Rx:

Therapeutic: Begin treatment when function is impacted; Parkinson sx fluctuate from hour to hour and day to day; thus evaluate med adjustments over days to weeks; seek family, staff observations over 24-h periods (Fig 4-1)

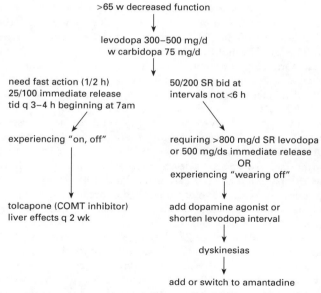

Figure 4-1. Flow sheet for medications for Parkinson disease. (Adapted from Stacy M. Parkinson's disease: therapeutic choices and timing decisions in patient management. Interview by Wayne Kuznar. Geriatrics 1999;54:44–9.)

L-dopa: effective, but because of adverse effects sometimes saved for more advanced disease; carbidopa/levodopa precipitates oxidation that further damages the substantia nigra and eventually spreads disease progression (J Am Geriatr Soc 1997;45:233); give w carbidopa (Sinemet) to limit breakdown (need at least 75–100 mg/d of carbidopa and do not exceed 200 mg/d); start with 25/100 one-half tab bid, increasing dose q wk by one-half to 1 tab daily (2–8 tabs/d); L-dopa requirement for most pts is 500–1000 mg, so may need to add 10/100 mg tabs to increase L-dopa but keep down carbidopa; painful dystonia upon awakening is a good indication that L-dopa should be increased; give 2nd dose in afternoon to avoid insomnia; major side effects: hallucinations, psychosis; dyskinesias usually mean there is too much dopamine; take controlled release (CR) with food and increase total dose of L-dopa by 30% because not as bioavailable as short-acting (Nejm 1993;329:1021); CR 50/200 mg bid 8 am and 3–4 pm (J Am Board Fam Pract 1997;10:412); breaking tablets in 1/2 speeds absorption and action, tid or qid; combine dosing CR night with multiple small doses during day (25/100 mg CR); use 50/100 mg CR for motor fluctuations (Am Fam Phys 1996;53:1281); diphenidol for nausea (does not block dopamine receptors as other antinausea medications do); avoid supplements that contain high doses of B_6 (50–100 mg) because reduces activity of carbidopa; transdermal L-dopa under investigation (Nejm 1993;329:1021)

Dopamine agonists: may want to start rx w dopamine agonist to delay or minimize use of carbidopa/L-dopa and also to avoid anticholinergic drugs, but demented patients prone to sedation, orthostasis, psychiatric side effects; pramipexole not as effective as L-dopa in initial rx of Parkinson (Jama 2000;284:1931); pt does not need to avoid protein in diet because does not affect absorption of dopamine; titrate slowly; may be neuroprotective (Mayo Clinic Proc 1966;71:659) (Med Let 2001;43:57)

Bromocriptine (Parlodel) at 20–30 mg moderate effects on bradykinesia; can be added to L-dopa to reduce the dose needed of L-dopa; start at 1.25 mg/d and increase over several days to weeks (q wk by 1.25–2.50-mg/d increments); side effects: nausea, vomiting, dry mouth, orthostasis, confusion, hallucinations; ropinirole and pramipexole not expected to have side effects of bromocriptine; alter overall symptomatic course of Parkinson by binding selectively to D_2-like receptors (Jama 1997;278:125; Med Let 1997;39:102)

Selegiline (Deprenyl): MAO-B inhibitor may delay onset Parkinson by 1–3 yr (Nejm 1989;321:1364); may not be so good for early Parkinson (multicenter British study in BMJ 1995;311:1602); $1400–1500/yr; not active in gut so no tyramine effect; selegiline in doses of 2.5–10.0 mg/d blocks metabolism of CNS dopamine, thus enhancing L-dopa, may also be antioxidant; other newer agents may act in similar manner, eg, catechol O-methyltransferase (COMT) inhibitors which in conjunction with L-dopa/carbidopa lengthens L-dopa's duration of action by inhibition of the conversion of L-dopa to 3-OMD; best for wearing off phenomenon; better in setting of confusion (J Am Geriatr Soc 2000;48:692); may be better than dopamine agonists (Lancet 1997;350:712); can be adjusted downward if dyskinesias appear (Tolcapone 100–200 mg/d); metabolized by liver, monitor liver function × 6 mo; or entacapone 200 mg w each dose interval of carbidopa-levodopa; allows reduction of L-dopa dose (Ann LT Care 1998;6f:1); selegiline sometimes used in advanced disease for reducing wearing-off effect; adverse effects include insomnia, confusion, dyskinesias, GI distress; do not combine w tricyclic antidepressants, selective serotonin reuptake inhibitors because of severe risk of hypertensive reaction; serious drug interactions w meperidine (Demerol); acts as MAO-A at >10 mg/d

Propranolol 160 mg/d (controlled release) first choice for tremor (Arch Neurol 1997;44:921)

Parkinson tremor may be coexistent with familial tremor—propranolol-responsive (20–320 mg) (Arch Neurol 1986;43:42); high dosing may worsen depression and sleep disturbance

Anticholinergics: generally toxic and minimally useful; benztropine 0.5 mg/d increasing slowly to 2 mg bid; trihexyphenidyl 2 mg/d increasing slowly to 5 mg tid; ethopropazine HCl (Parsidol) 50 mg/d gradually increasing to 600 mg/d for tremor; for drug induced dyskinesias

Amantadine: influences the release of dopamine; adverse effects: confusion, hallucinations, edema, livedo reticularis (purplish mottling of skin); modest short-lived efficacy; pts may respond again when reintroduced; more effective for rigidity and bradykinesia than tremor

Antioxidants (vit E), selegiline might help

Pergolide (Permax) when bromocriptine not effective, both expensive (Mayo Clin Proc 1988;63:969); pergolide better than bromocriptine (Neurol 1995;45:522); 0.05 mg tid w meals increasing q3–5d to 3–6 mg/d as mono Rx or 1.5–3 mg/d as adjunct to levodopa therapy

High drug costs and variable drug effectiveness over time mandate regular reviews, including trials off drugs, with careful, comprehensive, detailed observations to ascertain drug effectiveness implied

Muscle relaxants for pain and cramping

Clozapine (Clozaril) for hallucinations so can keep on using L-dopa and selegiline; drug-induced psychosis typified by visual hallucinations w insight, psychotic depression or dementia associated w auditory hallucinations; olanzapine not well tolerated, risperidone small doses, quetiapine (Neurol 2000; 55:727)

Depression responsive to nortriptyline—mild anticholinergic effects, also helps movement disorder, sialorrhea, tremor; serotonin reuptake inhibitors helpful as well, but have also been known to cause akathisia (β-blockers rx of choice for this side effect); both tricyclics and serotonin reuptake inhibitors can cause myoclonus, which can be controlled w clonazepam, citralopram, setraline, paroxetine; identify and monitor specific "target" depression sx; may not require chronic antidepressants—review useful

Sexual dysfunction: sildenafil (Viagra)

Seborrheic dermatitis may be relieved by L-dopa, ketoconazole (Nizoral) plus careful attention to hygiene

Stereotactic pallidotomy: long-term risks/benefits not established, complications include visual field deficits, contralateral paralysis, and speech problems (Med Let Drugs Ther 1996;38:107)

Fetal cell transplantation: postop sleep disturbance and mental status change more common and profound in older pts (Ann Neurol 1988;24:150)

Team Management:

Front-wheeled walker for Parkinson avoids retropulsion and tripping

Restricted protein diet—limit to protein meal at dinnertime; investment in long-term work w family and staff education vital to quality management; pain, fatigue, depression, strained family relationships—referrals to home health, social service, counseling, Parkinson support groups (J Am Geriatr Soc 1997;45:844)

Nausea: trimethobenzamide or diphenidol 25 mg q 6 h does not block dopamine receptors as other antinausea medications do (Chlorpazine, metoclopramide) but may cause confusion and ataxia.

Constipation: senna alkaloid 1–4 tabs at hs

Daytime sleepiness: stimulants, eg, methylphenidate (Ritalin), dextroamphetamine (Dexedrine), pemoline (Cylert) (J Am Board Fam Pract 1997;10:412)

4.3 SEIZURES

J Am Geriatr Soc 1998;46:1291; Nurs Home Med 1995;3:4b; Nejm 1990;323:1468

Cause: In 85–90% of new-onset seizures, there is identifiable brain lesion; vascular disease 50% of time (33% occur w onset embolic event which is predictive of future epilepsy (Neuro 1996;46:35), 33% occur during rehab phase, 33% are recurrent); focal seizure usually caused by brain tumor (cause of seizures in 12% of elderly population); brain abscess; previous head trauma; generalized seizure associated w h/o meningitis, encephalitis; 25% of pts w late-stage Alzheimer have generalized seizures; metabolic; hypoxia; abrupt withdrawal from benzodiazepines; other drugs lower threshold, eg, phenothiazines, tricyclics, meperidine, new-generation quinolones, theophylline

Epidem: Occur 2–3 times more frequently than in younger pts; complex partial seizures common; fewer than 20% of NH pts on anticonvulsants actually have a seizure diagnosis (Nurs Home Med 1995;3:4b)

Sx: "Don't feel myself, something's happening"

Si:

- Generalized tonic-clonic motor (grand mal) most common type of seizure in elderly v.s. partial more common (Mayo Clin Proc 2001;76:175)
- Complex partial sz: "tune out": intermittent confusion, disorientation, staring; repetitive motor acts: patting, rubbing, smacking lips, rarely wandering or disrobing

Table 4-6. Treatment of Seizures

Seizure Type	First-Choice Antiepileptic Drug	Second-Choice Antiepileptic Drug
Simple partial, complex partial, secondarily generalized	Carbamazepine, phenytoin lamotrigine, levetiracetam, oxcarbazine (Mayo Clin Proc 2001;76:175)	Gabapentin, felbamate, primidone, phenobarbital, tiagabine, topiramate, valproic acid
Absence	Ethosuximide	Valproic acid
Myoclonic	Valproic acid	Clonazepam
Primary generalized tonic-clonic	Valproic acid, phenytoin	Felbamate, phenobarbital
Atonic	Valproic acid, clonazepam	Felbamate

Reproduced by permission from Sirven JI. Epilepsy in older adults: causes, consequences and treatment. J Am Geriatr Soc 1998;46:1291–301.

Cmplc:
- Fractures, states of confusion, aspiration pneumonia
- R/o early dementia or late dementia behaviors can be confused w partial complex seizures (behaviors ranging from mutism to hallucinations); focal seizures can be confused w TIAs

Lab: No LP unless suspect meningitis

Noninvasive: EEG if confusing differential; most diagnostic value during event, periodic epileptiform discharges (occur in elderly w any acute CNS injury)

Xray: MRI best for small structural lesions; CT only in emergency r/o bleed or MRI contraindicated; contrast with both

Rx:

Therapeutic: See Table 4-6, Table 4-7

Because of high rate of recurrence of seizure in elderly, start antiepileptic drug after first seizure unless obvious metabolic cause (Lancet 1988;1:721); more likely to be recurrent if partial sz, post-ictal paralysis, FH, positive EEG, abnormal neurological exam; adverse effects of neuroleptics: gait disturbance, sedation, tremor; folate deficiency predisposes pts to neurotoxicity

Carbamazepine (Tegretol): for focal seizures, 100 mg bid–tid; anticholinergic side effect; pts with heart block can have conduction abnormalities; induces cytochrome P450 system, so interacts with drugs metabolized with this system, eg, antidepressants; can cause hyponatremia, neutropenia

Table 4-7. Advantages and Disadvantages of Antiepileptic Drugs

Antiepileptic Drug	Advantages	Disadvantages
Felbamate	Broad spectrum of coverage Efficacy	Serious idiosyncratic side effects Expensive
Gabapentin	Few side effects No drug interactions Easy to dose Renal excretion	Limited efficacy Multiple daily doses Expensive
Lamotrigine	Broad spectrum of coverage Well tolerated Twice a day dosing	Slow to initiate Rash Expensive
Topiramate	Broad spectrum of coverage Twice a day dosing Limited drug interactions Mostly renal metabolism	Cognitive adverse effects Expensive
Tiagabine	Well tolerated Limited drug interactions	Multiple daily doses Cognitive adverse effects Expensive
Vigabratin	Well tolerated No drug interactions Renal excretion	Multiple daily doses May exacerbate underlying psychiatric disorder Expensive

Reproduced by permission from Sirven JI. Epilepsy in older adults: causes, consequences and treatment. J Am Geriatr Soc 1998;46:1291–301.

NEUROLOGY

Valproate: for generalized seizures, 250 mg bid–3 gm/d; inhibits hepatic drug metabolizing enzymes so raises levels of benzodiazepines; pts may develop increased bleeding time, GI side effects

In pts w long-standing epilepsy on phenobarbital (>60 mg not usually tolerated, resulting in severe mental, behavioral effects; may also get osteopenia secondary to altered vit D metabolism) or phenytoin (Dilantin, 200–400 mg usual dose); drug need not be changed unless experiencing side effects (hirsutism, gum hyperplasia, folate deficiency, osteopenia secondary to impaired calcium absorption)

Effective phenytoin level = Phenytoin level/[0.2 (albumin + 0.1)]

The lower the albumin, the more free drug fraction, the higher the effective level of phenytoin; thus NH pts usually have a 25–50% higher "effective" phenytoin level than reported

Neuroleptics (especially phenothiazines/antidepressants) lower seizure threshold, especially w h/o alcoholism

CNS stimulants such as methylphenidate (Ritalin), pemoline (Cylert), oral decongestants, pentoxifylline (Trental), theophylline can provoke seizures (Nurs Home Med 1995;3:4b)

Enteral feedings, milk, supplements, and antacids reduce absorption of phenytoin and should be dosed several hours away from antiepileptic drug

Diarrhea can reduce the amount of anticonvulsant

Consider discontinuation of seizure med if long seizure-free period and normal EEG (Ger Rev Syllabus Suppl 1994;1:127S)

Gabapentin (Nejm 1996;334:1583; Neurol 1994;44:787) (GABA agonist) for partial seizures; lipid-soluble; does not affect concentrations of other seizure meds

Lamotrigine (Lamictal, a phenyltriazine derivative)—decrease the dose if given w other seizure meds (Nurs Home Med 1996;4:6b)

Some advantages to newer drugs: less drug interaction; lamotrigine single daily dose, less ataxia and cognitive impairment

Withdraw seizure medication slowly over months (reduce phenobarbital by 30 mg/mo)

Team Management: Educate family and staff on recognition and responses

4.4 SLEEP PROBLEMS

Am Fam Phys 2000;62:110; J Am Geriatr Soc 1998;46:700; Alessi C, Geriatric Intensive Review Course UCLA 1/96; Am Fam Phys 1994;51:191

Cause: Transient: stress, new bed, change time zone; chronic: depression, fear of death, substance abuse, pain, paresthesia, dyspnea, GE reflux, anxiety, delirium, myoclonus, restless legs, sleep apnea; drugs: alcohol, antihypertensives, antineoplastics, β-blockers, caffeine, diuretics, L-dopa, selegiline, nicotine, oral contraceptives, phenytoin (Dilantin), serotonin reuptake inhibitors, protriptyline (Vivactil), corticosteroids, stimulants, theophylline, thyroid hormone

Types:

1. Difficulty initiating or maintaining sleep (insomnia or dyssomnias)
2. Excessive sleep
3. Sleep-wake cycle problems
4. Parasomnias occurring during sleep-wake transitions; characterized as behaviors that intrude into sleep but do not change sleep architecture, eg, nocturnal leg cramps
5. Sleep disorders associated w Alzheimer: increased duration, increased frequency of awakenings; decreased REM, stages 3 and 4 sleep; daytime napping; sleep apnea in later stages
6. Sleep disorders associated w depression: more nighttime wakefulness and decreased slow-wave sleep; early morning awakening; more REM sleep earlier in night; community-dwelling elderly have decreased latency (number of minutes to fall asleep)
7. Sleep apnea: repeated cessation for ≥10 sec w oxygen saturation ≤80%

    Central: simultaneous cessation of breathing effort and nasal and oral airflow, as well as cessation of effort by diaphragm muscles

    Obstructive: airflow stops while thoracic respirations persist, cyclic snoring interrupted by occlusive apneas (Sci Am 1999; Respiratory medicine chapt. VI Ventilatory control during wakefulness and sleep. Iber C, Ingram RH.

    Mixed: (features of both) most common

    - Periodic leg movements: characterized by debilitating, repetitive, stereotypic leg movements occurring in non-REM sleep
    - Restless leg syndrome: uncontrollable urge to move one's legs at night, "creepy-crawling" sensation

Epidem: 50% of community have sleep problems, 90% of NH pts; 70% of caregivers cited sleep problems as reason for admitting relatives to NH; NH residents awake on average q 20–25 min during the night; psychoactive meds dampen normal diurnal variation in sleep, eg, sleep during day, not at night

Increased mortality when oxygen saturation <85% and >20 episodes apnea/night

Pathophys: Normal changes in sleep pattern with age: sleep latency increased; sleep efficiency decreased (ratio of time asleep to time in bed); earlier bedtime; earlier morning awakening; more arousals during night; more daytime napping

Changes in sleep structure w age:
- Stages 1 and 2 (light sleep) remain the same
- Stages 3 and 4 (deep sleep, slow high-amplitude delta-wave sleep) decreased
- Total REM sleep decreases
- Earlier-onset REM sleep and it does not increase in duration throughout the night as in young people

Sx: Loss of concentration and memory, dysphoria, malaise, irritability, daytime napping, fatigue, interference w ADLs, headaches on awakening

Si: Sleep apnea: consider if pt has unexplained right-sided heart failure, decreased cognitive function; most severe episodes occur in REM sleep

Compl: Pulmonary HT, RV failure

Lab:

Noninvasive: Polysomnography in a sleep laboratory if sleep apnea, narcolepsy, periodic leg movements

Rx:

Preventive:
- Screening questions: Is pt satisfied w his/her sleep? Does sleep or fatigue intrude w daytime activities? Does bed partner notice snoring, interrupted breathing, leg movements?
- Sleep hygiene: bed at same time each night; bedroom environment conducive; avoid excessive napping or before bedtime exercise; early day exercise helps in community dwelling elderly but not in NH elderly (Jama 1997;277:32; J Am Geriatr Soc 1995;43:1098); comfortable levels—temperature, light, noise; if can't get to sleep in one-half hour, get out of bed and participate in nonstimulating activity and return to bed when sleepy; light snack; relaxation techniques for those who ruminate; light therapy if a symptom of seasonal affective disorder (Jama 1997;277:990)

Therapeutic: See Table 4-8
- Chronic insomnia: intermittent dosing (2–4 weekly) (Nejm 1997; 336:341)
- Most OTC hypnotics are antihistamines w sedating properties; they also have anticholinergic properties and should be discouraged in elderly
- If elderly pt on low-dose barbiturates, glutethimide or chloral hydrate for years, may be reasonable to continue if pt very resistant to stopping it or may need to consult w psychiatrist (Ger Rev

Table 4-8. Benzodiazepines—Onset and Elimination Characteristics

Examination	Fast Onset	Intermediate Onset	Slow Onset
Past (6 h)	Zolidem (Ambien) Zolpidem Zaleplon	Triazolam (Halcion), oxazepam (Serax)	—
Intermediate (15 h)		Lorazepam (ativan), alprazolam (Xanax)	Temazepam (Restoril)
Slow (30–72 h)	Diazepam (Valium), clorazepate (Tranxene)	Chlordiazepoxide (Librium), flurazepam (Dalmane), clonazepam (Klonopin)	Prazepam (Centrax)

Syllabus 1996:175); sedating antidepressants such as doxepin, amitriptyline (Elavil) and trazodone may help w sleep, especially w underlying depression, bruxism, and fibromyalgia

- Choral hydrate 500 mg/hypnotics for 2–4 wk; tolerance develops unless dosed q 3 nights; increases warfarin metabolism; gradual tapering rather than abrupt discontinuation following prolonged use of agent (Drugs 1993;45:44); fatalities have occurred w as little as 4 gm ingestion of chloral hydrate (Med Let 2000;42:71)
- Benzodiazepines: work on GABA pathway, highly protein-bound; highly lipid-soluble; active metabolites prolonged in obese pts, except oxazepam (Serax) and lorazepam (Ativan) which are altered to inactive metabolites; many undergo oxidative hepatic metabolism: alprazolam (Xanax), chlordiazepoxide (Librium), clorazepate (Tranxene), diazepam (Valium), prazepam (Centrax); levels are increased by meds that inhibit liver metabolism: cimetidine, contraceptives, disulfiram, fluoxetine (Prozac), INH, valproic acid
- Clonazepam (Klonopin): for nocturnal myoclonus
- Flurazepam (Dalmane): has long half-life (85 h); accumulates; do not use in elderly
- Temazepam (Restoril): effective for 6–8 h but has 2–3 h onset
- Triazolam (Halcion): psychosis and violent behavior in doses over 1 mg (maximum dose prescribed = 0.5 mg)
- Quazepam (Doral): metabolite w a 72 h half-life

- Zolpidem (Ambien): not a benzodiazepine, no anticonvulsant or myorelaxant properties; as yet very few side effects reported: no withdrawal effects, no rebound insomnia, no tolerance; effectiveness lasts a year; rapid onset; lasts 2–4 h; can use w warfarin; start at 5-mg dose (cognitive impairment at higher doses); fewer falls; twice as expensive as triazolam (Halcion); side effects: nightmares, agitation, headache, dizziness, daytime drowsiness, impaired memory, and unsteady gait in the middle of the night (Med Let 2000;42:71)
- Zaleplon (Sonata): an imidazopyridine, does not decrease premature awakenings or increase total sleep time, but appears to have a low risk of next-day residual effects, even w middle-of-the-night use (Med Let 2000;42:71)
- When withdrawing from short-acting benzodiazepines, decrease drug by 50% first week and then by 12% for each of the next 4–8 wk
- Alleviation of insomnia w timed exposure to bright light (J Am Geriatr Soc 1993;41:829)
- Melatonin mg 2 po improves sleep efficiency 75–85% (Lancet 1995;346:541)
- Trazodone 25 mg, nefazodone, mirtazapine (Remeron) single dose hs not just for depressed pts (J Clin Psychiatry 1999;60(suppl 17):28)

For obstructive sleep apnea: tricyclic antidepressants reduce REM sleep and therefore ameliorate apnea; progesterone helps by increasing respiratory drive (Nejm 1990;323:520); dental prostheses; tracheotomy

CPAP (5–20 cm H_2O 50–70% successful) for central and mixed sleep apnea

For nocturnal myoclonus: avoid caffeine, tricyclics; clonazepam 0.25 mg hs increasing by 0.25 mg q 2 wk to maximum of 2 mg; trazodone 50–150 mg hs; L-dopa 100–200 mg, carbamazepine

For restless leg syndrome: avoid caffeine, tricyclics, antipsychotics, antihistamines; vit E 800–1200 IU/d, quinine, L-dopa or dopamine agonist antiparkinsonian drug, clonazepam, temazepam, carbamazepine, gabapentin, clonidine (Am Fam Phys 2000;62:110); cautious use of narcotic analgesics

Team Management: Nonpharmacologic sleep protocol in NH w massage, relaxation tapes, warm drinks (J Am Geriatr Soc 1998;46:700)

4.5 NEUROLEPTIC MALIGNANT SYNDROME (NMS)

Med Clin N Am 1993;77:185

Cause: Idiosyncratic reaction involving dopamine blockade, neuroleptic-induced hypothermia via dysregulation of hypothalamus and basal ganglia and muscle rigidity related to myonecrosis (Med Clin N Am 1993;77:185)

Epidem: Rare with incidence 0.02–3.23%; risk factors: increased age, high-dose/high-potency neuroleptics, eg, haloperidol, thiothixene, fluphenazine, and trifluoperazine; may also see increased incidence with depot meds, lithium, antidepressants or multiple neuroleptics (low-dose/low-potency), carbidopa/L-dopa and withdrawal of amantadine; increased incidence in pts with h/o NMS, dehydration, lyte imbalance, thyrotoxicosis, elevated ambient temperature (Med Clin N Am 1993;77:185), underlying CNS impairment (J Am Geriatr Soc 1996;44:474)

Pathophys: Precipitated by any med that acts as D_2 dopamine receptor antagonist; severe dopamine blockade-induced parkinsonism with resulting muscle rigidity, then myonecrosis; autonomic thermogenic dysregulation via dopaminergic input also postulated (Emergency Medicine Clinics of North America 2000;18:317)

Si: Hyperthermia w diaphoresis in 98% of pts, but can be lacking in elderly; rigidity 97%; other movement disorder less often; mental status changes vary from clouded consciousness to coma; autonomic instability, tachycardia, hypotension 97%; tachypnea secondary to metabolic acidosis, pneumonia, or pulmonary embolism (Med Clin N Am 1993;77:185; Clin Pharmacol Ther 1991;50:580)

Crs: High mortality if untreated; 10–20% mortality with treatment; usually occurs soon after initiating neuroleptic treatment or with dose increases; recovery usually within 10 d, 97% by 30 d (Med Clin N Am 1993;77:185)

Cmplc: Cerebellar or other brain damage secondary to hypothermia; fatal arrhythmias; metabolic acidosis; pulmonary emboli; pneumonia; respiratory arrest

R/o encephalopathies, tumors, CVA, seizures, infections, endocrinopathies (thyrotoxicosis, pheochromocytoma), SLE, heat injury, toxins, drugs (Med Clin N Am 1993;77:185; Psych Ann

1991;21:130), polymyositis, mesenteric vascular occlusion, rheumatoid arthritis; cancer of prostate, colon, lung (small cell); chronic renal disease; myoglobinuria (67%)

Lab: EKG, CBC (leukocytosis common), CPK occasionally extremely elevated, TSH, LDH, transaminases and aldolase may also be elevated from myonecrosis; metabolic acidosis, and hypoxia may be present; cardiac monitoring

Rx: Discontinue all neuroleptics and other centrally acting anti-dopaminergics; bromocriptine 7.5–60.0 mg daily po or via NG tube; dantrolene, initially 1–2 mg/kg IV, then 10 mg/kg daily, may have synergistic effect; other useful meds: amantadine, benzodiazepines to lessen agitation; electroconvulsive therapy for refractory cases, but can also lead to NMS when given to pts exhibiting extrapyramidal adverse effects

Team Management: Observe carefully for early signs in elderly when using neuroleptics

5 Psychiatry

5.1 DEPRESSION

Jama 1997;278:1186; 1997;278:1186; Am J Ger Psychiatry
1994;2:193; 1993;1:421; Nejm 1989;320:164

Cause: Often situational (losses, functional disability, illness, family
stress, caregiver stress, raising grandchildren) (Arch Fam Med
1997;6:445); hypothalamic-pituitary-adrenal axis and circadian
rhythm disruption; hypokalemia, hyponatremia, MI, COPD,
pernicious anemia, cancer, stroke involving either hemisphere,
especially close to the frontal pole (Aging 1994;6:49); other
dysfunction of frontal brain system, vascular disease (Am J Psychiatry
1997;154:562); drugs including alcohol, amantadine, antipsychotics,
cimetidine (within several wks of beginning therapy), clonidine,
cytotoxic agents, digoxin, α-methyldopa (occurs w higher doses,
mild, occurring within wks of initiation of drug and lasts several wks
after cessation of drug), propranolol and other β-blockers, sedatives,
steroids, NSAIDs (Nejm 1984;320:164), reserpine (may be severe w
suicidal behavior and sometimes does not clear w cessation of
reserpine, necessitating antidepressant therapy or ECT) (Jenike MA.
Geriatric psychiatry and psychopharmacology: a clinical approach.
Chicago: Year Book Medical, 1989); other risk factors are hx of
prior episodes, family hx, alcoholism, personality disorders

Epidem: Prevalence of depressive symptom syndromes is 13–27% in
the geriatric population and 30–45% in the medically ill and in
nursing homes (Jama 1997;228:1186), 8–10% in nonagenarians
(Br J Psychiatry 1995;167:61); major depression 2–4% of elderly
community-dwelling pts (Clin Ger Med 1998;14:33); third leading
cause of injury-related death in the elderly; proportion 2:1 F/M
(Mmwr 1996;45:3)

Diagnosis missed in as many as 86% of cases in primary care setting; reasons include pt and physician denial or minimization, therapeutic nihilism, limited access to care, medical comorbidities

Risk Factors: Hx of prior episodes; family hx of depressive disorder; hx of suicide attempts; female gender; comorbid medical illness; negative, stressful life events; active alcohol or substance abuse

Pathophys: Hypothalamic-pituitary-adrenal axis and circadian rhythm disruption; theorized that monoamine transmitters and neural pathways involving prefrontal cortex, amygdala, and hypothalamus axis involved; MAO activity increased in brains of elderly (Am J Psychiatry 1984;141:1276); cytokines involved in increased cortisol production and immune system activation (Am J Ger Psychiatry 1996;4:1)

Sx: Heterogeneous; careful hx is key to dx; ask directly about depressed mood; somatic complaints common, as is a complaint of fatigue; DSM-IV criteria for dx of major depression requires 2 wks of depressed mood or anhedonia and 4 more of following for major depression: impaired sleep often w early morning awakening, depressed mood, decreased interest in usual sources of pleasure (anhedonia), feelings of guilt, decreased energy, altered concentration, decreased appetite, psychomotor retardation or agitation, suicidal ideation; late-life depression more often associated with medical and neurologic illness and dementia (DSM IV); always ask directly about depressed mood; current elderly cohorts may resist dx because of ageist expectations, sense of shame or self-blaming

- Delusional depression more common in late-life; delusions more common than hallucinations; most common are somatic delusions followed by delusions of guilt or persecution
- Less typical presentations: hypochondriasis, pain syndromes, shoplifting, alcoholism, depressive dementia, malnutrition, passive suicide, non-dysphoric depressions (J Am Geriatr Soc 1997;45:570), anxiety/agitation (J Am Geriatr Soc 1989;37:458); watch especially for depression as earliest presentation of mild cognitive losses of Alzheimer
- Pseudo-depression in frontal lobe syndromes: pts present as avolitional, apathetic, without energy, psychomotor retardation but no low mood or irritability
- Bipolar illness in the elderly: paranoid delusions, circumferential speech; may be as many as 10 yr between first depressive and manic episode; predominance of depressive symptoms; irritability and

Choose the best answer for how you felt over the past week.

1. Are you basically satisfied with your life?	yes/**NO**
2. Have you dropped many of your activities and interests?	**YES**/no
3. Do you feel that your life is empty?	**YES**/no
4. Do you often get bored?	**YES**/no
5. Are you in good spirits most of the time?	yes/**NO**
6. Are you afraid that something bad is going to happen to you?	**YES**/no
7. Do you feel happy most of the time?	yes/**NO**
8. Do you often feel helpless?	**YES**/no
9. Do you prefer to stay at home, rather than going out and doing new things?	**YES**/no
10. Do you feel you have more problems with memory than most?	**YES**/no
11. Do you think it is wonderful to be alive now?	yes/**NO**
12. Do you feel pretty worthless the way you are now?	**YES**/no
13. Do you feel full of energy?	yes/**NO**
14. Do you feel that your situation is hopeless?	**YES**/no
15. Do you think that most people are better off than you are?	**YES**/no

Score bolded answers. One point for each of these answers. Cut-off: normal (0–5); above 5 suggests depression.

SOURCE: Courtesy of Jerome A. Yesavage, MD. Reprinted with permission.

For additional information on administration and scoring refer to the following:
1. Sheikh JI, Yesavage JA. Geriatric Depression Scale: recent evidence and development of a shorter version. Clin Gerontol 1986;5:165–172.
2. Yesavage JA, Brink TL, Rose TL, et al. Development and validation of a geriatric depression rating scale: a preliminary report. J Psych Res 1983;17:27.

Figure 5-1. Short form Geriatric Depression Scale.

anger more common; greater duration of episodes, mortality rate higher for bipolar than unipolar
- Rapid cycling more common in elderly women on antidepressants or with thyroid disease: 4 or more distinct episodes of mania, hypomania, or depression within a 12-mo period

Si: Tearfulness, stooped posturing, frequent sighing, increased response latency, low volume of speech, poor eye contact, poverty of movement, hand wringing, weight loss

Dx: Depression scales (Fig 5-1) (J Psych 1983;17:37); Dementia Flow Sheet (Fig 5-2)

Diff Dx: Alzheimer dementia grief reaction (beginning within 3 mos of loss and lasting 1 yr); dysthymia (not free of depression for >2 mo over a 2-yr period); secondary dysthymia (from chemical dependency, anxiety, stress, and physical illness); schizophrenia (bizarre delusions and hallucinations); drug reactions

PSYCHIATRY

Crs: If untreated, lasts 6–14 months; relapse rate is increased compared to younger (Convuls Ther 1989;5:75; J Am Geriatr Soc 1987;35:516); poorest prognosis: recent bereavement, delusions (50% of the time in the elderly), panic disorders; will respond better to antidepressants if have early am awakening or shorter period of depression; late-life depression with cognitive impairment reversed by antidepressants may predict development of irreversible dementia (Jama 1997;278:1186); depression with first appearance in late life often becomes chronic and often has vascular neuropathology

Cmplc: Increased 1-yr mortality rates (8–15% vs 5%); major depression increases risk for MI and risk of death from ischemic heart disease (Circ 1996;943:3123); suicide, fastest growing rate in U.S.; completed suicides M > W; suicide—20% fatal; rate of suicide in white men >84 yr is 6 times higher than general population; depression increases functional disability and reduces rehab effectiveness; longer hospital stays; multiple depressive sx associated with 2 times increased mortality; women with depression at increased risk of falling (Sci Am Med 2000;13:2)

Lab: TSH, B$_{12}$ level, lytes, CBC

Rx:

Medications:

General Considerations:

- Start LOW, Go SLOW, Go ALL the way
- Begin one-third usual adult doses (demethylation is decreased in the elderly), increase monthly, and use smallest effective dose (Table 5-1)
- Agitated depression responds less well than melancholic (vegetative) depression
- Minor depression responds well to treatment
- Biologic symptoms improve before mood (insomnia in first few days)
- Familial response good predictor of individual success w an antidepressant
- May discontinue antidepressant after 9 mo if no previous episode of depression in 2.5 yrs, reduce the dose by one-half, then taper by 25 mg/wk to avoid cholinergic hyperactivity w abrupt withdrawal (malaise, chills, muscle aches, coryza); maintenance doses of antidepressants should be as high as doses for acute treatment; if seasonal affective disorder (SAD) pattern, take into consideration

Table 5-1. Dosage Standards for Antidepressant Medications

Antidepressant	Minimal Dose Standard in mg/day	'Probably Adequate' Dose in mg/day
Tricyclics		
Amitriptyline	75	150
Clomipramine	75	150
Desipramine	75	150
Doxepin	75	150
Imipramine	75	150
Nortriptyline	40	75
Protriptyline	20	40
Trimipramine	75	150
Heterocyclics		
Amoxapine	100	150
Bupropion	225	225
Maprotiline	100	150
Trazodone	100	200
SSRIs		
Fluoxetine	10	20
Paroxetine	10	20
Sertraline	25	50
MAOIs		
Isocarboxazid	30	45
Phenelzine	30	45
Tranylcypromine	30	45

Reproduced by permission from Unutzer J, Simon G, Belin TR, et al. Care for depression in HMO patients aged 65 and older. J Am Geriatr Soc 2000;48:871–8.

when planning discontinuation; if recurrent episode, treat 12 mo; if 2 episodes, may need indefinite maintenance treatment

- Efficacy is similar across and within class; most decisions based on side effect profile and h/o of prior response

SSRIs: Efficacy same as tricyclics: 60–80% respond; risk of falls in frail elderly may be similar to tricyclics despite decreased hypotension (Lancet 1998;351:1303; Nejm 1998;339:875), but may not be as effective as tricyclics in melancholic elderly hospitalized pts (Am J Psychiatry 1994;151:1735); not sedating, do not produce anticholinergic side effects, are not cardiotoxic, do not produce hypotension; useful in obsessive-compulsive disorder, panic attacks as well; some may cause overstimulation and worsen anxiety sx, but are being used in low doses for anxiety; not effective in neuropathic pain (Nejm 1992;326:1250)

PSYCHIATRY

Adverse effects are nausea, diarrhea, headache, anxiety, more sexual dysfunction than other antidepressants (Geriatrics 1995;50:S41) especially inhibition of orgasm, pseudoparkinsonism, SIADH, bradycardia, interaction w β-blockers, 1c antiarrhythmics, some benzodiazepines (Am J Psychiatry 1996;153:311); SSRI + tramadol (Ultram), St. John's wort, sumatriptan, can cause serotonin syndrome (Am Fam Phys 2000;61:1745); hypertensive crisis with MAO inhibitors, so 14-d washout before giving MAO inhibitor, except 5-wk washout for fluoxetine; less effective in postmenopausal women than younger women; withdrawal can occur with SSRIs (Sci Amer Med 2000;13:9); mania in 1% general population on SSRIs and more common in bipolars; paranoia, psychosis; extrapyramidal occasionally (Nejm 1994;371:1354); skin rash

Preferred SSRIs are citalopram and sertraline due to fewer drug interactions, safer half-life and side effect profiles; paroxetine also has a favorable half-life and fewer drug interactions but is associated with a greater risk of extrapyramidal symptoms

- Citalopram (Celexa): half-life = 33 h, 10–40 mg qd (*favorable response in elderly to 10 mg*) (Mosby's Genrx 2000: a comprehensive reference for generic and brand drugs. 10th ed. St. Louis: Mosby-Year Book, 2000); rare drug interactions due to no CYP enzyme inhibition, may increase level of metoprolol (Postgrad Med 1999;106:236); well-tolerated with side effects similar to other SSRIs; not sedating; change dose at monthly intervals; only SSRI with significant renal clearances (about 10%) adjust dose in those with renal impairment.
- Sertraline (Zoloft): half-life = 25 h, 25 mg po qd [qod], target 50–125 mg; adjust dose on wk basis to minimize side effects and find lowest effective dose; increases warfarin, diazepam, tolbutamide, Tegretol, codeine (Postgrad Med 1999;106:236); not sedating; can produce more nausea and diarrhea than other SSRIs
- Paroxetine (Paxil): half-life = 18–24 h; 10–40 mg po qd; start at 10 and raise slowly (Postgrad Med 1999;106:236); increases digoxin, tricyclics, warfarin, codeine; the most sedating of the SSRIs; produces constipation and sexual dysfunction somewhat more than other SSRIs.
- Fluoxetine (Prozac): long half-life = 4–6 days, 10 mg po qod-20 mg po qd, increase q 2–4 wk; takes 5 wk to washout before adding MAO inhibitor; more drug interactions than other SSRIs because

potent inhibitor of multiple CYP enzymes, thereby increasing concentrations of cyclic antidepressants, class Ic antiarrhythmics, β-blockers, calcium channel blockers, chlorpromazine (Thorazine), codeine, risperidone (Risperdal), carbamazepine (Tegretol), phenytoin (Dilantin), alprazolam, triazolam, warfarin (Postgrad Med 1999;106:236; Psychiatry Drug Alerts 1996;10:65); serotonin syndrome from combination fluoxetine and trazodone (Psychosom 1995;36:159); less GI side effect than other SSRIs (Clin Ger Med 1998;1:33); more anxiety, nervousness, anorexia than other SSRIs (J Clin Psychiatry 1994;55:S10); can give low-dose trazodone (Desyrel) 25 mg or clonazepam (Klonopin) 0.5 mg hs for insomnia (Am J Psychiatry 1994;151:1069); avoid in polypharmacy due to long half-life and widespread interactions

- Fluvoxamine (Luvox): half-life = 15 h, most rapid onset of the SSRIs, 50–200 mg po q hs, dose bid at higher dose; potent inhibitor of cytochrome P450 enzymes; increases propranolol, warfarin, theophylline, carbamazepine, tricyclics, haloperidol (Haldol), phenytoin, caffeine, alprazolam, triazolam, diazepam, non-sedating antihistamines, eg, terfenadine, astemizole; avoid in polypharmacy due to widespread interactions; GI side effects more pronounced than sexual dysfunction or headache; labeled for treatment of obsessive compulsive disorder only

Atypical Antidepressants: Norepinephrine and Serotonin Effects:

- Venlafaxine (Effexor) half-life = 5–10 h; start 25 mg bid, go to 25–125 tid (extended release available); interacts with MAO inhibitors; well-tolerated with few side effects: nausea or diarrhea at start, increased diastolic BP and sexual dysfunction at higher doses (Clin Ger Med 1998;14:33); withdrawal symptoms can occur so taper (Sci Amer Med 2000;13:II)
- Mirtazapine (Remeron) half-life = 20+ h; 15–45 mg qhs; insignificant drug interactions except MAO inhibitors and additive sedation with diazepam; somnolence common side effect (30–50%); increased appetite; few GI effects; rare agranulocytosis; no sexual dysfunction
- Nefazodone (Serzone): half-life = 3 h; start 25–50 mg po bid, increase q 1–2 wk up to 150–300 mg bid; inhibits cytochrome P450 so decreases clearance of triazolam, alprazolam, digoxin antihistamines; not interactive w MAO inhibitors; sedating but less than trazodone; some anorgasmia; rarely used because ineffective at tolerable doses

Serotonin Effects: Much more sedating than SSRIs and therefore are used in agitated depression (Am Fam Phys 1997;55:1692)

- Trazodone (Desyrel): half-life = 3–9 h; 50–100 mg qhs as hypnotic for sleep disturbance caused by stimulatory antidepressants (Sci Am Med 2000;13:11); not as effective for depression; useful in agitated depression; no interactions w MAO inhibitors; increases digoxin levels; significant orthostatic hypotension as well as nausea and vomiting; rare priapism

Dopamine Effects:

- Bupropion (Wellbutrin) half-life = 10 h; 50 mg bid up to 150 tid; divided doses obviate seizures but lowers threshold so contraindicated in seizure disorder; well-tolerated and not sedating; may use trazodone, clonazepam for insomnia as w fluoxetine; no significant drug interactions (Sci Am Med 2000;13:10) but at high doses avoid other drugs which lower seizure threshold (Postgrad Med 1999;6:245); no cardiotoxicity; may exacerbate preexisting HT; no sexual dysfunction or headache; extrapyramidal side effects uncommon

Norepinephrine and Dopamine Effects: Most reliable drug levels obtained 12 h after last dose w the following meds: imipramine (therapeutic level = 125 ng/mL), desipramine (therapeutic level = 225 ng/mL), nortriptyline (therapeutic level = 50–150 ng/mL) (Am J Psychiatry 1985;142:155) (Table 5-2)

- Amoxapine (Asendin): (metabolite of loxapine, an antipsychotic) rarely used; 25–50 mg qhs; has a methylphenidate-like effect on appetite stimulation within the first few days of administration (Table 5-3); may use calorie counts to gauge its efficacy; moderately anticholinergic; increases digoxin levels; quinidine-like effect;

Table 5-2. Tricyclic Levels

Levels Increased by	Levels Decreased by
Aging	Smoking
Weight loss	Hyperlipidemia
Inflammatory disease	Barbiturates
Antipsychotics	Anticholinergics
Increased urine pH	Decreased urine pH
Morphine sulfate	
Cimetidine	
Steroids	

Table 5-3. Antidepressants and Appetite

Antidepressants That Increase Appetite	Antidepressants That Decrease Appetite
Amoxapine	SSRIs
Amitriptyline (sweet craving)*	Imipramine
Doxepin (sweet craving)*	Desipramine
	Trazadone

* Talley JH, Family Practice audiotape. Chapel Hill, NC, 1989.

increased QRS, QT, decreased T amplitude, LBBB, 2nd-degree AV block; ventricular arrhythmias as with tricyclics; extrapyramidal side effects; lowers seizure threshold

Tricyclics and Heterocyclics: Avoid tertiary amine tricyclics because of increased anticholinergic side effect (Mayo Clin Proc 1995;70:999), cardiotoxicity (bundle branch block a contraindication) and potent β-blocker activity producing postural hypotension (may not improve w dose reduction); except in the following situations:

• Imipramine (Tofranil) up to 150 mg po qd in pts w depression and urge incontinence

• Amitriptyline (Elavil) up to 75 mg po qd in post-stroke depression and pseudobulbar crying

• Doxepin (Sinequan) in pts w PUD (doxepin is somewhat less sedating than the other tertiary amines and is a potent histamine antagonist)

• Clomipramine (Anafranil) up to 75 mg po qd for obsessive-compulsive disorder when SSRIs not an option

Secondary Amine Tricyclics: Have fewer anticholinergic side effects but beware of additive effects w other anticholinergic meds (even at therapeutic doses) producing anticholinergic syndrome (anxiety, confusion, assaultive behavior, paranoia, hallucinations), which can lead to coma and death; drugs w anticholinergic side effect include antispasmodics, antidiarrheal agents, low-potency antipsychotics, antiparkinsonian meds, antihistamines, drugs for vertigo and OTC sleep meds; tricyclics block effects of clonidine (Catapres) (American College of Psychiatrists, Update Psychotropic Drug Interaction 1993;13:1); quinidine and carbamazepine (Tegretol) increase tricyclic levels; tricyclics cause more impotence while SSRIs cause more anorgasmia; can cause mania (Am J

PSYCHIATRY

Psychiatry 1995;152:1130); baseline EKG before prescribing tricyclic antidepressants

- Nortriptyline (Pamelor, Aventyl) 10–35 mg po qhs, titrate up by 10 mg watching blood levels, higher plasma concentrations correlate w greater cognitive impairment (Drugs Aging 1994;5:192); good for agitation; least hypotensive effects; avg half-life 43 h
- Desipramine (Norpramin) start 20–25 q hs to 25–150 mg po qd; less sedating than "snortriptyline," not as effective in the elderly (J Clin Psychopharmacol 1995;15:99); avg half-life 76 h

TCA overdose: Only prescribe 1 gm of tricyclic antidepressants (TCAs) at a time to avoid overdose (2 gm w trazodone) because potentially fatal

Treatment: Recognize anticholinergic side effects of excitation/restlessness w paradoxical progressive sedation, tonic-clonic seizure, flushed-dry skin, pupils dilated, bowel sounds decreased, urinary retention, tachyarrhythmias, hypotension

QRS >0.10 sec predictive of life-threatening ventricular arrhythmia and seizure (Nejm 1985;313:474); R wave in aVR >3 mm best predictive value for seizure or ventricular arrhythmia (Ann EM 1995;26:196)

Treat cardiac arrhythmias w propranolol; avoid digoxin, procaine, physostigmine; monitor for several days

Initial therapy: Pills radiopaque; lavage w charcoal (effective for a prolonged time after overdose because of paralytic ileus due to overdose), alkalinize urine w sodium bicarbonate; cannot remove w hemodialysis because protein-bound

- Methylphenidate (Ritalin) [0.25–1.00 mg po bid-tid (without antidepressant)]: 5 mg bid at 7 am and noon, increase gradually to 10 bid (Am J Psychiatry 1995;152:929); rapid improvement in medically ill or psychomotor retardation; low-dose adjunct in moderate to severe depression
- St. John's wort (Hypericum) inhibits uptake serotonin, norepinephrine, dopamine, and binds to GABA (Med Let 1997;39:107); no good data on efficacy or side effects to date, but trials underway (Sci Am Med 2000;13:14)

Resistant Depression: 30% of depressions; increase dose stepwise, and if no response at full therapeutic dosage for 4–6 wks, change drug class

May use nortriptyline in combination w SSRI (Br J Psychiatry 1992;161:562) or do ECT; elderly not a contradiction to ECT

Enhancers: If partial effect seen, augment with lithium, bupropion, mirtazapine, or occasionally thyroxine or methylphenidate

- L-Thyroxine 0.025 mg po qd
- Lithium (Nurs Home Pract 1995;3:17) trial for 2 wk (Arch Gen Psychiatry 1994;50:387); up to 300 mg po tid (follow 12-h post dose levels); obtain levels q 5 d (maximum initial therapeutic dose at trough = 1.2–1.5 mEq/L, then 0.8–1.2 mEq/L to prevent toxicity); in elderly half-life = 36 h; check TSH, BUN, Cr q 6 mo; withdrawal of caffeine may cause lithium toxicity (Biol Psychiatry 1995;37:348); carbamazepine increases neurotoxicity of lithium: lethargy, ataxia, muscle weakness, tremors, hyperreflexia

Early toxic effects: flu-type aching joints, sniffles, stiffness

"Benign" toxic effects: nausea, vomiting, diarrhea, polyuria, polydipsia, fine tremor, weight gain, edema

Acute toxicity: persistent vomiting, uncontrollable diarrhea, hyperactive DTRs, dysarthria, lethargy, somnolence, seizures, coma, death

Chronic toxicity: manifested as goitrogenic hypothyroidism, DI, tubular necrosis; lithium can be lowered by urinary alkalinization; if need diuretic, use amiloride instead of thiazide because lithium competes w sodium reabsorption at the proximal tubule; increased lithium levels from <2 gm/d sodium diet, thiazides, NSAIDS, ACE inhibitors

MAO Inhibitors: 3rd or 4th line due to toxic food and drug interactions causing hypertensive crisis; increase storage of norepinephrine, epinephrine, serotonin; tranylcypromine (Parnate) 10 mg bid and up to 40 mg/d; use tranylcypromine because reversible in 24 h; used for atypical depression as well: hyperphagia, hypersomnia, panic attacks; safer than tricyclics for heart block, ventricular arrhythmias; most common side effects are sedation, thus do not give before 4 pm, and orthostatic hypotension 3–4 wk into rx course because there is an accumulation of dopamine at the sympathetic ganglion; hypertensive crisis with tyramine-containing foods such as wine, cheese, aged meats, fermented foods and with sympathomimetic drugs and catecholamine precursors; affects all catecholamine precursors; L-dopa, pseudoephedrine, OTC cold remedies; interaction with SSRIs causes serotonergic syndrome consists of rigidity, diaphoresis, hyperthermia, coma, death; meperidine (Demerol) increases serotonin release; MAO-B

PSYCHIATRY

inhibitors have same effects as MAO-A inhibitors when given at higher doses (30 mg)

Electroconvulsive Therapy: (Am J Ger Psychiatry 1993;1:30) very effective in the elderly (Nejm 1984;311:163), efficacy 80% (J Am Geriatr Soc 2000;48:560); clear explanation to pt and family because of historical perception of "violence" of rx (Sci Am 2000;13:13)

Indications: drug-resistant or intolerant pts, delusional depression, pts w life-threatening behavior (suicidal, catatonic, stuporous); psychotic depression responds rapidly; usually 6–8 rx spaced 1–2 days apart; 3/wk more rapid recovery; minimize side effects by placing both stimulus electrodes to nondominant side, brief pulse, minimal duration of stimulus, mortality = 1/10,000, relapse rate 10–20% w maintenance drugs

Relative contraindications: increased intracranial pressure, MI in last 3 mo, severe osteoporosis; <1 mo s/p CVA (J Am Geriatr Soc 2000;48:560; Convuls Ther 1989;5:75; J Am Geriatr Soc 1987;35:516); β-blocker for known ischemic heart disease prevents cardiac complications; should also monitor for arrhythmias, bronchospasm, signs of aspiration; most common side effects are delirium, transient amnesia, cardiac (J Am Geriatr Soc 2000;48:560); if delirium occurs early in the course of ECT, do w/u; delirium common in vascular depression (J Am Geriatr Soc 2000;48:560); dementia not contraindication to ECT; f/u maintenance therapy required, either ECT or antidepressant

Depression Associated w Parkinson: Nortriptyline, desipramine, bupropion; ECT transiently improves tremor, rigidity, bradykinesia

Psychotic Depression: More common than in younger people; rx with antidepressants and antipsychotics or ECT

Mania: Carbamazepine (side effects: rash, sedation, memory problems, decreased WBC), valproate (side effects: GI upset, transient hair loss, tremors); lorazepam and haloperidol 0.5–1.0 mg qd early to control agitation

Team Management: If med intolerant, psychotherapy alone helps; also good for those with stressful situations and low social support; short-term group therapy (12 wk) using reminiscent therapy, cognitive therapy, behavioral therapy, and limited to small groups (about 6–10 pts) improves self-esteem, insight, social interaction, compliance, and decreases somatization; psychotherapy plus med more effective in maintaining remission in recurrent depression (Jama 1999;281:39)

- Model goal setting w family
- Music therapy: improvement in depression scores even after 9 mo f/u period (J Gerontol 1994;49:P265)
- Nurse-based outreach program reduces psychiatric sx in persons w psychiatric disorders (Jama 2000;283:2809)
- Nursing home: Nurses provide important dx information about non-major depression (J Am Geriatr Soc 1995;43:1118)
- Individual therapy or group therapy can help in situations involving caregiver stress

5.2 ANXIETY

NA Med 1998;6:2211; Am J Psychiatry 1994;151:640; J Clin Psychiatry 1994;55(suppl):5; Am J Psychiatry 1993;1:46

Cause: Primary anxiety or mood disorders, medical illness/treatment, psychosocial stressors, drug withdrawal

Epidem: Estimates of anxiety prevalence may be falsely low because it may not be admitted by the elderly or adequately recognized by caregivers; DSM-described anxiety disorders less common in elderly, 3.5–5.5% in those >65 yr old

Anxiety disorders and phobias: most common (30%) of all anxiety states (Ger Rev Syllabus 2001:175); agoraphobia with the highest prevalence of onset late in life; attributed to exaggerated fears of physical illnesses, falls, or muggings; <11% of agoraphobics have coexisting panic disorder; rate of phobias no different in 65–74 yr olds than those >75 yr old in the community

New-onset panic disorder: uncommon (0.3%) in old age; virtually all are women; associated w CAD, COPD, GI problems

Obsessive-compulsive disorder: may occur for the first time in old age in women; obsessive-compulsive and panic disorders more likely to persist in old age

Post-traumatic stress disorder: 70% early-onset persisting into old age (Am J Psychiatry 1994;2:239)

PSYCHIATRY

Parkinsonian pts much higher rates of anxiety than pts w arthritis or MS; anxiety in medical pts much less common in old (2–13%) than in young (10–40%)

Pathophys: Serotonin abnormalities resulting in depression, anxiety (J Clin Psychiatry 1994;55:2); medical illnesses (thyroid disease, COPD) or meds/drugs that may induce or exacerbate anxiety (aminophylline, L-dopa, prednisone, caffeine, OTC decongestants, alcohol, or benzodiazepine withdrawal)

Sx: Tachycardia, tremulousness, flushing, restlessness, unsteadiness, light-headedness, and sleep disturbances; somatic and anxiety-related complaints often mask depression

Si: Hyperventilation, depressed mood

Crs: R/o dysmorphic disorder (fear of going outside because of perceived physical deficit, rx w SSRIs; are also good for social problems, possibly PTSD)

Cmplc: Panic disorder: increased mortality, CVD, smoking, drug, and alcohol abuse

Lab/Xray: TSH, T_4, possibly CBC, lytes, chest xray and EKG for evidence of organic disease; hx, mental status exam, and physical exam (eg, BP) may suggest further studies such as urine metanephrine, 5HIAA or head CT (Mayo Clin Proc 1995;70:1999)

Rx: Identify and eliminate stressors when possible; provide support and companionship; instruction in muscle relaxation techniques; possible cognitive psychotherapy; if pharmacotherapy added, always consider risk of side effects vs benefit of treatment; treat depression if present

- Trazodone can cause orthostatic hypotension; nefazodone (Serzone) very effective
- Tricyclics, eg, nortriptyline and desipramine, are secondary amines with less anticholinergic effects
- β-Blockers reduce physical sx but not necessarily emotional sx
- SSRIs have low overdose risk; may either decrease or increase anxiety, insomnia; fluvoxamine (Luvox) approved for obsessive-compulsive disorder symptoms; takes higher doses and longer for SSRIs to work for OCD than for depression; down-regulation of receptors w chronic use of SSRI causes eventual improvement of sx; fluvoxamine most studied for anxiety; sertraline qd; paroxetine not sedating
- Risperidone, thioridazine (Mellaril) useful as first-line treatment of agitated, anxious pts with dementia or psychosis; antihistamines may induce confusion

- Buspirone HCl: 6–8-wk trial period may be effective at very low dose 2.5 mg qd to decrease anxiety/agitation in demented pts
- Lorazepam available im, IV; oxazepam and temazepam rather than those with long-acting breakdown products if possible; wean benzodiazepines slowly over several mos to avoid acute withdrawal sx in elderly

Team Management: Discover reversible etiologies; behavioral therapies; short-term cognitive therapy (5 sessions); long-term exposure therapy (exposure to anxiety precipitant); observe carefully for benefits or negative effects of rx

5.3 ALCOHOL MISUSE

Am Fam Phys 2000;61:1710; J Am Geriatr Soc 2000;48:985; Jama 2000;284:963; Int J Addict 1995;30:1819

Cause: Reduced tolerance, lower body water for a given amount of alcohol resulting in more pronounced effects; used inappropriately for sleep, pain, loneliness; health professionals may reinforce denial because of unexamined stereotypes; atypical presentation delays diagnosis

Epidem: Prevalence of ETOH abuse in elderly >65 yrs is 3% in the community, 10:1 M/F (Jama 1993;270:1222), 18% of general medical inpatients and 44% of psychiatric inpatients; Medicare claims data show 1.1% of all hospitalizations in geriatric pts are for alcohol-related dx (Am Fam Phys 2000;61:1710)

Pathophys:
- Proportion of total body weight that is fat increases with aging; decreased volume of distribution in elderly increases blood ETOH concentration per unit dose of ETOH; moderate drinking in elderly should be defined as no more than 1 drink qd
- Increase permeability of blood–brain barrier leads to greater medical morbidity in the elderly alcoholic
- 66% of elderly alcoholics have had lifelong problems with ETOH ("early onset" defined as onset by 25 yrs); 33% develop habits later in life ("late onset" defined as onset >60 yr)

Sx:

- Drinking 5–6 d/wk, 4–5 drinks per occasion; confusion (10% of dementias alcohol-related); self-neglect; self-reported rates of consumption may not accurately indicate impact on elderly lifestyle
- CAGE and MAST screens have decreased sensitivity in the elderly; better when also ask about quantity and frequency (Jama 1996;276:1964); MAST-G (geriatric version) under evaluation (J Am Geriatr Soc 2000;48:985–995)
- Sx tend to be nonspecific: "failure to thrive," insomnia, diarrhea, incontinence, repeated falls, loss of libido, increased metabolism of some drugs, eg, tolbutamide (Orinase), phenytoin (Dilantin)
- Have high index of suspicion if hospitalized pt develops new-onset seizures, agitation, confusion, anxiety

Si: Lab abnormalities: nonspecific high MCV, abnormal LFT, multiple spider nevi, hypoalbuminemia, fluctuations in INR

Crs: Improved prognosis w late age of onset of alcoholism, social and family support, absence of dementia; drug withdrawal can take longer

- Watch for ETOH-med interactions, especially CNS depressants: benzodiazepines, barbiturates, diphenhydramine (Benadryl), psychotropics; ETOH interacts with 50% of most commonly prescribed meds!
- Can precipitate hypoglycemic episodes in IDDM
- HT, afib, stroke, Wernicke encephalopathy, Korsakoff syndrome, GI bleeding can all result
- First year after dx of cirrhosis 50% mortality in individuals >60 yrs compared w 7% of those <60 yrs

Cmplc:

- Alcoholic women have 4 times risk for CAD
- Increased cancer risk (liver, esophagus, larynx, nasopharynx, colon, prostate, breast)
- Thrombocytopenia, hyponatremia

Preventive:

- Pt education to help elderly understand that habitual use of alcohol as aging advances may interfere with achievement of optimal health and functioning in context of increasing chronic disease conditions
- Avoid trap that the pt has only a few years left, so why not enjoy?
- Emphasize negative effect of alcohol on sleep pattern, nutrition, energy

Therapeutic: (Clin Ger Med 1993;9:197; Prim Care 1993;20:155)

Sx: Can see onset of withdrawal delayed 2–10 d, presenting w confusion, hallucinations; may continue for wks to mos (Drugs Aging 1999;14:405)

Treat withdrawal w

- Thiamine and MVI
- One-third to one-half average adult benzodiazepine dose reducing by 10%/d; long-acting benzodiazepine may be better for withdrawing from high-mg-potency benzodiazepines
- Ensure hydration; detoxification may take mos
- Postpone w/u of cognitive loss several wks
- *Do not* prescribe disulfiram (Antabuse) because elderly susceptible to disulfiram reaction w resultant cardiac complications
- Naltrexone has been approved for rx of alcoholism by FDA (Am J Med 1997;103:447)
- Ondansetron (Jama 2000;284:963) being investigated; both naltrexone and ondansetron are indicated for the rx of early onset ETOH abuse; their role in the rx of older alcoholics is being established

Watch for reactive depression and treat w SSRI; when depression coexists with alcoholism ("dual diagnosis"), both must be treated to achieve success (Int J Addict 1995;30:1819)

Team Management:

- Rehab units 1–3 wks; Alcoholics Anonymous (about 33% AA participants >50 yr old) or social situations that help elderly pursue an abstinent lifestyle
- AA meetings located at senior centers
- Involve pt pharmacy to monitor prescription refills; outreach program
- Pt education: alcohol affects medical conditions (eg, can worsen DM, CHF) and interacts with 50% of meds; informed pts can change behavior
- Explore family constellation: enablers, scapegoats

5.4 SUBSTANCE MISUSE

J Am Geriatr Soc 2000;48:985

Cause: Increased need to treat emotional and physical pain, most commonly for arthritis and sleep; increased risk of drug–drug interaction because 4 OTC drugs daily, and if chronically ill, 10–15 drugs daily (women prescribed more than men)

Epidem: 5% of older adults abuse drugs; 80% drug reactions are from minor tranquilizers and sedatives—propoxyphene (Darvon), diazepam (Valium), chlordiazepoxide (Librium); abuse of narcotics is rare among elderly unless previous h/o abuse at younger age

Pathophys: Reduction of renal and hepatic function; decreased body water and increased fat proportionally; displacement of one drug from protein-binding site by another makes drug–drug interaction more common and complex to treat

Sx: "Doctor shopping," "lost pills," anxiety, amnesia, memory loss, depressed mood, agitation, falls, abdominal pain or constipation, personal hygiene deterioration, confusion, obtundation

Crs: Drug withdrawal longer in older pts; benzodiazepine withdrawal mortality higher

Lab: Drug levels in abuse or w enzyme-competing drugs; LFTs may be elevated

Rx: Treat drug withdrawal in medically monitored setting due to risk of hyperautonomic syndrome, delirium or convulsion; lipid-soluble benzodiazepines cause more difficult withdrawal (diazepam, chlordiazepoxide); may take mos; less lipid-soluble, cut one-half dose for 2 wk, next one-fourth dose for 1 wk, then last one-fourth over 1–2 wk, and monitor vital signs; sedative hypnotic withdrawal 10–21 d; opioids halved over 5–10 d, then gradual reduction over weeks; use alternative pain relief

Team Management: Groups specific for older people; chronic pain groups; chemical-dependency units especially important for elderly withdrawal of sedative/hypnotics; consider NA/AA; psychosocial issues need addressing; abuse/misuse may be self-treatment of stresses or losses of late life; pt education of potential for interaction of complex med regimen and its enhanced effect in elderly

5.5 DEMENTIAS

Jama 1997;278:1363; Sci Am 1997;11:xi; Nejm 1996;335:330;
Cummings JL, Intensive Geriatric Review Course, UCLA, 1/96;
Clin Ger Med 1994;10:239; Med Clin N Am 1994;78:811; Ann
IM 1991;115:122; Nejm 1986;314:964
See Figure 5-2
See Table 5-4

Cause: 20–40% genetic transmission.

Early onset (<60 yr old):
- Amyloid percussor protein gene on chromosome #21
- Presenillin single gene
- Presenillin two gene type

Late (>60 yr old):
- Apolipoprotein E gene, E4 allele hetero/homozygotes on
  chromosome #19 (Nejm 2000;343:450)
- Chromosome #12 autosomal dominant (Jama 1997;278:1237)
- Chromosome #10 affecting beta-amyloid linked to late onset AD
  (Science 2000;290:2302)

Family hx imparts 3–4 times risk of general population; head trauma
imparts 3 times risk of general population; most are acquired and
of unclear cause; toxins, eg, carbon dioxide, carbon monoxide;
elevated risk of subsequent strokes in older persons w cognitive
impairment suggesting CVD plays important role in causing
cognitive impairment (J Am Geriatr Soc 1996;44:237); low
linguistic ability in early life strong predictor of poor cognitive
function and Alzheimer in late life (Jama 1996;275:582); smoking
imparts increased risk (Lancet 1998;351:1840)

Epidem: Prevalence = 5% at 70 yr, 20% at 80 yr, 50% at 90 yr (Jama
1995;273:1354) vs doubles q 5 yr from 1% at 60 yr to 40% at 85 yr
(Neurol 1998;51:S2; Nejm 1999;341:1670); 50% incidence in family
members of late-onset Alzheimer pts (Geriatrics 2000;55:34); M = F;
100% of Down syndrome pts >35 yr (Science 1992;258:668; Ann IM
1985;103:526); nondemented elderly w depressed mood more at risk
for developing Alzheimer dementia (Arch Gen Psychiatry 1996;
53:175)

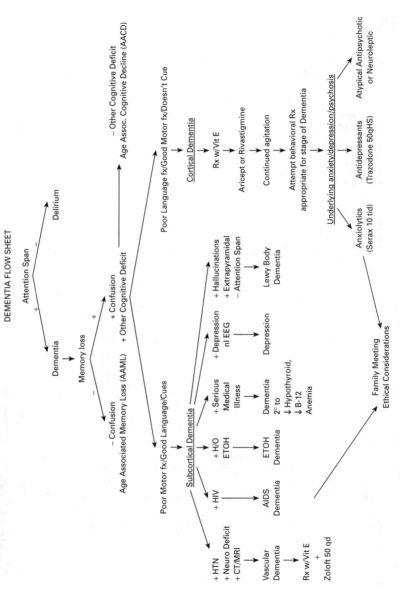

Figure 5-2. Dementia flow sheet.

40+% of elderly dementia is purely Alzheimer, the rest is vascular multi-infarct type predominantly (Nejm 1993;328:153); 70% of NH pts have Alzheimer dementia; "mixed dementia" felt to be common

Associated w E4 allele of apolipoprotein E (Nejm 1996;334:752; Jama 1995;273:1274) which facilitates β-amyloid protein deposition in neurofibrillary tangles (Nejm 1995;333:1242), high concentration of neurofibrillary tangles associated w cognitive decline (Jama 2000;283:1571,1615); higher mortality in pts w dementia and apolipoprotein E phenotype (J Am Geriatr Soc 1998;46:72); E2 allele protective against the development of Alzheimer (Jama 1996;275:1612)

Higher antioxidants: ascorbic acid and β-carotene plasma levels associated w better memory performance (J Am Geriatr Soc 1997;45:718)

Pathophys: Structural changes most severe in hippocampus and association cortex of parietal, temporal, frontal lobes; atrophy of corpus callosum differentiates Alzheimer from healthy elderly and incipient dementia (J Am Geriatr Soc 1996;44:798); neurofibrillary tangles are paired helical filaments that contain tau and ubiquitin proteins associated w intracellular microtubules (Nejm 1991;325:1849); unknown relation to deficiency of acetylcholine vs glutamate (Jama 1999;281:1401,1433)

Neuronal dropout; decreased acetylcholine synthesis (Nejm 1985;313:7), hence anticholinergics worsen (Nejm 1985;313:7); serotonin and norepinephrine deficit as well (Geriatrics 2000;55:34); whether plaques are a consequence of altered metabolism or are primary causative lesions (Neuron 1996;16:921)

Sx: Loss of social skills and memory usually unacknowledged by pt unless early stages; depression related to insight into cognitive losses

Si: Abnormal mental status (Psychiatr Clin N Am 1991;14:309) w memory loss >6 mo + 2 other cognitive function impairments for definition of dementia according to National Institute of Neurological and Communicative Disorders and Stroke-Alzheimer Disease and Related Disorders (NINCDS-ADRDA); these criteria produce 90–100% accuracy (Neurol 1993;43:250); DSM-IV only requires one cognitive deficit for definition of dementia, producing 80–85% accuracy (American Psychiatric Association, DSM IV, 1994:142);

Table 5-4. Dementias

	Delirium—Infecting, Metabolic, etc.	AD (60%)	Frontal Lobe Dementia (10%), Pick (1–2%)	Subcortical (2–3%) Huntington's, Wilson's, SNP, NPH, Parkinson	Vascular Dementias (15%) (Multi-infarct, Binswanger's Cortical Infarctions)	Wernicke-Korsakoff
History Onset, duration	Sudden, hours-days (CJD-dementia die within 1 yr)[a]	Insidious, month–years; 8–10 yr AD	2–10 yr	—	Acute, stepwise[a]	—
Mental status Attention	Fluctuating[a]	—	—	—	—	—
Memory Learning, recall, and recognition	Impaired by poor attention	Amnesia early	Amnesia late[a]	Forgetful[a] (retrieval deficit)	—	—
Language Comprehension, repetition, naming	Normal or mild anomia, misnaming, dysgraphia, may be impaired	Aphasia	—	Normal[a]	—	—
Speech	Slurred	Normal	Stereotyped speech, terminal mutism	Abnormal (hypophonic, dysarthric, mute)	—	—
Perception Visual spatial skills, constructional apraxia	Hallucination	Visual spatial	Visual spatial disturbance late	Impaired	—	—

Cognition Calculation, abstraction, judgment	—	Abnormal[a] (acalculia, poor judgment, impaired abstraction)	Calculations spared early	Abnormal (slowed), dilapidated		Confabulation early, antegrade memory loss[a]; can't learn new things
Executive skills Drive, programming response control synthesis	Very poor	—	Impairment of initiation, goal setting, planning	Problems with executive skills	—	—
Mood affect	Fear, suspiciousness may often be prominent	Paranoid delusions, 25% disinterested or uninhibited	Personality change early[a] Klüver-Bucy[b] syndrome, apathy, irritability, jocularity, euphoria, loss of fear	Abnormal (apathetic or depressed), blunting, emotional withdrawal	Preservation of personality; emotional lability	Placid, congenial
Motor Posture, tone, movement, gait	Postural tremor, myoclonus, asterixis; AIDS: psychomotor slowing, focal neurologic signs	Normal into final stages (then increased tone and flexed posture)	—	Posture-stooped,[a] SNP (extended or flexed) (Parkinson's) tone, increased, tremor, bradykinesia, chorea, dystonia, abnormal gait	Multifocal defects in lacunar disease, rigid, EPS, pseudobulbar palsy	Nystagmus, ataxia (detectable in late stages)

AD = Alzheimer; CJD = Creutzfeldt-Jakob disease; AIDS = acquired immunodeficiency syndrome; SNP = supranuclear palsy; EPS = extrapyramidal syndromes.

[a] Most characteristic findings.

[b] Klüver-Bucy—blunted emotional response, hypersex, gluttony.

Modified from tables in Cummings, Benson, and Loverme, 1980; Sultzer/Cummings intensive course in geriatric medicine, 1/96.

proper interpretation of Mini Mental State Exam (MMSE) requires knowledge of pt reading level (J Am Geriatr Soc 1995;43:807)

Family key to earliest dx if can be encouraged to share information; spousal denial and covering of sx of losses common; retrospective hx suggests 3–4 yr of sx before presentation to health professional

- Memory, recent much worse than remote; including orientation to time (d, mo, yr) (day of week is 53% sens, 92% specif) (Ann IM 1991;115:122); recall 3 items associated w medial temporal lobe-hippocampus, mammillary bodies, hypothalamus
- Perceptive/spatial disorientation, eg, answers to "How do you get there from here?"; clock-face drawing; copy interlocking pentagons associated w parietal, frontal, occipital
- Language impairments: anomias/paraphasias/aphasias which often result in neologisms or circumlocutions, fluent aphasia (posterior L brain-Wernicke); use of automatic phrases and clichés; as pt progresses, ask questions that only require short answers to demonstrate comprehension: "Point to the light," "Do you put your shoes on before your socks?", "Is my wife's brother a man or a woman?", "The lion was killed by the tiger. Which animal is dead?"
- Abstraction impairments: "What does it mean to give someone the cold shoulder?"; categorization; calculations
- Scoring: <21 on the MMSE is abnormal for 8th-grade education, <23 is abnormal for high school education, <24 abnormal for college education, 18–24 mild cognitive impairment, 0–17 severe cognitive impairment; MMSE insensitive to noncortical dementias; Hachinski scale helps discriminate other dementias from Alzheimer dementia
- Executive skills (Lancet 1999;354:1921): motivation, ability to initiate activity, ability to recognize patterns, generate motor programs and the ability to plan and execute a strategy; alternate square and triangle pattern (frontal lobe) (Exp Aging Res 1994;20:73); highly correlated w the appearance of problem behaviors in Alzheimer dementia (Exp Aging Res 1994;20:73)
- Affect changes and poor judgment: neuropsychiatric findings with other assessment tests (J Fam Pract 1993;37:599)
- Impairment of verbal memory and category naming associated w incipient dementia (Neurol 1995;45:957)
- Pupillary dilatation not si of dementia (Arch Neurol 1997;54:55)

Crs: Slowly progressive; mean survival from first sx = 10 yr, shorter for more severe cases (Ann IM 1990;113:429); average decline = 3 points per year on the MMSE, poor prognosis w extrapyramidal signs or psychosis (Jama 1997;277:806); stages (Am J Psychiatry 1982;139:1136) 1 and 2, forget familiar names and places; stage 3, family and coworkers aware; stage 4, difficulty w finances; stage 5, need assistance dressing; stage 6, incontinence, delusional; stage 7, grunting, nonambulatory

- Personality changes (from progressive passivity to marked hostility) can develop before cognitive impairments (J Ger Psychiatry Neurol 1990;3:21)
- Delusions (50%) of paranoid type most common; accusations of theft, infidelity; hallucinations, usually visual in 25% of pts, early in course predict rapid decline (Am J Psychiatry 1996;153:1438)
- Depression in 40%; orbital frontal (irritability), mediofrontal (apathy) early in Alzheimer dementia; dorsal frontal (aphasia, apraxia, agnosia) occur later (J Am Geriatr Soc 1997;45:891)
- Lewy body variant: intraneural inclusion bodies on histopathology, cortical-type cognitive impairment, extrapyramidal signs (Neurol 1990;40:1)
- Clinical characteristics of atypical dementia syndromes (Nejm 1996;335:330): those w language, constructional apraxia out of proportion to memory loss progress less rapidly
- Agitated behavior occurs sometime during course of disease in one-third to one-half of pts w Alzheimer, not predictive of rapid decline
- Fever common in progressive dementia, most pts recover regardless of antibiotics, little benefit in advanced dementia (Jama 1990; 263:3168)

Cmplc:

R/o: *Age-associated memory impairment* (AAMI), also termed *benign*, and if more severe, *malignant senescent forgetfulness*, may be an early monosymptomatic stage of Alzheimer dementia; lower N-acetyl-acetate in AAMI and DAT brains than in normal aging brain (J Am Geriatr Soc 1996;44:133)

Age-associated cognitive decline (AACD), a transitional state between normal aging but does not meet criteria for global cognitive deficit of dementia; no memory impairment

R/o: *Delirium*, if acute, in which attention span is most prominent deficit; test by serial 7s; serial digits up to 7, eg, phone numbers; spell "world" or repeat days of week backward; associated w increased mortality (J Am Geriatr Soc 1992;40:759; Jama 1990;263:1097); if decline on MMSE is >3–4 pts/yr or score of 15 after only 3 yr h/o dementia, must r/o other problems; rx w Haldol 0.5 or Ativan 0.5 in hospital (J Am Geriatr Soc 1992;40:829); sitters, reorienting routines helpful

Independent risk factors for developing delirium in hospital include preexisting dementia, >80 yr, fx on admission, symptomatic infection, male gender, use of antipsychotic or narcotic med; septic encephalopathy (Jama 1996;275:470): severity of Glasgow Coma Score correlates w BUN, bilirubin, bacteremia

Other risk factors include single or multiple drugs (6%); toxins like occult solvent/paint exposure may cause peripheral neuropathy, myopathy, cerebellar signs; elevated blood or urine levels of Pb, As, Hg, manganese, thallium

R/o: *Other reversible cortical or type I dementias* notable for posterior cortical features; test w ability to draw, not copy, clock (Geriatrics 1998;53:49; Nejm 1986;314:1111; Ann IM 1984;100:417)

R/o: *Other irreversible cortical or type I dementias* notable for posterior cortical features (amnesia, aphacia, agnosia, anomia, apraxia); see Table 5-5 (J Am Geriatr Soc 1998;46:98)

Pick disease (1–2% cases, argentophilic inclusion bodies or Pick body on histopathology); if no histopathology, then frontal-temporal dementia (J Am Geriatr Soc 1997;45:579) similar to Alzheimer

Table 5-5. Dementing Illnesses Arranged by Qualitative Subtypes

Type 1 Dementias	Type 2 Dementias
Alzheimer disease	Frontal types/Pick disease (early)
Atypical AD cases	Alcoholic dementia
Frontal types/Pick disease (late)	B_{12}/Folate deficiency
Creutzfeldt-Jakob	Dementia of depression
Cortical Lewy body disease	Dementia pugilistica
Some vascular dementia	Huntington disease
	Hypothyroidism
	Normal pressure hydrocephalus
	Parkinson dementia
	Polypharmacy
	Vascular dementia (most cases)

Reproduced by permission from Yeager BF, Farnett LE, Ruzicka SA. Management of the behavioral manifestations of dementia. Arch Intern Med 1995;155:250–60.

but much younger onset with less memory impairment and more behavioral change (apathy, irritability, jocularity, euphoria, *Klüver-Bucey syndrome* = emotional blunting, loss of fear, oral exploratory behavior, change in eating habits, altered sexual activity); disordered executive function (impairment of initiation goal setting planning); inability to refrain from touching objects and/or shoplifting; rx w Risperdal, Zoloft; 2–10 yr duration; no praxis or visuospatial deficit as w Alzheimer; language-abundant unfocused speech, echolalia, palilalia; is rare and anatomic changes are isolated to frontal and temporal lobes; other frontal lobe dementias comprise 10% of dementias (frontal lobe degeneration of the non-Alzheimer type, progressive subcortical gliosis, amyotrophic lateral sclerosis [ALS] dementia syndrome); MMSE may be nl w early frontal lobe, Lewy body, Pick dementias

Creutzfeldt-Jakob (CJD), rare, slow virus, prior incubation period several years; no known cure; progresses rapidly once active, death within 1 yr; cerebellar and extrapyramidal signs, startle myoclonus, asymmetric slowing or periodic polyspike discharges on EEG

R/o: *Reversible type II subcortical dementias* which affect frontal systems (at frontal cortex or subcortical level) while sparing posterior cortical regions; executive control functions in three main systems are affected: dorsolateral (abstraction and hypothesis generation), orbitofrontal (emotional control), mediofrontal (apathy, impaired goal directed attention); impaired pt can draw clock but cannot indicate 1:45 on clock (the hands point to the 1, the 4 and the 5 instead of the 1 and the 9)

Hypothyroidism (depression, irritability, mental slowing); myxedema (4%), thyrotoxicosis less common, psychomotor retardation, apathy, less anxiety, tremor, tachycardia that is characteristic of younger pts; both hypothyroidism and hyperthyroidism can present w frank psychosis

Vit B$_{12}$ deficiency: irritability, psychosis, delirium, amnesia, slowing of thought processes may also occur; peripheral neuropathy, optic atrophy, older pts symptomatic at higher levels of vit B$_{12}$ (low NL) than younger pts (J Am Geriatr Soc 1996;44:1355)

Subdural hematoma (2%), results from cerebral atrophy and shearing of already stretched bridging veins during trauma

Wernicke-Korsakoff syndrome w anterograde memory loss, alcohol hx; may recover partially over 1 yr (Nejm 1985;312:16)

Depression pseudodementia: more "I don't know" answers than the "guesses" of DAT; lack of progression of sx; preserved awareness of deficits; preserved language skills; cued recall nl; impaired problem-solving and word-list generation; also often both depression and dementia occur together; more likely to respond to antidepressant if MMSE >21; rx of apathy responds to stimulant such as amphetamine; depression associated w significant memory deficit may be in fact preclinical dementia (J Am Geriatr Soc 2000;48:479)

Syphilitic dementia: meningovascular (2–10 yr, sometimes 30–40 yr after initial infection); inflammatory arteritis that can result in stroke and vascular dementia; general paresis (7–12 yr after initial infection); delusions, hallucinations, mood disorders often present; pseudobulbar palsy; poor coordination; hyperreflexia or hyporeflexia; pupillary abnormalities; signs of posterior column dysfunction (taboparesis); VDRL and rapid plasma reagent nonreactive in one-fourth of pts w late neurosyphilis; fluorescent treponema antibody (FTA) more sensitive but remains positive even after treatment

AIDS: psychomotor slowing, focal neurologic signs, frontal lobe cell loss

Frontal/temporal tumor

R/o: *Nonreversible causes type II or subcortical dementias* (Ann IM 1984;100:417) which show forgetfulness, executive dysfunction (J Am Geriatr Soc 1997;45:386) and motor findings early (Arch Neurol 1993;50:873) unlike the amnesia and early language deficits in DAT: eg, Parkinson (slowing of cognition), less agnosia and more apathy than w cortical dementias

Diffuse Lewy body disease (DLBD): see Table 5-6; vivid recurrent visual hallucinations that are recognized as unreal occur earlier, and extrapyramidal dysfunction more mild than w Parkinson and appear w onset of dementia; alteration in alertness, attention resembling confusional states, transient loss of consciousness (J Am Geriatr Soc 1998;46:1449, Neurol 1996;47:111), sensitive to neuroleptics, may be life-threatening w malignant neuroleptic syndrome, even Risperdal; consider olanzapine instead (Nejm 1998;338:6031); minor response with L-dopa (Neurol 1997;48:376); relative serotonergic dominance; ondansetron (Zofran), a 5-HT3 receptor antagonist, used for delusions and hallucinations

Table 5-6. Clinical Diagnostic Criteria for Diffuse Lewy Body Disease

1. The central feature is progressive cognitive decline amounting to dementia; deficits on tests of attention, fronto-subcortical skills, and visuospatial ability may be especially significant.
2. Two of the following are required for a probable, and one for a possible diagnosis of DLB:
   a. Fluctuating cognition with pronounced variations in attention and alertness
   b. Recurrent visual hallucinations that are typically well formed and detailed
   c. Spontaneous motor features of parkinsonism
3. Features supportive of the diagnosis are:
   a. Repeated falls
   b. Syncopes or transient losses of consciousness
   c. Neuroleptic hypersensitivity
   d. Systematized delusions
   e. Hallucinations in other modalities
4. DLB is less likely in the presence of:
   a. Stroke disease, revealed by focal neurological signs or brain imaging
   b. Evidence of any other physical or brain illness that may account for the clinical picture

Progressive supranuclear palsy (axial rigidity, vertical gaze palsy) may respond to amitriptyline 10–40 mg bid (J Am Geriatr Soc 1996;44:1072); spinocerebellar degenerations, Huntington, Wilson, olivopontine degeneration and NPH (obstruction of CSF flow around the convexity of the brain, impaired absorption into the sagittal sinus, gait abnormalities initial symptom w small shuffling steps w feet set down at variable force, postural instability, difficulties w fine hand movements, lack of initiative and slowness of thought, best outcomes of shunt done earlier in disease, may be partially reversible, not without substantial morbidity, see "Normal-Pressure Hydrocephalus"); systemic diseases: end-stage renal failure, CHF, COPD, DM (subcortical microvascular lesions and hippocampal damage from hypoglycemia)

Multi-infarct dementia: stepwise crs, emotional lability prominent, and h/o HT, CVA, or ASHD; features of mixed cortical/subcortical dementia, see "Vascular Dementias"

Alcohol-related dementias: 10–15-yr drinking hx; apathy and noncortical features predominate; irritability; may have nl MMSE; partially reversible w abstinence; direct toxic effect of alcohol has not been established

PSYCHIATRY

R/o: *Paraphrenia:* hallucinations and delusions out of proportion to intellectual dysfunction

Lab: Cost-effectiveness of w/u for reversible dementias questionable (J Neurol 1995;242:446)

- Brain histology at postmortem shows neurofibrillary tangles, senile plaques with eosinophilic amyloid
- CBC
- T_3, T_4, chem panel, lytes if acute, vit B_{12} level, folate, UA
- VDRL, perhaps HIV antibody if young; dementia occurs in 20% HIV pts
- EEG occasionally helpful to distinguish DAT (slow waves) from depression (nl), toxic, metabolic; or partial complex seizure and CJD
- Obtain CSF in subacute cases
- APOE (genotyping for E allele) positive predictive value very high but negative predictive value nil, only recommend in combination w clinical criteria (Nejm 1998;338:506); cholinergic markers not present until relatively late in the course of Alzheimer dementia (Jama 1999;281:1401)

Xray: Head CT or MRI distinguishes from multi-infarct dementia—periventricular hyperintensities on T2-weighted images w multi-infarct dementia and in deep white matter w Alzheimer (Neurol 1993;43:250); only if si of subdural or rapid onset (Ann IM 1984;100:417); very low yield of reversible disease, eg, <1/250; CT, MRI not helpful unless focal findings present (Ann IM 1994;120:856)

If motor dysfunction, eg, rigidity, reflex asymmetry, abnormal reflexes, then obtain MRI to detect stroke and ischemic changes (J Am Geriatr Soc 1995;43:138); MRI better than CT for subcortical pathology

PET, SPECT: Decreased cerebral blood flow and glucose metabolism in parietal, temporal, frontal association cortex bilaterally (Arch Neurol 1995;52:773); mostly a research tool at this point; as early treatment evolves these will become more clinically applicable tests; low sens and specif of SPECT in Alzheimer (J Am Geriatr Soc 1997;45:15)

Rx:

Preventive:

- Apolipoprotein E screening not appropriate (Jama 1997;277:832); pts with extensive social networks protected against development of dementia (Lancet 2000;355:1291)

- NSAIDs may decrease risk (Neurol 1997;48:626); large studies only epidemiological, not controlled
- Screening for preventive rx of other diseases limited to account for overall prognosis (Jama 2000;283:3230)

Therapeutic:

- Memory aids (J Fam Pract 1993;37:6)
- Acetylcholine esterase inhibitors: improvement in non-cognitive items: cooperation, delusions, pacing (Arch Neurol 1997;54:836; J Ger Psychiatry Neurol 1996;9:1), also decreased behavioral problems (Am J Psychiatry 2000;157:4), increased word-finding and memory of important names and events, improved ADLs; Rivastigmine may also help w Lewy body dementia (Neurology 2000;54(suppl 3):A450); more likely to have clinically relevant response to tacrine if mild to moderate dementia; w relative preservation of language and praxis; reduces necessity of other psychotropic meds (Ann LT Care 1998;6(suppl):92)
- Donepezil (Aricept) 5 mg po (Med Let 1997;39:53; Neurol 1998;50:135; J Clin Psychiatry 1996;57:30), which may be increased to 10 mg after 6 wk, like tacrine has similar MMSE improvement, does not affect liver function but has GI side effects, eg, nausea, vomiting, diarrhea; avoid if hx PND, sick sinus syndrome, pulmonary disease, bladder outflow problems; give in am to avoid nightmares; Aricept helps for 6 mo–2 yr, 8-wk trial suggested; Rivastigmine (Exelon) 1.5–6 mg/bid, side effects nausea, vomiting, diarrhea, weight loss, interacts w P450 drugs (Med Let 2000;7:28;2000;42:93)
- Metrifonate good in drug company reports only (Neurol 1998; 50:1203,1214,1222); rivastigmine and galantamine similar GI side effect profile but not the myalgias associated w donepezil (Clin Ger Med 2001;17:346) (Med Let 2001;43:53)
- Vasodilators like ergoloid mesylates (Hydergine) 2 mg tid 6 mo no value (Nejm 1990;323:445; Ann IM 1984;100:896)
- New drug rx being developed: pharmacologic interventions against the amyloid cascade, neuroprotective agents such as glutamate antagonists, antioxidants; huperzine A (a compound first isolated from traditional Chinese herbal medicine), a potent inhibitor acetylcholinesterase, may also protect neurons (Jama 1997;277:276); injection of neurotrophic agents into ventricular system to retard neural degeneration (Nurs Home Med 1995; 3:3E)

PSYCHIATRY

- Estrogen protective (Horm Metab Res 1995;27:204; J Am Geriatr Soc 1996;44:865); NSAIDs protective (J Am Geriatr Soc 1996;44:1025,1307); promotes cholinergic and serotonergic activity, favorable lipoprotein alterations, prevents cerebral ischemia (Jama 1998;279:688); vs data on estrogen-preventing memory loss limited by inconsistency of associations, specificity, lack of stepwise graded association, lack of temporality, no prevention or reversibility data, age confounder, compliance and misclassification bias (J Am Geriatr Soc 1998;46:918); vs ERT not protect against age-related decline in cognitive function (Jama 2000;283:1007) but education does (J Am Geriatr Soc 1999;47:159,518); relationship between ERT and cognitive functioning must be measured by long-term randomized controlled trials which are under way—Women's Health Initiative Memory Study to study ERT relationship w development of dementia (J Am Geriatr Soc 2000;48:588, Control Clin Trials 1998;19:604) and Women's Health Initiative Study of Cognitive Aging to study ERT relationship w subtle changes in memory w aging (Neurol 1997;48:1516)
- Vit E up to 2000 IU delayed death, institutionalization, loss of ADLs and progression of dementia; monoamine oxidase-B inhibitors, eg, selegiline 5 gm po bid may have neurotropic effects as well (Nejm 1997;336:1216,1245; Science 1997;276:675)
- Ginkgo biloba modest improvements cognitive function without adverse effects, 6 mo–1 yr (Jama 1997;278:1327), but not a blinded study (Med Let 1998;40:63)

Of agitated behavior: See Table 5-7

- Antipsychotic drug uses: anti-aggressive effects of antipsychotics may take up to 8 wk to appear; pts w severe dementia do not respond as well; agitation may result from benzodiazepine withdrawal (Am J Hosp Pharm 1994;51:2917)
- Government-approved indications for antipsychotic drug use in *NH:* biting, kicking, scratching or other aggressive behaviors presenting as danger to self or others; functional impairment caused by continuous crying out, screaming, pacing, hallucinations, paranoia or delusions; documentation of frequency and duration necessary (Omnibus Nursing Home required, Federal Register 1992;57:4519)
- Phenothiazines, in order of increasing extrapyramidal and decreasing sedation/anticholinergic/hypotensive effects (Table 5-8): Mellaril (thioridazine), Thorazine (chlorpromazine), Navane

Table 5-7. Medications for Agitated Demented Patients

Insomnia, Anxiety, Fear, Tension	Depressed Mood, Crying	Hostile, Assaultive, Psychotic
Benzodiazepine, oxazepam up to 10 mg qid, or propranolol up to 40 qid plus buspirone	Antidepressant, trazodone 25 mg up to 200 mg/d or SSRIs	Carbamazepine 25 tid mg to 400 mg/d (level = 7), or risperidone 0.5 mg or antipsychotic

Adapted from Royall DR, Polk M. Dementias that present with and without posterior cortical features: an important clinical distinction. J Am Geriatr Soc 1998;46:98–105.

Table 5-8. Antipsychotic Drugs

Antipsychotic	Side-Effect Profile	
	Hypotension, Sedation, Anticholinergic	EPS
Mellaril ("my")	+++++	+
Thorazine ("troubles")	++++	++
Navane ("now")	+++	+++
Haldol ("have")	++	++++
Prolixin ("passed")	+	+++++

EPS = extrapyramidal syndrome.

(thiothixene), Haldol (haloperidol), Prolixin (fluphenazine)—mnemonic = "My Troubles Now Have Passed"; 20–25% dose used in younger person

- Extrapyramidal side effects (EPS): acute dystonic reactions rare in the elderly (Consult Pharm 1992;7:921), treated w diphenhydramine (Benadryl); parkinsonian signs treated w benztropine mesylate (Cogentin) or anticholinergic or amantadine for 3 mo or switching to lower-potency antipsychotic; akathisia: 20% prevalence, anticholinergics not as effective at treating as benzodiazepines or β-blockers for effects on GABA (Am J Hosp Pharm 1991;48:1271); also w amantadine, diazepam (Valium); tardive dyskinesia: prevalence as high as 40% and more severe w age (J Am Geriatr Soc 1987;35:233); 2 times more frequent in blacks than whites; increasing antipsychotic dose when this sx first appears will eliminate it temporarily (supersensitization of dopaminergic receptors after prolonged receptor blockade, abnormal movements can paradoxically worsen when the dosage of the antipsychotic is first decreased); anticholinergics often exacerbate it; greatest risk first 2 yr of treatment; adding lithium to antipsychotic may lead to neuroleptic malignant syndrome (NMS) (J Clin Psychopharmacol 1993;54:35); 5–40% tardive dyskinesia eventually remit, can rx w carbamazepine, dopaminergic and Gaba drugs (valproic acid and Depakene)

- Orthostatic hypotension: blockade of β_1-receptors more common w low-potency antipsychotics, aliphatic phenothiazines and clozapine; weight gain also w these drugs

Clozapine: Avoid extrapyramidal sx; no tardive dyskinesia, but causes agranulocytosis in 1–2% pts, which can be fatal; thus weekly monitoring and report agranulocytosis to national registry; older pts at greater risk for leukopenia, hypotension, and seizures can continue med and rx seizures w valproic acid; average dose 37 mg/d; optimal duration of clozapine trial 6 wk–12 mo (Am J Ger Psychiatry 1995;3:26; Am J Hlth Syst Pharmacol 1995;52:S9; Can J Psychiatry 1995;40:208; Neurol 1995;45:432; Drug Topics 1994;138:30; J Ger Psychiatry Neurol 1994;7:129; Med Let Drugs Ther 1994;36:33; Neurol 1994;44:2247; Med Let Drugs Ther 1993;35:16)

Clozapine significantly reduces gastric acid secretion, resulting in decrease in gastric ulcers (Am J Psychiatry 1995;152:821)

Clozapine overdose: somnolence, tachycardia, aspiration pneumonia, hypotension, seizures; no cases of agranulocytosis reported with overdose; death rare (J Emerg Med 1995;13:199)

Drug interactions: clozapine and tricyclic antidepressant may produce delirium due to additive anticholinergic effects; cimetidine induced toxicity because of inhibition of cytochrome P450

Kinetics: cleared mostly through hepatic enzyme metabolism; start w 6.25 mg to avoid bradycardia (J Clin Psychiatry 1995;56:180)

First Choice Antipsychotics:

- Risperidone: decreases neg (depression, social withdrawal, apathy) as well as pos (delusions, hallucinations, paranoia) sx of schizophrenia; diminishes depression through its antagonism of 5-HT2 receptors (American Medical Directors Association 19th annual symposium, New Orleans, LA, 3/7/96); also better than other phenothiazines for Lewy body dementia (Nurs Home Med 1995;3:300); not anticholinergic; rarely causes sedation at low doses; starting dose 0.5 mg qd or bid w slow titration avoids hypotension (J Ger Psychiatry Neurol 1995;8:159); few drug interactions; when tapering clozapine and beginning risperidone, watch clozapine levels carefully (Psychiatry Drug Alerts 1996;2:9); extrapyramidal side effects dose-dependent (>10 mg/d); no tardive dyskinesia or agranulocytosis reported; may see elevation of prolactin, weight gain, sexual dysfunction

Kinetics: well absorbed from GI tract; unaffected by food; more rapid onset of action than clozapine, producing clinical response after 1 wk; extensively metabolized by the liver, excreted in urine, partly in feces; elimination half-life = 20 h; available in 1-, 2-, 3-, 4-mg tabs; cost comparison: haloperidol (Haldol) = $21–79, risperidone = $237, clozapine = $308

• Olanzapine: serotonin-dopamine antagonist w few EPS, but side-effect profile otherwise very much like clozapine, 5–20 mg qd (30-h half-life), 2.5 mg in NH pts (Nurs Home Med 1997;5 (suppl 7F); check baseline LFTs

Other Atypical Antipsychotics:
• Sertindole
• Quetiapine (Seroquel) 150–750 mg/d, 25 bid × 1 wk, 50 mg bid × 1 wk, 100 bid × 1 wk, 200 bid × 1 wk; may be used for sexually inappropriate behavior (J Am Geriatr Soc 2000;48:707); dyspepsia, weight gain, abdominal pain w increased doses; does not induce P450, may need more w hepatic enzyme inducers, eg, phenytoin, tegretol, barbiturates, rifampin, glucocorticoids

Second Choice Antipsychotics:
• Mood stabilizers/anticonvulsants (limbic kindling phenomena): carbamazepine effective in treatment of agitation, aggressiveness, impulsivity, and sexually inappropriate behaviors; 25 mg po bid up to 200 tid to a level of 6–7 mg/dL, following CBC and LFTs (J Clin Psychiatry 1990;51:115); carbamazepine levels decreased by warfarin, theophylline, haloperidol, divalproex sodium, carbamazepine (auto induction); levels increased by macrolides, cimetidine, propoxyphene, INH, fluoxetine, calcium channel blockers; valproic acid may reduce aggression, temper outbursts, and agitation (J Neuropsychiatry Clin Neurosci 1995;7:314); ASA may increase valproic acid levels, can cause diarrhea
• Benzodiazepines for anxiety but not for chronic use, eg, oxazepam (Serax) 10 mg po tid or lorazepam (Ativan) 0.5–1.0 mg qid; diminished effect after several months; agitation can be a result

of benzodiazepine withdrawal; clonazepam stimulates serotonin production and may lessen aggressive behavior, hyperactivity, social intrusiveness, and impulsivity

- Azaperone when given w neuroleptic drugs decreases severity of tardive dyskinesia, improves akathisia and parkinsonism, eg, buspirone 60 mg/d (Buspar); switching from benzodiazepine to azaperone: change short- or intermediate-acting benzodiazepine, eg, alprazolam (Xanax) to long-acting, eg, clonazepam (Klonopin), add azaperone 5–10 mg 3 × a day up to 30 mg/d; schedule taper of benzodiazepine over 60–90 d; takes 2–3 wk for azaperone to take effect (Am Fam Phys 1996;53:2349)
- Trazadone is beneficial in treatment of sleep deprivation, aggression, and hostility (J Clin Psychiatry 1995;56:374; Neurology 2000;55:1271); give hs because of hypotension
- Propranolol 40–120 mg (Med Clin N Am 1994;78:814)
- Estrogen 1.25 mg qd for sexual aggression in elderly men (J Am Geriatr Soc 1991;31:1110); ethics of treatment questionable (Am J Psychiatry 1981;138:5); rx hypersexuality, paraphilias w SSRI—most safe; then consider antiandrogens, eg, medroxyprogesterone (Ann LT Care 1998;6:248; J Clin Psychiatry 1987;48:368) which causes sleepiness, mild DM, increased appetite and weight gain, loss of hair, hot flashes, decreases ejaculatory volume, depression; estrogen causes thromboembolism, vascular risk; GnRH analogue which causes hot flashes, erectile dysfunction, decreased libido, and have to use continuously (J Am Geriatr Soc 1999;47:231)

Team Management:

See Tables 5-9, 5-10, and 5-11

Meeting w the family (Am Fam Phys 1984;29:149): important that pt be included in initial family meeting, may not remember content but will remember being included and taken seriously

Encourage catharsis about family's burden to explain or cover up Alzheimer secret; the family's loss of social roles and identities; violence from pt catastrophic reactions; being accused of malevolent motives by the pt; guilt regarding reflex anger to physical abuse by pt; blaming themselves for pt irritability and withdrawal; difficulties w having to constantly supervise pt

Facilitate learning of family about differences between memory loss and attention deficit; stages of dementia; compliment family and pt for recognizing the problem and dispel myths (pt not lazy, crazy; dementia is not caused by stress or vit deficiency and not

Table 5-9. Alzheimer Disease Assessment Tool

Group	MMSE Mean (±SD)	Characteristic Function and Cognitive Deficit	Approximate Age Function Acquired	Characteristic Function Preserved	Adjuvant Psychological Features	Major Treatment Concerns	Prognosis During 4-yr Follow-up
Forgetfulness (Stage I)	29.6 (±0.7)	None	—	All	None	—	—
Forgetfulness (Stage II)	28.9 (±1.3)	Subjective c/o word finding, forgetting familiar names, normal performance at work	Adult	No objective Memory deficit on clinical interview	Anxiety	Reassurance Treat anxiety	Most will not develop AD but only mild forgetfulness Predicted life expectancy in AD is 8–10 yr
Confusion Stage III	24.6 (±3.5)	Disorientation to time. Clear-cut memory and cognitive deficit Withdrawal from challenging situations (work) Word and name finding deficit	Young adult	Normal ADL and IADL Routine activity well preserved Driving to familiar area	Anxiety Depression	Prevent conditions that increase anxiety Treat depression	80% deterioration in cognitive function Predicted life expectancy 6–8 yr
Dementia Stage IV	20.0 (±3.8)	Disorientation to place Decreased ability to handle finances, perform complex tasks, and remember recent events Decreased driving ability: gets lost, unable to interpret signs	8 yr	Might be oriented ×2 Able to drive to familiar places Able to stay in the community	Denial Paranoid thoughts	Strategy to approach patient with denial Handling finances Use of a notebook as a memory aid Control driving location	25% in nursing home 25% remain in the community Predicted life expectancy 4–6 yr

PSYCHIATRY

Table 5-9. (cont'd)

Group	MMSE Mean (±SD)	Characteristic Function and Cognitive Deficit	Approximate Age Function Acquired	Characteristic Function Preserved	Adjuvant Psychological Features	Major Treatment Concerns	Prognosis During 4-yr Follow-up
Dementia Stage V	14.3 (±3.4)	Require assistance choosing attire Forget to bathe Not able to stay in community without assistance	5–7 yr	Able to dress Able to bathe alone	Agitation Reserved sleep patterns	Full home assistance Day care Prepare for long-term care facility	Most in nursing homes Persistent gradual deterioration Predicted life expectancy 3–4 yr
Dementia Stage VI	8.3 (±4.8)	Not remembering names of spouse, child Require assistance bathing Require assistance dressing Require assistance toileting Urinary incontinent Fecal incontinent	5 yr 4 yr 3 yr 2 yr	Language impaired Walk with small steps	Violent psychosis, eg, hallucination	24-h home help Nursing home Treatment for agitation and psychosis	Most will die or be in a nursing home
Dementia Stage VII	0 (±0)	Dramatic deterioration in: Speech activity Ambulation Sitting Smile Body posture/ head Neurologic cortical signs	15 mo 12 mo 8 mo 4 mo 2 mo	None	None	Soft food diet NG or PEG tube	14% will die from unknown etiology Possible due to defect in the regulation of vital signs, eg, respiratory function

MMSE = Mini-Mental State Exam; c/o = complains of; PEG = percutaneous endoscopic gastrostomy; AD = Alzheimer. From Am J Alzheimer Dis Rel Disord Res 1995;10:4.

Table 5-10. Behavior of Demented Patients During Late Stages (Usually in Nursing Home Setting)

Stage V/VII:

Usually placed in NH; aware of surroundings but not aware of their purpose; "all dressed up with nowhere to go"; very unhappy when have to interact w unkempt, aggressive patients; eg, stage VII/VII patients; enjoy opportunity to look after needy cooperative patients (stage VI/VII)

State VI/VII:

Not sure where or who they are; need constant reassurance; "Velcro stage"; get along well w stage V/VII patients; like being led around by them; don't mind stage VII/VII patients; not aware enough to be bothered by them

Stage VII/VII:

If still ambulatory, will follow retreating stimuli; they stop following people when others have stopped moving; tend to follow visitors out of the door of the NH, but are easily redirected

From lecture by Lucero M, Lewiston, ME, 1994.

amenable to repetition; pts can still feel embarrassment and shame)

Send letters to family members who are geographically separated, who may not have recognized subtle changes in the pt and who may think the primary caregiver is exaggerating the problem

Have family read Alzheimer material and return for a f/u without the pt: identify where guilt has led to self-sacrificing caregiver behaviors; acknowledge their fears for the future and support them in decisions they must make that may be unacceptable to their afflicted parent or spouse, eg, NH placement (explore cultural values and family conflicts)

Help family draw up a day-to-day care plan for the pt that will provide a predictable environment and repeated reassurance; learn from family as much as possible about the successful approaches and accomplishments to this stage of disease; acknowledge importance of individualized approach for the pt and spouse and assure that care plan will integrate their prior work; create a "team" w family and health professionals; emphasize importance of family's continuing role

Encourage family to participate in support group, continue to meet their own individual needs; reinforce that they are developing expertise that is of value to the community at large; support political advocacy when it is suggested by the family

Table 5-11. Phases of Family Adaptation to Alzheimer Disease

Phase	Issue	Intervention
1. Predx	• Ambiguity, splitting "mom's OK" "she is not OK" • Break down taboos and talk about it to gather info	• Information/education

2. Dx	• Won't seek painful dx until crisis (part of family may disengage)
	• Hard to accept dx if process sends them back to predx phase
		• Families need to process together (1½ hours)
		• Keep pt within family boundary
		  —Who are going to tell—essential
		  —Marker of acceptance—starting to organize

3. Role change	• Repeated losses as patient less like him/herself • Ambiguity about when and how to make major role transformation; eg, driving • Danger = loss of all expectation, pt becomes non-person	• Change expectations rather than take away role—see the possibility in role—eg, co-driving • Relationship work with demented family member and family
4. Chronic care giving	• 36-h day for daughter-in-law while others critique or cheerlead (efficient but overwhelming)	• Change boundaries—who can be counted on to help • Change of structure: roles—Hands-on care, Phone calls, E-mail • Maintain family vitality, normal family life—rituals like Thanksgiving; and adolescent fights (conspiracy of happiness = a problem)
5. Shared care giving	• Services not a commodity. Home health means developing new relationships	• New relationships require that culture of caregiver meshes with family's basic values—eg, autonomy vs safety • Nurses look so proficient that family may react by withdrawing or be critical of care
6. Long-term care	• Almost always traumatic (guilt/failure/marginalized)	• Families need a role and expectations of them or else they become a non-entity [hx and biography providers] • Families need to be partners, not consumers, need collaborative atmosphere

7. End of life	• Ambivalence, relief, guilt, conflict	• Anticipate death early—talk about the good death (pt comfortable, family around, generativity) so family can move along smoothly and with legitimacy
		• Life review
		  —Feel as though pt that died is still present
		  —Family emerges whole

Adapted from AMDA Lecture, March 5, 1999, Orlando, Florida. Wayne Caron, PhD, & James Pattee, MD, CMD-R.

Behavioral management: look for precipitants of difficult behavior (what, where, why, when, who); reassurance and redirection effective, do not "reality orient" pts w cortical dementia, may result in "catastrophic reaction"; however, reality orientation and prompting very important techniques in subcortical dementias; otherwise pts may become depressed when caregivers assume pts are less capable than they are

Hallucinations, delusions = poor prognosis (J Am Geriatr Soc 1992;40:768); pts may often conceal, so ask subtly: "How are you getting on with other relatives? Neighbors? Are they annoying in any way? Are they deliberately trying to annoy you? Often when one is elderly, other people are unsympathetic—is that a problem?"

Sundowning (increased confusion and agitation in the late afternoon secondary to disturbances in circadian rhythm and REM sleep, deterioration of suprachiasmatic nucleus of hypothalamus): restrict daytime sleep, expose to bright light during the day, low-stress activity schedules (J Psychol Nurs 1996;34:40; Acta Psychiatr Scand 1994;89:1), provide routine, be sure pt has glasses and functional hearing aid, avoid sedative hypnotics, place familiar objects on pt bed or bedside to help assure safety

Wandering: "goal-directed" (disguise exit signs, place stop signs), "aimless wandering" (provide more structure, investigate possible discomfort)

Repetitive speech: group singing, reminiscing activities

Resistance to care: "good cop, bad cop" intervention in which pt is rescued from purposely overbearing caregiver by gentler caregiver so that the pt will follow the second caregiver and perform a task they usually resist

Caregivers should be encouraged to recognize their own stress; "36-h day" daycare center

In NH, wandering can also be managed by "wandering areas," posted signs, pictures of residents on resident room doors, tape barriers on floors and across doors, half-doors, coded locks

Screaming: hearing augmentation devices may prevent hard-of-hearing elderly from yelling (Nurs Home Med 1997;4:515)

Driving: score on MMSE and visual tracking can be used to stratify which cognitively impaired pts can drive safely (J Am Geriatr Soc 1997;45:949; Jama 1995;273:1360; Clin Ger Med 1993;9:279); not at night, not in traffic, but w someone else, on familiar roads;

take driver's test w copilot (J Am Geriatr Soc 1996;44:815); emphasize family's need to develop clear plan for driving cessation—a necessary eventual goal; predictive of car accident: visual field testing, falling in past 2 wks, poor near vision acuity, limited ROM of neck, visual attention (J Am Geriatr Soc 1998;46:556,562); mildly cognitively impaired individuals have as many car crashes as controls but the accidents result in more injury and involve failure to yield (J Am Geriatr Soc 2000;48:18)

Ethical considerations: if demented pts unable to carry out decisions and manage the consequences, the presumption in favor of maintaining autonomy may need to be reconsidered (J Am Geriatr Soc 1995;43:1437); 80% of elderly want to be told about their dx of Alzheimer disease vs 92% want to be told of a terminal illness of medical origin (J Am Geriatr Soc 1996;44:404)

Discussion w pt and family including advanced directives (living will, Durable Power of Attorney for Health Care) early on; refer to local Alzheimer chapter (J Gerontol Nurs 1983;9:93); at end stage of disease: discuss "do not resuscitate" (DNR), hospice; reassure that DNR does not mean "do not treat" (Clin Ger Med 1994;10:91); be certain to establish who has DPOA-HC and family "communication tree" in crisis; aim for acute illness care plan that is NH-centered as much as possible, emphasizing risk issues w hospitalization (worsening of cognition, disorientation, lack of understanding by hospital staff); tube feeding does not help prevent aspiration and is risky (Nejm 2000;342:206; Jama 1999;282:1365)

NORMAL-PRESSURE HYDROCEPHALUS

Jama 1996;44:445; Nejm 1985;312:1255

Cause: Idiopathic, postsurgical, trauma, subarachnoid hemorrhage, infectious meningitis, small-vessel disease

Pathophys: A "communicating hydrocephalus" (in contrast to foraminal or aqueductal) and obstruction is therefore at cisterna; hence, 4th ventricle may dilate causing cerebellar compression

Sx: First, trouble walking (ataxia with initiation and spasticity in lower extremity, leading to "magnetic gait," feet grip floor, only lifted with difficulty), progressive dementia and incontinence; dementia includes psychomotor slowing, impaired ability to concentrate, mild memory difficulties

Si: Horizontal nystagmus, normal disks, spasticity, frontal lobe si

Crs: Progressive dementia

Lab: CSF: transient but consistent improvement with removal of 50 mL (Acta Neurol Scand 1987;75:566) 1–3 in 1 wk; some neurosurgeons now not doing shunt unless see improvement with this first; Miller Fisher test—objective gait assessments before and after removal 30 mL CSF (Acta Neurol Scand 1986;73:566)

Xray: CT scan shows enlarged ventricles (100%); cisternogram shows delayed or no movement of dye out over hemispheres, but there are false-neg results

Rx: Surgical shunt, 80% success (Nejm 1985;312:1255)

Cmplc: Infections in 3–5%; factors associated with pos outcomes from shunting: short duration, known cause (trauma, hemorrhage), gait disturbance before onset of dementia or incontinence, presence of high-amplitude waves on intracranial pressure monitoring (Jama 1996;44:445)

VASCULAR DEMENTIAS

Cause:

1. Multiple subcortical (lacunar) or cortical infarctions (MID)
2. Ischemic demyelinization of subcortical white matter—Binswanger disease—clinical picture similar to MID
3. Single infarction; stroke not always leads to dementia (J Neurol Sci 1968;7:331); generally takes large amount brain tissue destruction (J Neurol Sci 1970;11:205)

Epidem: Estimates of prevalence vary:

- 15% of all postmortem diagnosed dementias are vascular dementias; more common in blacks, Japanese (Neurol 1995; 45:1161); MID over-diagnosed, needs more neuropathic correlation (Neurol 1993;43:243); stroke frequently coexists w Alzheimer or Parkinson dementia (Arch Neurol 1989;46:651); estimated number of vascular dementias inflated when Hachinski index (point system based on presence of neurologic and atherosclerotic disease) used (47–60%) (Nejm 1993;328:153)

- Low prevalence MID 25% (Alzheimer Dis Assoc Disord 1992;6:35; J Neurol Sci 1990;95:239; Psychol Med 1990;20:881; Jama 1989;262:2551; Ann Neurol 1988;24:50)
- 50% of community-dwelling demented elderly have vascular dementia (Nejm 1993;328:153)

Pathophys: Amyloid deposits in walls of small cerebral blood vessels

Sx: Subcortical infarctions (basal ganglia, internal capsule, thalamus): slowness, forgetfulness, apathy, executive skill deficit; depression, anxiety; behavioral retardation more severe in pts w vascular dementia than in Alzheimer

Si: Need temporal relationship between stroke and dementia to make dx vascular dementia (Nejm 1993;328:153; Neurol 1993;43:250; 1992;42:473); mixed 10–20% of time

Erkinjuntti criteria for vascular dementia (NINDS-AIREN in Fortschr Neurol Psychiatrie 1994;62:197):

1. Focal neurologic signs + imaging findings: multiple lacunae (multiple motor and sensory deficits, rigidity, extrapyramidal signs, pseudobulbar palsy), extensive white matter lesions, multiple large-vessel infarcts strategically placed (angular gyrus, thalamus, basal forebrain, bilateral infarcts, left hemisphere infarcts)
2. Neurologic deficit and confusion occur within 3 mo of each other
3. Stepwise progression: unknown dx utility of a hx of "stepwise progression," eg, episodic behavioral complications of Alzheimer, eg, UTI may cause deterioration in behavior (Am J Psychiatry 1990;147:435)

Crs: Mortality from vascular dementia is higher; as more older people have strokes and survive, prevalence will increase

Xray: CT: lacunar infarcts 50% of time w MID; MRI: Binswanger: confluent deep white matter hyperintensities, periventricular white matter lesions (in nl aging too); central atrophy, 3rd ventricle enlargement marker for vascular dementia (Neurol 1995;45:1456)

Rx:

Preventive: Prevent and postpone atheromatosis and embolization through dietary changes and smoking cessation, aspirin, unknown effectiveness pentoxifylline; ticlopidine; HT control may actually reverse cognitive impairment by treating preexisting HT (J Am Geriatr Soc 1996;44:411); β-blockers better than calcium channel blockers and diuretics resulting in better MMSE score and improved white matter findings on MRI (J Am Geriatr Soc 1997;45:1423); DM, afib management (Nejm 1993;328:153), anticoagulants;

metabolic enhancing agents have not produced consistent benefits; Galantamine

5.6 SCHIZOPHRENIA (PARAPHRENIA)

Nurs Home Med 1995;3:248; Schizophr Bull 1993;19:701,817; J Am Geriatr Soc 1980;8:193

Cause: Sensory impairment debatable

Epidem: 0.1% in pts >65 yr; 2–12% of NH pts carry the diagnosis of new-onset schizophrenia; two-thirds of early-onset schizophrenic pts are left w mild symptoms by old age; M/F = 1:10 in elderly

Pathophys: Dorsal lateral prefrontal cortex, superior temporal gyrus, hippocampus, basal ganglia

Sx: Pos or neg sx lasting for more than 6 mo; pos: delusions, hallucinations, distorted language and communication patterns, disorganized or catatonic behavior; neg: restriction in range and intensity of emotional expression, changes in fluency and productivity of thought and speech, changes in initiative; 5 categories: paranoid, disorganized, catatonic, undifferentiated, residual type; associated with schizoid premorbid personality, few surviving children, deafness, low socioeconomic class, female

Si: Difficulty focusing attention, formulating concepts, slowing in reaction time; cognitive impairments in memory and construction typical of Alzheimer dementia not usual w paraphrenia

Crs: Paranoid delusions w or w/o hallucinations, usually with preservation of personality and affective response

Cmplc: R/o dementia, intracranial masses, thyroid disease, infections, liver disease, substance abuse, NPH, delirium, mania, depression

Xray: CT, MRI: ventricular enlargement, cortical prominence, decreased temporal and hippocampal size, increased basal ganglia size; 5–10% have lesions due to stroke

Rx:

Therapeutic: Responsiveness to neuroleptics may be more favorable than in younger schizophrenics, risperidone 0.25–2 mg bid

Team Management: Nursing Home: Make sure to obtain psychiatric records (should be a requirement for admission); identify neuroleptics taken within 2–4 wk; refer to Alzheimer management

PSYCHIATRY

6 Infection

6.1 LUNG

PNEUMONIA

Cause: Community acquired: often more than one pathogen; streptococcal pneumonia still most common; TB in pts >60 yr old often with co-pathogens: *Streptococcus pneumoniae, Staphylococcus aureus, Haemophilus influenzae*, aerobic gram-neg bacilli, aerobes and anaerobes (aspiration), *Moraxella catarrhalis, Legionella pneumophila*

NH-acquired organisms of aspiration: *S. pneumoniae, Klebsiella pneumoniae, S. aureus, H. influenzae, Escherichia coli, M. catarrhalis, Mycobacterium tuberculosis; Chlamydia pneumoniae* cause of rapid spread of respiratory infection (Jama 1997; 277:1214)

Hospital-acquired infection: aerobic gram-neg including *Pseudomonas aeruginosa, S. pneumonia, S. aureus, H. influenzae, Legionella* (Am Rev Respir Dis 1993;148:14118); *S. aureus* and *S. pneumoniae* most common co-pathogens with influenza

Epidem: Pneumonia is the leading cause of death from infectious disease in the elderly (Geriatrics 1991;46:25); 11% pneumonia cases, but 85% pneumonia deaths in pts >65 yr old (Mmwr 1991;40:7); age alone doubles risk of complications and death; risk increases w each additional comorbid factor, especially CHF, COPD (Ann IM 1991;115:428; Am J Med 1990;88:1N)

Pathophys: Age-related changes: decreased immunity, decreased cough and gag reflexes, decreased ciliary activity, increased colonization with resistant gram-neg organisms; comorbid diseases (stroke, etc.) affect ability to swallow and increase risk of aspiration pneumonia; 25% of all clinically septic pts (not just from pneumonia) are afebrile due to modified IL-1 response, hypothalamic alterations

Sx: Shaking chill, fever, cough; decreased function (including cognition), falls, anorexia, 10% no symptoms; <35% typical presentation (J Am Geriatr Soc 1989;37:867); 50% of febrile geriatric pts presenting to ER w no other physical signs have serious illness including pneumonia

Si: Rhonchi, rales, tachypnea; confusion (33% in community-acquired pneumonia vs 53% in NH) (J Am Geriatr Soc 1986;34:697), tachypnea, dehydration, decreased function, anorexia, worsening of preexisting CHF or COPD

Crs: Dx may be delayed with "atypical presentation"; this and comorbidity may contribute to longer course of illness, longer hospitalization in the elderly

Cmplc: Delayed resolution, bacteremia (40% mortality), death, mixed infections; r/o other infections, COPD, pulmonary embolus (PE), malignancy, drug reactions, myelodysplastic syndrome

Lab:

- CBC—important to compare w WBC baseline but be aware 20–40% of all septic pts do not develop leukocytosis (Ger Rev Syllabus 1996:264)
- Electrolytes
- Oxygen saturation (use early and often in NH) to assess severity; if requiring hospital admission, then consider ABGs, blood culture, sputum Gram stain and culture (often impossible to obtain adequate sample; <50% can produce dx specimen) (Am J Med 1990;88(5N):1N; J Am Geriatr Soc 1989;37:867)
- EKG

Xray: Chest film with infiltrate, though may not be obvious in setting of chronic lung changes

Rx: See Table 6-1; about 66% will require hospitalization; may be able to avoid hospital with risks of delirium, depression, and nosocomial infection if there is adequate NH or home care and the pt is hemodynamically stable; in some cases, the elderly and their families elect to have no hospital care; consult advance directives for rx guidance; antibiotics, initially empiric broad-spectrum and then treat appropriate organism if becomes known; oxygen if indicated by decreased oxygen saturation or by clinical respiratory distress

Preventive: Influenza vaccine annually; pneumonia vaccine q 6 yr

Therapeutic: Oral outpatient or NH regimens include erythromycin, azithromycin, clarithromycin, amoxicillin–clavulanic acid, TMP/SMZ,

Table 6-1. Treatment Guidelines for Pneumonia

Treatment in the Nursing Home	**Treatment in the Hospital**

Treatment in the Nursing Home

1. *Route (PO or IM) of Initial Therapy*: Treatment with a parenteral (im) agent should be considered if:
   a. there is no response to an oral agent
   b. vital signs are abnormal
   c. resident has an acutely altered mental status and is unable to take oral medications (tube feeding not avaliable)
2. *Choice of Parenteral Agent*: Ceftriaxone 500–1000 mg IM qd or Cefotaxime 500 mg im q 12 h
   In the penicillin allergic patient the type of hypersensitivity (rash, hives) should be considered in making a treatment decision.
3. *Timing of Switch to an Oral Agent*: Residents given im treatment should be switched to an oral agent when they achieve clinical stability. In most (75%) residents this will occur on day 3–5 of treatment. Clinical stability is defined as all of the following being present:
   a. improvement in signs and symptoms
   b. afebrile (<100.5°F) for ≥16 hours
   c. no acute cardiac or other life-threatening event in the first 3 days of treatment
   d. resident is able to take oral medication
4. *Oral Antibiotic Regimens*:
   Amoxicillin
   Amoxicillin/clavulanate
   2nd or 3rd generation oral cephalosporin
   In the penicillin allergic patient, Levofloxacin 500 mg po qd can be prescribed.
5. *Duration of Therapy*: 7–10 days

Treatment in the Hospital

1. *Choice of Empiric Therapy*:
   Ceftriaxone 500–1000 mg IV qd
   Cefotaxime 500 mg IV q 8–12 h
   Ampicillin/sulbactam 1.5 gm IV q 6–8 h
   Cefuroxime 750 mg IV q 8 h
   In the penicillin allergic patient the type of hypersensitivity (rash, hives) should be considered in making a treatment decision. An alternative to consider is Levofloxacin 500 mg IV qd
   IV erythromycin should be avoided because of the adverse effects such as pain and phlebitis and increasing resistance of pneumococci to macrolides.
2. *Timing of Switch to an Oral Agent*: When the resident achieves clinical stability (day 4–6), switch to an oral agent:
   Amoxicillin
   Amoxicillin/clavulanate
   2nd or 3rd generation oral cephalosporin
   In the penicillin allergic pts one of the following agents can be used:
   Levofloxacin 500 mg po qd
   Erythromycin
3. *Duration of Therapy*: 7–14 days

BSJ Naughton BJ, Mylotte JM. Treatment guideline for nursing home-acquired pneumonia based on community practice. J Am Geriatr Soc 2000;48:82–88. Reprinted by permission of Blackwell Science, Inc.

or a 2nd- or 3rd-generation cephalosporin or TMP/SMZ (up to 24% *S. pneumoniae* resistance)

If pt hypoxic, serious underlying illness, or lives alone, cover *S. aureus* and gram-neg bacilli w IV ceftriaxone or im in NH pts w no IV access, along with oral or IV erythromycin or azithromycin for initial broad coverage; clindamycin is used when suspicion of anaerobic organisms is high

Hospital-acquired infection: IV β-lactam-β-lactamase inhibitor combination, or 3rd-generation cephalosporin and clindamycin or piperacillin

S. pneumoniae sens: 100—vancomycin; 99.2—ceftriaxone, doxycycline, levofloxacin; 99—imipenem; 98.8—erythromycin; 97.2—ofloxacin; 96.2—ciprofloxacin; 95—cefuroxime; by 1994 increasing resistance developed including against penicillin (14%), ceftazidime (12%), and TMP/SMZ (24%) (Jama 1996;275:194; Nejm 1996;335:1445); if *Pseudomonas* endemic in NH use ceftazidime, if not ceftriaxone (Ann LT Care 1998;6(suppl E):7)

Team Management: Caregiver awareness of baseline to recognize changes; community and institutional efforts to provide appropriate vaccinations and chemoprophylaxis for influenza and pneumonia; use acute crisis to focus future advance directive discussions, particularly w NH pts

INFLUENZA

Cause: Influenza virus, types A, B, C

Epidem: Worldwide, 90% of deaths associated with influenza are among those >65 yr old

Pathophys: RNA single-stranded viruses spread by respiratory droplets

Sx: Cough, fever, malaise, sore throat, aches

Si: Cough; geriatric: exacerbation of cardiopulmonary or chronic illness, changes in behavior/cognition

Crs: Incubation time only 1–2 d, symptoms usually last 5–6 d, malaise up to 2 wk

Cmplc: Primary influenza pneumonia, secondary bacterial pneumonia and exacerbation of cardiopulmonary and other chronic illnesses result in increased hospitalization and death

Lab: Serology on first few cases to establish the type and strain of an outbreak; QuickVue (immunoassay that uses monoclonal antibodies to detect viral nucleoprotein) easiest and fastest test for rapid diagnosis of influenza A and B; however, negative tests do not exclude influenza (Med Let 1999;41:121)

Xray: Chest film if secondary pneumonia suspected (threshold should be low to xray)

Rx:

Preventive: Influenza vaccine annually for those >65 and/or working, or living in institutional settings, or in elderly community (Ann IM 1995;123:518); each trivalent influenza vaccine usually includes two inactivated A strains and one B strain chosen each year based on strains from the previous season; new vaccine combination is required each yr because of ongoing change (antigenic drift)

Pneumococcal vaccine should be given every 6 yr to those >65 yr old and should decrease incidence of secondary bacterial pneumonia; may give pneumococcal vaccine at the same time as influenza vaccine without problems

Flu vaccine better at preventing death due to influenza than infection; in NHs, influenza vaccination prevents an estimated 50–60% of hospitalizations and pneumonia and 80% of deaths; influenza vaccine can decrease the hepatic metabolism of drugs including theophylline and warfarin by 50% for up to 1 wk; for those with contraindications to influenza vaccine (allergy to eggs or other vaccine components) use amantadine or rimantadine prophylactically during peak influenza season

Start amantadine or rimantadine at first indication of influenza A outbreak in NH, for at least a 2-wk course or until 1 wk after the outbreak is over; this prophylaxis decreases the infection rate of influenza A by 70–80%

Therapeutic: Approach to fever in NH: fever >100°F (37.7°C) for all infections including influenza (J Am Geriatr Soc 1996;44:74); antiviral-resistant strains have emerged and can be shed as soon as the end of one rx course; dosages for those >65 are the same for prophylaxis and rx:

• Amantadine 100 mg po qd for those with Cr clearance >50; adjust as per package insert for Cr clearance <50

- Rimantadine 200 mg po qd, 100 mg po qd for Cr clearance <10 or liver disease; observe carefully and decrease dose if CNS side effects noted; may increase seizure activity
- Neuroaminidase inhibitors: inhaled zanamivir (Jama 1999;282:31) or oral oseltamivir started within 30 hours after onset of influenza can shorten duration of sx and possibly decrease incidence of complications, but zanamivir associated with bronchospasm in pts with underlying lung disease (Jama 2000;284:2847); neither a substitute for vaccination (Med Let 1999;41:91)

PULMONARY TUBERCULOSIS

Am Fam Phys 2000;61:2673; MacLennan WJ, Watt B, Elder AT. Infections in elderly patients. London/Boston: E. Arnold/Little, Brown, 1994

Cause: Reactivation, cross-infection in NH

Epidem: 8% conversion rate in 2.5 yr in NH (Nejm 1985;312:1483); more at risk for reactivation w DM, alcoholism, smoking, cancer, partial gastrectomy, corticosteroids

Pathophys: Inhaled droplets deposited in alveoli, replicate slowly, spread to regional lymph nodes, then hematogenous spread; may have bronchopneumonia w initial infection but more often pts develop asx nodule (Ghon complex); TB reactivation occurs at sites w high oxygen concentration (upper lobes) because TB is an obligate aerobe, but middle and lower lobes can be involved in NH pts

Sx: May not have fever or night sweats; weight loss, cough, shortness of breath more common; extrapulmonary sx include mental status changes, back, abdominal pain

Si: Pleural effusion

Crs: ARDS if miliary spread occurs; segmental atelectasis upper lobe; involvement of lingula or middle lobe can be mistaken for tumor

Complc: 10% of primary infections may progress to chronic TB or death (ascribed to antibiotic-unresponsive pneumonia); dissemination bone marrow, liver, GU tract, bone (spine = Pott's disease)

Lab: PPD is negative in active TB 10–15%; polymorphonuclear leukocytosis, normocytic anemia, elevated ESR; examine 3 sputum samples for AFB, may take up to 12 wk to grow on culture medium (may be inhibited by ciprofloxacin, gentamicin, and amoxicillin-clavulanate [Augmentin]); ribosomal DNA/RNA in sputum if have clinical suspicion w negative AFB; pleural effusions may not reveal organisms

Xray: Delayed resolution of supposed bacterial infiltrate; classic findings of apical cavitary lesions less common; opacities of middle and upper lobes in isolation or w apical lesions more common; cavitation less common because of decreased cellular immunity

Rx:

Preventive: For screening, see 2.3 Infection Control, Tuberculosis

Therapeutic: Treat NH residents w INH (300 mg/d) and rifampin (600 mg/d) for 9 mo because no multidrug resistance; drug therapy (INH + rifampin + pyrazinamide) reduces rx duration from 9 to 6 mo; first 2 mo:

- INH (300 mg): 5% develop hepatitis; 100 mg pyridoxine to avoid peripheral neuropathy; multiple drug interactions; do not give Tylenol concurrently
- Rifampin (450 mg if pt <50 kg, or 600 if pt >50 kg): 3% hepatitis; 8% hepatitis when taken in combination w INH; skin rash, GI sx; thrombocytopenia (uncommon); optic neuritis; induces hepatic microenzymes
- Ethambutol (15 mg/kg): modify dosage in renal impairment to avoid retrobulbar neuritis (reduced visual acuity, scotomata, red/green color blindness); good synergistic action w rifampin against resistant mycobacteria
- Pyrazinamide (1.5 gm if pt <50 kg, or 2 gm if pt >50 kg): 2–6% hepatitis (dose-related), arthralgia, anorexia, nausea, photosensitivity, gout
- Streptomycin: high toxicity (vestibular, renal)
- Treat in hospital until smear is neg
- New therapies being developed: compounds that can inactivate enzyme isocitrate lyase, critical in protecting *M. tuberculosis* against macrophage attack (Nature 2000;289:1123; 2000;406:683)

6.2 HEART

ENDOCARDITIS

Jama 1995;274:1706

Cause: Etiology of septicemia found in <50% of pts; prosthetic valves; pacemakers; *S. aureus* can cause dz in a preexisting healthy valve

Epidem: More than one-half of pts w endocarditis are elderly because they have more prosthetic valves, hospital-acquired bacteremia, rheumatic valvular lesions

Pathophys: Alteration in endothelial surface, deposition platelets and fibrin, vegetation where there is increased turbulence; *Streptococcus* 25–70%, *Streptococcus bovis* 25% (associated w GI malignancy, especially colon cancer), *Staphylococcus* 20–30%, *Enterococcus* from GU 25%, *Streptococcus viridans* less common than in younger pts; culture neg 10–20%

Sx: Aortic and mitral valve regurgitation most common, heart failure, systemic embolism, cerebral embolism (25% of time presenting as acute confusional state)

Si: Suspect in pts w pyrexia, high ESR, CHF, peripheral emboli, vaguely unwell after recent GI or GU procedure, changing cardiac murmur; still suspect w pos blood cultures despite no heart murmur; may see splenomegaly w *S. viridans*; Janeway lesions on palms and soles and Roth spots on fundi indicative of emboli; immune complexes produce Osler nodes, arthralgias, finger clubbing, petechiae, glomerulonephritis, hematuria

Crs: 50% mortality

Cmplc: R/o myocardial abscess if ESR does not normalize w rx, or w LBBB, or progressive lengthening of PR interval

Lab: 3 blood cultures separated in time establish cause in 95% of pts; *S. viridans* (30–45%), associated w dental procedure, not all penicillin-sens; *Staphylococcus* (10–30%) coagulase-neg associated w prosthetic valves, better prognosis than with *S. aureus*; other streptococci (10–15%) include enterococci (*S. bovis*)

Associated w colon cancer and diverticulosis, GU manipulation in men, varying resistance

ESR >100 mm/h, elevated C-reactive protein, 50% positive rheumatoid factor and positive ANA, normochromic normocytic anemia, elevated WBC

Induced:

Noninvasive: Echocardiography (transthoracic and transesophageal): vegetations on prosthetic valves, septal or annular abscess; two-dimensional echocardiography allows evaluation of chamber size and serial evaluations can be done if worsening valve dysfunction; if neg and still suspect clinically, recheck echocardiogram

Rx:

Preventive: For pts w cardiac disorders: highest risk w prosthetic valves, previous infective endocarditis, aortic regurgitation, aortic stenosis, mitral stenosis and regurgitation, s/p intracardiac surgery w residual hemodynamic abnormality (Med Let 1999;41:75; Nejm 1995;332:38)

For procedures involving mouth or respiratory tract: amoxicillin 2–3 gm po 1 h before procedure (Jama 1997;277:1794)

Manipulation of GU or GI tract (*Enterococcus*): 1 gm ampicillin and 1.5 mg/kg (not to exceed 120 mg) gentamicin IV 1 h before procedure and 6 h later (Jama 1997;277:1794); ampicillin l gm im/IV or amoxicillin 1 gm po; if penicillin-allergic, substitute 1 gm vancomycin

Prevent hospital-acquired infection

Prosthetic valves (*Staphylococcus*): use regimen for *Enterococcus*

Therapeutic: See Table 6-2; require doses that reach bactericidal concentrations; EKG to follow clinical course; surgery may be needed if worsening CHF, embolism, cardiac abscess, vegetations >10 mm or fungal infection; valve replacement delayed until residual infection of valve annulus, adjacent structures reduced; anticoagulation not much help

Table 6-2. Medical Treatment for Endocarditis

Infectious Agent	Drug	Dosage	Duration
PCN-susceptible *Streptococcus viridans* or other strep. (MIC <=0.1 µG/mL)	PCN G aqueous (preferred in the elderly) OR	12–18 million U IV/24 h continuously or divided q 4 h	4 weeks
	Ceftriaxone	2 g/day IV or im	4 weeks
PCN allergic	Vancomycin	30 mg/kg per 24 h IV in 2 doses (do not exceed 2 gm/24 h)	4 weeks
S. viridans, other strep. (MIC >=0.1)	PCN G aqueous PLUS	18–30 million U IV/24 h continuously or divided q 4 h	4 weeks
	Gentamicin* (use w/ caution in elderly)	1 mg/kg im or IV q 8 h	2 weeks
β-lactam allergy	Vancomycin	30 mg/kg per 24 h IV in 2 doses (do not exceed 2 gm/24 h)	4 weeks
Enterococci Screen all enterococci endocarditis for antibiotic resistance	PCN G aqueous PLUS	18–30 million U IV/24 h continuously or divided q 4 h	4–6 weeks
	Gentamicin OR	1 mg/kg im or IV q 8 h	4–6 weeks
	Ampicillin PLUS	12 gm IV/24 h continuously or divided q 4 h	4–6 weeks
	Gentamicin	as above	
β-lactam allergy	Vancomycin PLUS Gentamicin	as above as above	4–6 weeks 4–6 weeks
Staphylococci, no prosthetic material	Nafcillin or oxacillin PLUS (optional)	2 gm IV q 4 h	4–6 weeks
	Gentamicin	1 mg/kg im or IV q 8 h	3–5 days
PCN allergy	Vancomycin	30 mg/kg per 24 h IV in 2 doses (do not exceed 2 gm/24 h)	4–6 weeks
MRSA	Vancomycin	as above	4–6 weeks

Table 6-2. (*cont'd*)

Infectious Agent	Drug	Dosage	Duration
Staphylococci, with prosthetic material	Nafcillin or oxacillin PLUS	2 gm IV q 4 h	6–8 weeks
(Prosthetic material may need to be removed or replaced)	Rifampin PLUS	300 mg po q 8 h	6–8 weeks
	Gentamicin	1 mg/kg im or IV q 8 h	2 weeks
MRSA	Vancomycin PLUS	30 mg/kg per 24 h IV in 2 doses (do not exceed 2 gm/24 h)	6–8 weeks
	Rifampin PLUS	300 mg po q 8 h	6–8 weeks
	Gentamicin	1 mg/kg im or IV q 8 h	2 weeks
HACEK microbes	Ceftriaxone	2 gm IV or im/day	4 weeks

* Age over 65 is a relative contraindication for use of gentamicin.
Sources: Jama 1995;274:1706; Sci Am Med 1999;7:XVIII.

6.3 BONES AND JOINTS

OSTEOMYELITIS/SEPTIC ARTHRITIS/ JOINT PROSTHESIS INFECTION

Nejm 1997;336:999; MacLennan WJ, Watt B, Elder AT. Infections in elderly patients. London/Boston: E. Arnold/Little, Brown, 1994

Cause:
- Septic arthritis: chronic septic arthritis most often caused by *Staphylococcus*
- Joint prosthesis infection: *Staphylococcus*, gram-neg, anaerobes

Epidem:
- Septic arthritis: 25–33% in pts >60 yr old; impaired immune system; preexisting joint disease, eg, osteoarthritis and rheumatoid arthritis; *Staphylococcus*, *Streptococcus*, gram-neg bacteria; hematogenous spread from UTI, cellulitis, endocarditis, *Salmonella* bowel infections; predisposing factors: malnutrition, diabetes, chronic renal failure, hepatic cirrhosis, malignancy, alcoholism, corticosteroids

- Joint prosthesis infection: 1–2%, hematogenous spread from surgery; sources: gums, GI tract, GU tract

Sx:
- Septic arthritis: tenderness, redness, warmth; diabetics may not have pain or pyrexia; may only see uncontrolled blood glucose; normocytic normochromic anemia
- Chronic septic arthritis: may not have pyrexia or tachycardia

Si: Osteomyelitis, foot: metatarsal heads, proximal phalanges; close to ulcer discharging pus from a sinus; erythema and swelling over infected bone; fluctuant swelling; painful limitation of active and passive movement; usually febrile; difficult to dx w preexisting joint disease; masked in sternoclavicular, sacroiliac, hips and shoulder joints

Cmplc: Septic arthritis: osteomyelitis in adjacent bones, avascular necrosis, septicemia, high mortality; chronic septic arthritis: bacteremia common, giving rise to endocarditis, cholecystitis, cerebral abscess (mortality approaching 50%)

Lab: Osteomyelitis: blood cultures pos in 50% pts; culture discharging sinuses w sterile syringe; bone bx; elevated WBC, high ESR may not be present in the elderly

Septic arthritis: only 50% elderly have elevated WBC; ESR usually elevated; large-bore needle w heparin to prevent clotting for joint tap: WBC = 100,000, 90% polymorphonuclear leukocytes, elevated lactate, culture pos in 66% pts

Xray: Osteomyelitis: initial phases show soft tissue swelling over the diaphysis indistinguishable from changes w cellulitis; 2 wk after onset: translucency of the cortex of the diaphysis, radiopaque new bone formation under an elevated periosteum; sclerosis anytime after 3 wk

In elderly pts periosteum more likely to be adherent to cortex, so infection does not separate the bone layers; gallium scan to define areas of chronic or subacute infection; CT and MRI to distinguish osteomyelitis from soft tissue infection; MRI less useful in infections related to surgical hardware

Osteoporosis may mask areas of lysis; 95% MRI pos in vertebral osteomyelitis

- Septic arthritis: radionucleotide scan for less accessible joints: hips, sacroiliacs

- Joint prosthesis infection: translucency of surrounding bone; technecium and gallium scans helpful in late infection; US in detection of abscess

Rx:

Therapeutic:

- Osteomyelitis: ≥3 wk antibiotics to prevent progression to chronic osteomyelitis; oral therapy should be started 24 h before cessation of IV antibiotics
- Chronic osteomyelitis: treat for several months; methicillin-resistant *S. aureus* may respond to clindamycin, erythromycin, rifampin, but vancomycin may be required; gram-neg, eg, pseudomonas: quinolones (especially chronic); anaerobic osteomyelitis: metronidazole; osteomyelitis difficult to treat in areas w trauma or vascular insufficiency: often requires surgical intervention
- Septic arthritis: IV antibiotics for at least 6 wk; intra-articular injections of no benefit; benzylpenicillin and aminoglycoside do not achieve adequate levels in joints; surgical debridement and exploration may be needed, especially w hip involvement
- Joint prosthesis infection: early: 3 wk antibiotics may avoid losing the prosthesis; late: remove prosthesis, pack w antibiotic-impregnated cement and begin parenteral antibiotics 6 wk; persistent in 60% pts, may require joint fusion and new prosthesis

Preventive:

- Joint prosthesis infection: 24 h before surgery use prophylactic antibiotics (J Bone Joint Surg Am 1990;72:1); treat mouth, alimentary and GU (including asx UTI) infections before surgery

6.4 CENTRAL NERVOUS SYSTEM

MENINGITIS

See Table 6-3; symptoms of meningitis in elderly: confusion 57–96%, HA 21–81%; other symptoms include nausea, vomiting, seizures, weakness, and photophobia; fever is inconsistent, and pts can have hypothermia; nuchal rigidity is neither sens nor specif, is pos in only 57% cases and can be false-pos in pts with cervical spondylosis and Parkinson disease; CSF studies are necessary for a definitive diagnosis

Table 6-3. Meningitis

Organism	Epidem	Si/sx	Crs/Cmplc	Labs	Rx	Alternate Rx	Prophylaxis
Bacterial Unknown Ethiology	—	—	—	Increased PMNs, glucose >45 mg/dL, protein <45 mg/dL	Ampicillin + cefotaxime/ ceftriaxone	Add vancomycin if resistant pneumococcus suspected	—
Pneumococcus	17% cases bact. meningitis Mortality 19–26% Inc. mortality risks: basilar skull fracture, spleenectomy, DM, liver disease, ETOH, HIV	Pts often have concomitant/ preceding pneumonia, otitis, mastoiditis, sinusitis, or endocarditis Rapid coma, convulsions	Subdural empyema, cerebral vein thrombosis, middle cerebral arteritis causing hemiparesis; permanent memory deficit, NPH	See above	Pending sensitivities: vancomycin + 3 rd gen. cephalosporin MIC <0.1 Pen G or ampicillin MIC = 0.1–1.0 Ceftazidime or ceftriaxone MIC >= 2.0 Vancomycin + ceftazidime/ ceftriaxone	Ceftazidime or ceftriaxone Meropenem, vancomycin Meropenem, subs rifampin for vancomycin	Pneumovac- recommended age >65
Meningococcus	5% cases bact. meningitis peaks late winter/early spring Mortality 3–13% Inc. mortality risk: age >60, focal neuro. signs at admission, hemorrhagic diathesis	Septicemia, acute confusional state, agitation, aggression	Deafness often permanent, transient paralysis of 6th and 7th CN	See above	Pen G or ampicillin	Ceftriaxone or cefotaxime	Close contacts: rifampin within 24 h, alt. Ciprofloxacin single 500 mg oral dose

Table 6-3. Meningitis

Organism	Epidem	Si/sx	Crs/Cmplc	Labs	Rx	Alternate Rx	Prophylaxis
Listeria	0% cases bacterial meningitis Mortality 15–30% Inc. mortality risk: immunosuppression, renal failure, malignancy, organ transplant, older age	1° food borne transmission Rarely have meningeal signs	Seizures, CN abnormalities, focal neurological symptoms	See above Rarely + Gram stain	Ampicillin + Gentamicin	TMP-Sulfa	High-risk patients: avoid soft cheeses: Mexican style, feta, Brie. Reheated foods should be steaming hot
Aerobic gram-negative	11–25% cases of bacterial meningitis Mortality 35% nosocomial infections; 6–22% community acquired	Hematogenous spread from urosepsis, head trauma, or neurosurgical procedures	—	See above	Cefotaxime or ceftriaxone *Pseudomonas*: add tobramycin or gentamicin *Influenzae*: ceftriaxone	Ciprofloxacin	—
Staphylococci	4–11% cases bacterial meningitis Mortality 14–77%	Sequela to infection elsewhere, post-neurosurgical procedure, posttrauma, CSF shunt	—	—	Methicillin sensitive: Nafcillin +/- rifampin MRSA: vancomycin +/- rifampin	Vancomycin	—
Cryptococcus neoformans	4% meningitis Rarely life threatening	Usually immuno-compromised If present, HIV testing recommended	—	40–400 WBC per mm >50 lymphs, protein 40–150, normal glucose India ink stain, culture for definitive dx	Amphotericin B +/- flucytosine Prolonged rx with multiple agents often necessary	Miconazole, fluconazole	—

Viral meningoen-cephalitis HSV type 1	—	Primary or reactivation infection: headache, fever, neck stiffness; personality change; dysphagia; impaired temperature regulation, abnormal bladder function, postural hypotension	Stroke syndrome—ipsilateral middle cerebral artery to ophthalmic involvement	—	CSF: lymphocytosis up to 1000/μL, RBCs, nl glucose, protein mildly elevated; acute; convalescent titers; temporal lobe abnormalities on EEG, CT, MRI after 6 d obtundation, neurologic deficit	—	—
HIV	5–10% of HIV infected have an acute meningoencephal itis with initial infection						

Sources: Goldman 2000:1645; Geriatrics 1997:52:43; Neuro Clin 1999;17:711; Phys Postgrad Med 1993;93:153; Nejm 1997;336:708; Phys Postgrad Med 1998;103:102; Rosen 1998:2208; Mandell 2000:906; Rakel 2000;103.

6.5 SKIN

Young EM Jr, Newcomer VD, Kligman AM. Geriatric dermatology: color atlas and practitioner's guide. Philadelphia: Lea & Febiger, 1993.

Cause: Thinning epidermis, decreased sebaceous gland secretion compromises barrier between sc tissue and external environment; less effective T-cell immunity

Pathophys, sx, si, crs, lab, rx: See Table 6-4

6.6 GASTROINTESTINAL TRACT

See Table 6-5

6.7 EYE

CONJUNCTIVITIS

See Table 6-6

6.8 HUMAN IMMUNODEFICIENCY VIRUS INFECTION

J Gerontol Nurs 1999;25:25; J Am Geriatr Soc 1995;43:7; Arch IM 1995;155:184; J Comm Health 1995;20:383; Nurs Home Med 1995;3:265; Arch IM 1994;154:57; Geriatrics 1993;48:61; J Acquir Immun Defic Syndr 1991;4:84

Epidem: 10% of pts w AIDS are >50 yr old (J Acquir Immun Defic Syndr 1991;4:84); risk factors: homosexual sex, 49%; IV drug abuse, 17%; heterosexual sex, 11%; transfusion/hemophilia, 7%; other,

Table 6-4. Skin Infections

Disease	Pathophys/Sx/Si/Crs/Lab	Rx
Bacterial		
Cellulitis	Red, tender, warm, swollen, fever, elevated wbc, ESR; distinguish from DVT; often *S. aureus* or *S. pyogenes*	Amoxicillin or amoxicillin-clavulanate potassium to cover group A streptococci, *S. aureus*; metronidazole for anaerobes; warm compresses, elevation and drainage of fluctuant areas help expedite healing
Erysipelas	Variant of cellulitis w well-demarcated borders, patches of hemorrhage, exudates, and bullous eruption on leg. β-hemolytic strep, *S. aureus*; recur in 2–4 yr; higher risk w peripheral edema	Benzylpenicillin 600 mg im bid 2–3 d then po penicillin; dicloxacillin or amoxicillin-clavulanate potassium for *S. aureus*; prevent with good hygiene and correct predisposing factors
Furunculosis	Tender red nodule that develops into pustule, abscess in hair follicle, may recur in areas of excessive sweating, restrictive clothing; diabetes risk factor	Drain, antibiotics for *S. aureus*, occasional anaerobes, shampoo and bath w chlorhexidine; if nasal carrier of staph, use bacitracin or mupirocin
Impetigo	Cutaneous inflammation w honey-colored crusts; *S. aureus* or *S. pyogenes*	Topical tx w mupirocin 2% ointment (Bactroban) tid × 7 d; if topical fails, tx w PCN or anti-staphylococcal agent (dicloxacillin 250 mg qid, e-mycin 250–500 mg qid, cephalexin 250–500 mg qid, clindamycin 150–300 mg qid); recurrent infections tx w mupirocin 2% ointment in calcium base; treat *S. aureus* w dicloxacillin 250 mg qid or topically w mupirocin 2%
Fungal		
Candidiasis	Glazed red skin w satellite lesions; intertriginous; beneath condom catheters, around stomas, fistulas; spread to the fingers by scratching; chronic paronychia w loss of cuticle and brawny swelling	2% miconazole, clotrimazole, ketoconazole or nystatin; nystatin ointment or imidazole cream in nail fold tid; when topical tx fails, ketoconazole, fluconazole, or triaconazole po

Table 6-4. (*cont'd*)

Disease	Pathophys/Sx/Si/Crs/Lab	Rx
Fungal (*cont'd*)		
Onychomycosis	Thickening, irregularity and discoloration of toenails and fingernails; increased incidence assoc w aging secondary to slower growth of nail, increased trauma to nail plate, decreased circulation and changes in sizes and width of foot	Treat selectively; podiatry consult for mechanical improvements and to reduce nail mass; terbinafine po 125 mg bid, resolution in 6 mo, mild GI side effects (Lancet, 1990;1:636), griseofulvin: tx 4–6 mo for fingernails, 10–18 mo for toenails, ketoconazole 200 mg po qd × 4–6 mo for fingernails, × 10–18 mo for toenails; newer agents w shorter course: itraconazole approved by FDA
Tinea	Dermatophytosis—annular red brown patches on scalp, face, extremities; candidiasis—beefy red patches thick white coating; *T. versicolor*—white tan confluent macules on upper trunk; dermatophytid reaction—allergic vesicles on palm or finger after exposure to fungus	*T. pedis, cruris, corporis*: astringent aluminum acetate solution (Domeboro), 1% tolnaftate, clotrimazole, griseofulvin; *capitis, versicolor*: 2.5% selenium sulfide; barbis: fluconazole 2% × 2–3 d
Burns		1% Sulfadiazine-silver (Silvadene); dicloxacillin 250 mg po q 6 h for staph, strep; quinolone for *P. aeruginosa*
Pressure ulcers	Localized areas of tissue necrosis that develops when soft tissue is compressed between bony prominence and external surface for prolonged period of time; most common sites are sacrum, ischial tuberosities, greater trochanters, heels, and lateral malleoli	Prophylactic antibiotics produce resistant organisms; antiseptics, eg, Povidone-iodine, may be helpful; 0.5% acetic acid for wounds infected w *P. aeruginosa*; adjunctive tx includes pressure relieving support, wound debridement; moist dressing

Table 6-4. (*cont'd*)

Disease	Pathophys/Sx/Si/Crs/Lab	Rx
Herpes simplex virus	Small patch of blisters involving skin and mucosa, lip, gums, and hard palate, can present as eczema, can involve eye; herpetic Whitlow (fingers); rarely elsewhere on body	Acyclovir topically; acyclovir oral (400 mg tid × 7–10 d) may help with intermittent use; may try Valtrex 1 gm bid × 10 d; adjunctive tx inc compresses, emollients, antibx for bacterial infection
Zoster	Malaise, paresthesias affecting single root dermatome precede papular rash which becomes vesicular, sometimes hemorrhagic; reactivation of chicken pox virus: duration—many mo; trigeminal nerve distribution, cornea, iris; lesion of tip of nose = risk for ophthalmic involvement; overlapped dermatomes = disseminated; postherpetic neuralgia 50%; unpredictable resolution or persistence; pain can induce disruption of sleep, mood, and work	Rx within 72 h of onset w valacyclovir (1 gm tid × 7 d), famciclovir (750 mg tid × 7 d), or acyclovir (800 mg 5 × a day × 7 d); consider prednisone (60 mg/d) tapered over 21 d if no contraindication to corticosteroids; rx speeds recovery but effective only early in course, does not prevent postherpetic neuralgia; corticosteroids not help post-infective neuralgia; can try amitriptyline (Elavil) 10 mg, carbamazepine (Tegretol), capsaicin topical ointment, or TENS; not contagious once crusted over; extent of contagiousness debated, but caution and covering of active skin lesions advised

Sources: Kost, Straus. Nejm 1996;335:1; Elewski, Roderick. Clin Infect Dis 1996;23:305–13; Mathisen, Clin Infect Dis 1998;27:646–8; Kanj et al, J Am Acad Dermatol 1998;38:517–36; Ko et al, Med Clin N Am 1998;82:5.

16% (J Gerontol Nurs 1999;25:25); 5% of all newly reported cases of HIV infection are >50 yr old (J Midwife Women Hlth 2000;45:176); w rx, increasing prevalence in some cohorts to be expected

Risk Factors: Physicians not considering dx in elderly because pts thought not to be sexually active or assumed to be in monogamous heterosexual relationship; increased age risk factors for progression of disease (J Gerontol Nurs 1998;24:8; Int J Epidemiol 1997;26:1340);

Table 6-5. Gastrointestinal Infections

Disease	Cause	Sx/Si	Crs/Cmplc	Lab	Rx
Oral Parotitis	Xerostomia, anticholinergics, malnutrition, DM	Swollen tender parotid gland, red warm overlying skin; pus expressed from Stenson's duct; patient may not complain of pain because symptoms may be masked by other infections (pneumonia, abdominal abscess)	Cmplc: septicemia, osteomyelitis facial bones, facial nerve palsy, parotid abscess w rupture into pharynx or auditory canal, 10%–50% mortality	Commensal aerobic and anaerobic organisms in the floor of the mouth	IV cefuroxime w metronidazole or amoxiclavulinic acid until organism identified; hydration; discontinue anticholinergics; may need to drain w external excision
Candidiasis	Anemia, agranulocytosis; CRF; alcoholism; deficiency in riboflavin, nicotinic acid, ascorbic acid; DM, poor oral hygiene (dentures); antibiotics; steroids	Red, raw mucous membrane, w or w/o sheets of whitish pseudomembrane patches	—	Yeast budding cells and pseudohyphae on Gram stain	Nystatin pastilles 100,000 units qid or amphotericin lozenges 10 mg qid, or miconazole gel 10 mL qid p meals, retaining near lesion before swallowing; fluconazole 100 mg qd systemic therapy; chronic glossitis: coat dentures w nystatin ointment × 2 wk

Stomatitis	—	Medication side effect: furosemide, HCTZ, β-blockers, cholestyramine, desipramine, doxepine, ACE-inhibitors (J Am Ger Soc 1995;43: 1414)
Dental abscess	—	*Enterococcus* (endocarditis), *S. pyogenes* (glomerulonephritis), actinomycetes (cervicofacial, brain abscess)
Gingivitis	—	*Peptostreptococcus* (lung, brain abscess), gram negative rods (pneumonia, endocarditis) (J Am Ger Soc 1995;43:1414), calcium channel blockers
Peptic ulcer	—	*H. pylori*, atrophic gastritis, NSAIDs (see gastrointestinal diseases)

Table 6-5. (cont'd)

Disease	Cause	Sx/Si	Crs/Cmplc	Lab	Rx
Small-bowel overgrowth	Achlorhydria, jejunal diverticular disease; surgery leading to blind loops, overgrowth of bacteria causes more metabolism of vit B_{12} resulting in B_{12} deficiency	Malabsorption, weight loss, diarrhea	Severe overgrowth can lead to protein-energy deficiency; bacteria synthesize folic acid so may see increase in folic acid levels; bacteroides cause deconjugation of bile salts and reduce solubility and absorption of lipids	Macrocytic anemia, ostomalacia, culture jejunal contents	Broad-spectrum antibiotics including metronidazole; surgical intervention
Diarrhea	*Clostridium difficile* 25% of antibiotic-associated diarrhea (ampicillin, amoxicillin, cephalosporins most common)	Varying causes of loose watery or frequent stools When severe explosive watery w blood and mucus; pyrexia, dehydration, and shock	R/o noninfectious causes (diverticulosis, inflammatory bowel disease, ischemic colitis, bowel cancer, laxative, theophylline derivatives, NSAIDs, sulfa derivatives, iron supplements, levodopa, cimetidine, ranitidine, allopurinol	—	Rx: *C. difficile* w vancomycin 125 mg q 6 h for 10 d, $^1/_3$ recur, rx w metronidazole, single room precautions *Campylobacter* when severe, use erythromycin

Organism / source	Clinical features	Severity	Treatment
Campylobacter from inadequately prepared poultry	Incubation 2–3 d; colicky abdominal pain; diarrhea can be blood-stained	*Salmonella, Shigella:* may be severe (bacteremia, septicemia) in elderly because of heavy inoculum; lower gi not protected by stomach acidity (achlorhydria); *Salmonella choleraesuis* causes endocarditis	*Salmonella:* always rx w antibiotics: ciprofloxacin 500 mg bid ×7 d or 14 d if bacteremic; or 200 iv bid at first w nausea
Salmonella from egg products	Incubation 6–24 h; vomiting, colic-like pain; watery diarrhea w blood or mucus; sometimes severe dehydration		Rx of *dehydration:* oral (Dextrolyte, Glucolyte, Rehidrat) 2–3 Lt; may be difficult in elderly because of impaired thirst and decreased response of renal tubules to ADH; then give 0.9% sodium chloride 3 L/d; avoid D_5 if Na >160 mmol/L
Shigella, fecal oral route direct contact	Incubation 2–4 d, tenesmus; colicky abdominal pain; watery, *bloody* or mucus containing stool; elderly may get bacteremia		
S. aureus, heat-labile enterotoxin eg, cold meats not recooked	Incubation few hours; vomiting; diarrhea; self-limiting		
Norwalk, rotavirus	Vomiting, mild diarrhea 2–7 d self-limited; except rotavirus in NH can cause fatal dehydration		

Table 6-6. Conjunctivitis

	Itching	Tearing	Exudate	Periauricular Adenopathy
Viral	Minimal	+	Minimal (follicle formation) keratoconjunctivitis: subepithelial opacities in epidemics, 3–4 wk	+
Bacterial	Minimal	Moderate	+	Uncommon
Chlamydial	Minimal	Moderate	+	+
Allergic	+	Moderate	Minimal	None

+ = little or few.

pts not perceiving themselves at risk (Oncology 1998;12:749), thus less informed regarding risk status and modes of protection: pts age >50 1/6 as likely to use condoms; 1/5 as likely to get tested as at-risk younger adults; older women becoming infected at greater rate: no risk of pregnancy encourages sexual contact with no protection, atrophy of vaginal wall leads to increased susceptibility to micro tears and hence viral entry; likewise elderly males may have an increased incidence in anal mucosa tears during homosexual intercourse (J Emerg Med 1996;14:19; J Midwife Women Hlth 2000;45:176)

Pathophys: HIV infection leading to progressive decreased immune function and subsequent opportunistic infection often misdiagnosed as other chronic conditions in older adults; more rapid progression due to inability of older persons to replace functional T-cells that are being destroyed (Mech Age Dev 1997;96:137)

Sx/Si:

Early: Viral syndrome; wasting syndrome, candidiasis, HIV encephalopathy occur frequently; elderly often present with opportunistic infections; 5 most common opportunistic infections (J Gerontol Nurs 1999;25:25; J Am Geriatr Soc 1998;46:153):

1. *Pneumocystis carinii* pneumonia (PCP): gradual onset, fever, fatigue, weight loss, persistent dry cough, shortness of breath and dyspnea on exertion; median lifespan 9 mo vs 22 mo for young pts upon diagnosis

2. *Mycobacterium tuberculosis* (TB): fever, bloody sputum with cough, weight loss, night sweats, and fatigue

3. *Mycobacterium avium* complex (MAC): fever, night sweats, weight loss, nausea, and abdominal pain
4. Herpes zoster: fluid-filled blisters, painful rash skin, fever, fatigue
5. Cytomegalovirus (CMV): sx based on site of infection:
   - Retinitis: floaters, decreased visual acuity and peripheral vision, blindness
   - Colitis: loss of appetite, dysphagia, substernal and epigastric pain, weight loss, diarrhea, fever
   - Neuropathy: tingling and pain in hands or feet

Late: AIDS dementia–subcortical type, rapidly progressive; often associated with peripheral neuropathies, myelopathies

Crs: Faster progression in elderly due to delayed diagnosis and more rapid clinical deterioration (J Gerontol Nurs 1999;25:25) w disease-free period being much less than 11 yr (San Francisco cohort) along with more HIV comorbidity (J Midwife Women Hlth 2000;45:176); 37% >80 yr old die within 1 mo of dx vs 12% in younger population (J Emerg Med 1996;14:19)

Cmplc: Specific to opportunistic infection (most common: PCP, TB, MAC, herpes zoster, CMV); AIDS dementia complex: mild abnormal on psychometric tests, inability to perform demanding job tasks, can perform ADLs; progressing to need for cane, eventually paraplegia in end stages; inability to work, upper extremity weakness, progressing to double incontinence, mutism, and vegetative cognitive state in end stages

Lab: Initial w/u as with other age groups; AIDS dementia often associated with elevated protein levels and relative monocytosis in CSF

Xray: Disease-specific (eg, PCP—chest film, serum LDH, ABG)

Rx: Antivirals: nucleoside reverse transcriptase inhibitors, nonnucleoside reverse transcriptase inhibitors, protease inhibitors; for treatment guidelines refer to Department of Health and Human Services recommendations; older adults less likely to respond to treatment; controversy over aggressiveness of antiviral therapy: aggressive treatment because of rapid pt deterioration (Mech Age Dev 1997;96:137) vs therapy at smaller doses due to increased toxicity, increased SE, changes in absorption, distribution, renal clearance, and drug–drug interactions (J Gerontol Nurs 1999;25:25; J Emerg Med 1996;14:19); zidovudine (AZT) used as 2nd-line therapy due to hematological SE: anemia, granulocytopenia (J Gerontol Nurs

1999;25:25); ritonavir potent inhibitor of P450 so re-dose drugs, eg, tricyclics, coumadin, amiodarone

Preventive: Encourage condom use; health hx forms for older people that include risk factors of AIDS (J Gerontol Nurs 1998;24:8)

Team Management: Multidisciplinary; parenting by grandparents as a result of the AIDS epidemic is increasing

7 Hematology/Oncology

7.1 HEMATOLOGY

ANEMIAS

Ger Rev Syllabus 1996:314

Cause: Hypoproliferative is the most common in elderly: Fe deficiency
(blood loss), inflammatory diseases, marrow damage or dysfunction,
erythropoietin deficiency (renal, thyroid, nutritional)

Ineffective erythropoiesis: megaloblastic (vit B_{12}, folate), microcytic
(thalassemia, sideroblastic), normocytic

Hemolytic anemia: immunologic (tumor, drug, collagen vascular,
idiopathic), intrinsic (metabolic, abnormal hgb), extrinsic
(mechanical, lytic substance)

Epidem: >33% outpatients, after age 85 more common in men (44%)
(Mayo Clin Proc 1994;69:730)

Pathophys: Sequential changes in Fe deficiency begin w decrease in
serum ferritin, followed by low serum Fe and increase in TIBC, then
change in rbc indices and decreased hgb

Reduced erythropoietin secretion, decreased BP, and compensatory
increase in heart rate; 80% success w erythropoietin 50 units/kg
$3 \times$ wk (Ann IM 1994;121:181)

Myelodysplastic syndrome where hematopoietic precursors abundant,
but defective maturation and peripheral cells have shorter lifespan;
can develop into CML; caused by alkylating agents, RNA
virus, somatic mutations, radiation, environmental toxins;
20% in pts >65 yrs old and twice as common in men; anemia,
thrombocytopenia, leukopenia presenting w fatigue, exercise
intolerance, purpura, infection; hepatomegaly 5%, splenomegaly
10%, pallor 50%; find increased Fe stores, hemochromatosis,

basophilic stippling, monocytosis in 30%, elevated LDH; 3-yr
mortality, better prognosis if only erythroid dysplasia

Sx: Fatigue, worsening shortness of breath, angina, peripheral edema
related to underlying atherosclerotic heart disease; mental status
changes, dizziness, poor balance, pallor less noticeable; commonly
without sx if slow onset

Si: Fe deficiency causes atrophy of the tongue, buccal mucosa, angular
stomatitis, atrophic gastritis which can lead to achlorhydria and vit
B_{12} deficiency

Megaloblastic: glossitis, mild jaundice, paresthesias and abnormal
position and vibratory senses, dementia, depression, mania

Crs: Megaloblastic stages: first vit B_{12} <300 pg/mL; then hypersegmented
neutrophils; then anemia; neurologic damage and dementia seem to
occur before hypersegmented phase

Lab:

- <11% hgb
- Check stool guaiac
- If reticulocyte count high, consider hemolysis (warm-reactive IgG
  or more commonly cold-reactive IgM)
- Check vit B_{12}, folate if macrocytic, consider methylmalonic acid
  and homocysteine levels to detect subclinical B_{12} (Am J Med
  1994;96:239); previously Schilling test used to identify cause of
  inadequate absorption but high-dose oral vit B_{12} effectively treats
  deficiency regardless of cause (Am Fam Phys 2000;62:1565; Blood
  1998;92:1191)
- Check transferrin saturation if microcytic or normocytic; if
  transferrin nl (>20%), check hgb electrophoresis-fetal and $HgbA_2$
  (thalassemia); if transferrin <20%, check TIBC, ferritin; if TIBC
  <250 gm/dL, ferritin >100 ng/mL, anemia chronic disease, thyroid,
  renal; if TIBC >400 gm/dL, ferritin <20 ng/mL, Fe deficiency
  anemia; if TIBC 250–400 gm/dL, ferritin 20–100 ng/mL, check
  for ringed sideroblasts and Fe stores in marrow (Fig 7-1)
- Anemias may be "mixed" types in elderly (rbc distribution width
  elevated)

Rx:

Preventive: Dietary review routinely

Therapeutic:

- Chronic disease: erythropoietin 50–100 units/kg 3 ×/wk,
  increase dose to 150 units/kg if no response in 2–3 wk
  (Nejm 1997;336:933)

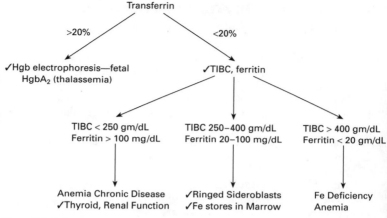

Figure 7-1. Laboratory tests for anemia.

- Fe deficiency: ferrous sulfate 325 mg tid; start w 1 tab/d and build up over 2 wk to avoid constipation; 6 mo needed to replenish Fe stores
- Fe replacement contraindicated in thalassemia because produces Fe overload
- Hemolysis: remove offending drug, eg, L-dopa, penicillin, doxepin, quinidine, thiazides; rx IgG (warm) w prednisone 60 mg/d, danazol, splenectomy, azathioprine, cyclophosphamide; transfusion if unstable; emergency—immunoglobulin 0.4 gm/kg/d × 5 d; rx IgM (cold) w transfusion, plasmapheresis
- Vit B_{12} 1000 μg/d orally until serum B_{12} >300 pg/mL (J Am Geriatr Soc 1998;46:1125; 1997;45:124; Nejm 1996;337:1441; Sci Am 1996;3:14; Jama 1991;265:94) or parenteral 1000 mg/d 1st wk then q mo; folic acid 1 mg/d
- Myelodysplasia: rx w washed rbc, granulocyte transfusion, antibiotics, blood cell products w hydroxyurea to keep WBC down
- Intermittent transfusion may be warranted occasionally, particularly in anemia of chronic disease; if pt otherwise stable, will improve quality of life

CHRONIC LYMPHOCYTIC LEUKEMIA

Ger Rev Syllabus 1996:319; Nejm 1995;333:1032

Cause: No genes have been identified; 50% have cytogenetic abnormalities: trisomy 12, chromosome 13 at band q14

Epidem: Most common form of leukemia in Western countries

Pathophys: Accumulation of neoplastic B lymphocytes in blood, bone marrow, liver, and spleen; monoclonal proliferation (Leukemia 1994;8:1610)

Sx: Fatigue; malaise; decreased exercise tolerance; exacerbation CAD, cardiovascular disease; abdominal pain; early satiety w splenomegaly; >25% asx

Si: Enlarged lymph nodes (cervical, axillary, supraclavicular); splenomegaly; hepatomegaly w disease progression; jaundice secondary to hemolysis or biliary obstruction from enlarged periportal lymph nodes (caloris node); ecchymoses, petechiae in late stages secondary to thrombocytopenia; fever in late stages may be secondary to the development of lymphoma

Crs: 60% diagnosed in asx phase; staging worsens in the following order: lymphocytosis >50,000/µL, lymph node enlargement, splenomegaly, hgb <11 gm/dL, thrombocytopenia (platelet count <10^5/µL); lifespan varies from nl to 5 yr w median survival 9 yr

Cmplc: Hypogammaglobulinemia chief cause of infection (Leuk Lymphoma 1994;13:203)

Lab: Criteria: 95% small mature lymphocytes; bone marrow confirms

Rx:

Therapeutic:

- Treat constitutional symptoms, bulky lymphadenopathy, splenomegaly causing compression, doubling of WBC in under 1 yr: chlorambucil 0.4–0.8 mg/kg body weight po q 2 wk for 8–12 mo yielding response rates of 40–70% vs chlorambucil does not prolong survival (Nejm 1998;338:1506); addition of prednisone no help; combination therapy does not prolong survival (Ann Oncol 1995;6:219) vs fludarabine cyclophosphamide (Med Let 2000;42:83; Ger Rev Syllabus 1999–2001); discontinue treatment when response has been achieved and restart w disease progression
- If no response due to gene mutation, try purine analogue, fludarabine (Blood 1994;84(suppl 1):461A)

- Treat pts w cytopenias w high-dose immunoglobulin, cyclosporine, splenectomy, low-dose radiation of the spleen
- Hypogammaglobulinemia not helped much by vaccines that produce a suboptimal response
- Neutropenia from chemo rx can be treated w hematopoietic growth factors
- International Bone Marrow Transplant registry: probability 3-yr survival = 46% (Bone Marrow Transplant 1995;15(suppl 2):S11)
- Monoclonal antibodies for minimal residual disease (Ann Oncol 1995;6:219)

7.2 ONCOLOGY

MULTIPLE MYELOMA

J Am Geriatr Soc 1994;42:653; Nejm 1997;336:1657

Cause: Proliferation of plasma cells and plasma cell precursors, usually monoclonal IgG or IgA; translocations 14 q 32 and chromosomes 11, 6, 16, 9, 18, 8; point mutations; monoclonal gammopathy representing first oncogenic event leads to multiple myeloma; in 1690 cases over 30-yr period, a second oncogenic event (Nejm 1997;336:1657)

Epidem: Mean age at diagnosis = 69.1 yr; black males highest incidence, 9.6 cases/100,000; increased risk w asbestos exposure, farming, atomic bomb survivors, radium dial workers

Pathophys: First loss of T-cell-mediated control of early B-cell development, then abnormal proliferation of multiple clones, followed by malignant transformation and accumulation of immunoglobulins; clinical manifestations result from tumor growth, accumulation of immunoglobulin chains and cytokines released from malignant plasma cells (bone resorption)

Sx: 60–70% of newly diagnosed pts have bone pain (Eur J Cancer 1991;27:1401); hypercalcemia: anorexia, nausea, vomiting, constipation, weakness, pain, confusion, and lethargy; new onset of DM

Crs: Prognosis for healthy old people same as for healthy young people (Am J Med 1985;79:316) (Table 7-1)

Table 7-1. Durie and Salmon Staging System

Stage	Criteria	Survival

I	All of following:
	  Hgb >10 gm/dL
	  Calcium <12 mg/dL
	  Normal bones or single
	    plasmacytoma
	Low M component
	  a. IgG <5 gm/dL
	  b. IgA <3 gm/dL
	  c. Urinary M-component
	    <4 gm/24 h
		46 mo

II	Neither stage I nor II	32 mo

III	Hgb <8.5 gm/dL
	Calcium >12 mg/dL
	Advanced bone disease
	High M-component
	  a. IgG >7 gm/dL
	  b. IgA >5 gm/dL
	  c. Urinary M-component
	    >12 gm/24 h
		23 mo

Subclassification		
A = serum creatinine <2.0 mg/dL		32 mo
B = serum creatinine >2.0 mg/dL		11 mo

Reproduced by permission from Gautier M, Cohen HJ. Multiple myeloma in the elderly. J Am Geriatr Soc 1994;42:653–64.

Cmplc: Renal failure: up to one-half of pts have renal insufficiency at the time of diagnosis; light chains precipitate in renal tubules, leading to obstruction, dilatation, and subsequent atrophy of the nephron; other mechanisms renal dysfunction: amyloid, infection, hyperuricemia

  Amyloid and hyperviscosity: results from deposition of immuno-globulin light chains in susceptible organs, eg, kidneys, GI tract, myocardium, peripheral nerves; manifestations of hyperviscosity: mucosal bleeding, retinopathy, CHF; sx may be absent in the setting of anemia, so use caution when deciding to transfuse

Hypogammaglobulinemia and infection: major cause of morbidity in multiple myeloma pts, increased risk w encapsulated organisms: *Streptococcus pneumoniae, Haemophilus influenzae, Staphylococcus aureus,* gram-neg rods (Semin Oncol 1986;13:282)

Lab: 10% atypical plasma cells in bone marrow, monoclonal immunoglobulin in serum, light chains in urine; hgb <12 gm/dL: normocytic, normochromic w few reticulocytes; rouleaux formation because of excess monoclonal protein; identify in tissue w Congo red stain

Prognostic tests: β_2-microglobulin <4 µg/mL better prognosis; plasma cell labeling index is a measure of DNA replication and reflects tumor growth (Blood 1988;72:219); IL-6 levels are higher w severe disease (J Clin Invest 1989;84:2008); follow M protein on SPEP, UPEP; proteinuria; follow recurrence w β_2-microglobulin tumor marker

Xray: Multiple osteolytic lesions throughout skeleton, pathologic fx and osteopenia on xray; scans not sens because not enough blastic activity in the lesions; MRI to evaluate cord compression

Rx:

Therapeutic: (Med Clin N Am 1992;76:371) Initial therapy: melphalan and prednisone (MP); little rationale for using interferon as initial therapy (Semin Oncol 1991;18:18); multi-agent chemo rx better for those w a poor prognosis (J Clin Oncol 1992;10:334); maintenance therapy: interferon prolongs remission (Semin Oncol 1991;18:37; Nejm 1990;322:1430); resistant disease: vincristine, doxorubicin, dexamethasone, watch for toxicity (Ann IM 1986;105:8); high-dose therapy not recommended for the elderly; pamidronate for pain, to decrease bone turnover, has antitumor effect (Ann IM 2000;132:734)

Supportive Therapy: Hyperviscosity: plasmapheresis; anemia: erythropoietin (Blood 1996;87:2675; Nejm 1990;322:1693), transfusions; hypercalcemia: bisphosphonates; immunization w Pneumovax recommended but frequently ineffective because of failure to induce antibodies

LUNG CANCER

Am Fam Phys Monograph 1995;191:26

Cause: 85–90% from smoking; 15 yr must elapse after cessation for risk to approach that of nonsmokers; also from radon, nickel, chromium, asbestos

Epidem: Most common cause of death due to cancer; greatest prevalence in the ≤65 yr group (Jama 1987;258:921); increasing incidence in women because of increased smoking in elderly women (Cancer Pract 1995;3:13; Radiol Clin N Am 1994;32:1)

Crs: Elderly have more localized disease at dx than do middle-aged pts; more squamous cell carcinoma and less adenocarcinoma; small-cell lung cancer decreases; thus, elderly have greater chance of resectable and, hence, curable lung cancer (Cancer 1987;60:1331)

90% of pts w recurrent lung cancer have distant metastases; most recurrences within 2 yr of primary lung cancer

Solitary nodule r/o metastasis, carcinoid tumor, granuloma, bronchiogenic cyst; dx of small-cell lung cancer in a nonsmoker should raise the question of misdiagnosis of lymphoma

Lab: Sputum cytology—90% accurate, but not for individual histopathology; fiberoptic bronchoscopy well tolerated by elderly (Chest 1989;95:1043); hgb and hct; pleural effusion: thoracentesis w or w/o pleural biopsy

Xray: Chest film; peripheral lesion needle bx or resection

CT: enlarged hilar nodes: bronchoscopy; if nodes present, obtain CT, bone scan for metastasis to liver, brain, bone; if mediastinal nodes enlarged, obtain mediastinoscopy to determine resectability

Rx:

Therapeutic: See Table 7-2, Table 7-3

Chemo rx: Non-small-cell: chemo effectiveness dismal, usually use experimental drugs, paclitaxel + cisplatin; small cell: cyclophosphamide, doxorubicin, vincristine, nitrosourea, etoposide, cisplatin (S.E. = n, v, renal) (Ger Rev Syllabus 2001:283)

Team Management: Determine if pt will tolerate surgery: FEV_1 >2.5: will tolerate pneumonectomy; FEV_1 >1.1: will tolerate lobectomy; controversial whether elderly have increased rate of mortality (Jama 1987;258:927; J Thorac Cardiovasc Surg 1983;86:654); function most predictive of postop outcome; poor prognostic signs include advanced disease, weight loss, nonambulatory for

Table 7-2. Non-Small-Cell (Adenocarcinoma, Large-Cell, Squamous Cell) Lung Cancer

Stage	Treatment	Median Survival
Stage I (not involving entire lung, no node involvement or metastases)	Lobectomy	60 mo w small lesion, 27 mo w large lesion
Stage II (ipsilateral peribronchial or hilar lymph node involvement)	Lobectomy or pneumonectomy (right lung particularly high risk in elderly (Clin Sym 1993; 45:20); postop chemotherapy may be helpful (cisplatin-based)	17–20 mo
Stage IIIA (entire lung without involvement of the carina, ipsilateral metastases to mediastinal, and subcarinal lymph nodes)	Surgery plus chemotherapy, and radiotherapy (Nejm 1990;323:940)	8–11 mo
Stage IIIB (invading mediastinum, pleural effusion, contralateral lymph nodes)	—	—
Stage IV (distant metastases)	Radiation for pain, obstruction, hemoptysis	6 mo

Table 7-3. Small-Cell Lung Cancer

	Treatment	Survival
Limited	Radiation primary tumor, and mediastinum +/– cranial irradiation (dementia can occur); if aggressive chemo rx cannot be tolerated, try VP-16 (Ger Rev Syllabus 1996; p. 327)	14–18 mo, 15–25% survive 2 yr and considered cured, high association w second primary cancers (Nejm 1992;327:1618)
Extensive	Oral etoposide (Semin Oncol 1990;17:49)	9–11 mo

non-small-cell lung cancer; increased age, elevated LDH, alkaline phosphatase, hyponatremia for small-cell lung cancer

Routine f/u after primary lung cancer treatment: history and physical examination (H+P) (pulmonary, abdominal, neurologic sx; cervical, axillary, and supraclavicular lymph nodes; edema of face and neck), and chest xray q 4 mo for 2 yr, then q 6–12 mo

BREAST CANCER

Am Fam Phys Monograph 1995:191; Surg Clin N Am 1994;74:145

Cause: Risk factors: breast cancer in 1st-degree relative (Jama 1993;270:1563), age >30 at birth of first child, late menopause, benign breast disease, heavy radiation exposure, conjugated estrogens, obesity, decreased bone mineral density (Jama 1996;276:1404), moderate alcohol use: 1–2 times that of healthy age-matched controls (Nejm 1992;327:319); dysplasia in 5–10% of benign bx specimens = 4 times risk; hereditary in 5%, usually younger women

Epidem: Most common cancer in women; incidence in women <50 has declined by 13%, but increased in women >50 by 7%; half of breast cancers occur in women >65 yr old

Pathophys: Elderly women more likely to have well-differentiated cancer; both estrogen and progesterone receptors present in 60–70% of elderly pts; biologically less aggressive than in younger women

Si: Masses more likely malignant in elderly women

Crs: Overall course more benign, more at risk for subsequent colon cancer (Am J Gastroenterol 1994;84:835)

Compl: Elderly more at risk for emergency complications, eg, hypercalcemia, spinal cord compression, symptomatic brain metastasis

Lab: CEA, CA27.29

Xray: May not see palpable lesion on mammography 20% of the time; palpable lesion in postmenopausal women requires bx; bone scans, CT of abdomen, pelvis, chest, and brain not called for in asx pts w nl physical exam findings; determination of presence of sentinel axillary lymph node reduces requirement for axillary node sampling (Ger Rev Syllabus 1999–2001:282)

Rx:

Preventive: See 2.2 Cancer, Breast Cancer

Therapeutic: Surgical rx w curative intent similar to that adopted in younger pts is appropriate for women >70 (J Am Soc Ger 1996;44:390)

Contraindications for breast-conserving surgery: tumor mass >5 cm, large breast size, subareolar lesion

Cancers >4 cm, preop chemo rx results in substantial tumor shrinkage, allowing for breast-conserving surgery (J Natl Cancer Inst 1991;82:1539)

Excision alone ("lumpectomy") for tumors <1 cm

Postoperative adjuvant radiation rx recommended for extensive cancers, eg, >4 pos lymph nodes; ER-pos more likely to benefit from tamoxifen (Eur J Surg Oncol 1994;20:207)

Frail pts w advanced localized lesions respond to tamoxifen (Jama 1996;275:1349) w 40–70% tumor shrinkage, but long-term survival unchanged (Arch Surg 1984;1:548); tamoxifen well tolerated: decreases bone loss, increases HDL levels; increases risk of DVT, endometrial cancer, visual loss

Megestrol acetate (Megace), anastrozole fewer side effects (Med Let Drugs Ther 1996;38:62); decrease recurrence rate w tamoxifen (Br J Cancer 1988;57:612)

Routine f/u of asx pts after primary breast cancer treatment: H+P (skin, chest, breast, abdominal exam) (Am J Clin Oncol 1988;11:451) q 3 mo × 2 yr, then q 6 mo × 3 yr, then annually after 5 yr; breast self-exam q mo for life; mammography q 6 mo × 2 yr, then annually

Adjuvant chemo rx survival benefit for healthy elderly women 70 yr old (Jama 1992;268:57); responses last 6–12 mo; paclitaxel (Taxol) for tumors overexpressing HER2 protein (Med Let 2000;42:83), see Ovarian Cancer; most cytotoxic drugs metabolized in the liver; altered metabolism only with major liver dysfunction; myelosuppression more common in the elderly; psychosocial adjustments to chemo rx better in the elderly than in the younger population (Hlth Serv Res 1986;20:961)

Metastatic breast cancer: median survival 2 yr; palliative rx for bone, skin, lymph nodes, pleural and pulmonary metastases; soft tissue and bone metastases will respond to hormonal therapy if they have responded before, eg, progestins, aromatase inhibitors, estrogens

Rx bone mets w clodronate (bisphosphate): decreases bone destruction, decreases tumor burden by inhibiting release of bone-derived tumor growth factors (Nejm 1998;339:357,398)

COLORECTAL CANCER

Epidem: Accounts for 14% of cancers in men and women; 3rd leading cause of cancer death after lung and breast; incidence 4–5 times higher in people >65 yr old; two-thirds of colon cancers occur in people >65 yr

Pathophys: Minimum of 5 yr for adenomatous polyp to become malignant; if polyp >2 cm, 40% chance of being malignant; pts w cancers confined to mucosal layers, Dukes stage A (just mucosal involvement), have 80–90% 5-yr survival; Dukes stage B (through bowel wall but no lymph node involvement) 60% 5-yr survival; Dukes stage C (involving lymph nodes) 40% 5-yr survival; Dukes stage D (metastatic) 5% 5-yr survival

Sx: Anemia, abdominal discomfort; hematochezia, pencil-thin stools, obstruction

Crs: 5-yr survival for overall colon cancer population is 57% and somewhat worse in geriatric age groups (CA 1992;42:9)

Colon cancer recurrence: most likely if tumor penetrated through colon wall; w poorly differentiated histology; presence of obstruction; elevated CEA; increased number of pos lymph nodes; rate of recurrence: 1st yr 50%, 2nd yr 20%, rare after 5 yr; 10% have second primary approximately 11 yr after initial colon cancer; pattern of recurrence: regional lymph nodes, then hematogenous spread to liver; 8% recurrence at site of original surgical anastomosis; local recurrence 25–40%, liver 40%, abdominal peritoneal implants 12–28%; solitary lung nodule has 50% chance metastasis and 50% chance of being primary lung cancer—thus, need tissue dx; sx of recurrence: abdominal or pelvic pain, lower GI bleeding, change in bowel habits, weight loss, cough, bone pain; associated cancers: breast, ovarian, endometrial (Prim Care 1992;19:607); CEA elevation associated w tumor recurrence in 85–90% of pts and may precede sx by 3–8 mo (Surg Clin N Am 1993;73:85)

Lab: CEA good to follow postop for recurrence; false-pos: smoking, liver disease, PUD, pancreatitis, diverticulitis, IBD

Rx:

Preventive: 10-yr regular aspirin use in doses similar to those recommended for prevention of cardiovascular disease substantially reduces risk of colon cancer (Nejm 1995;333:609); COX-2 inhibitors may prevent colon cancer (Jama 1999;282:1254)

Therapeutic: Surgical excision only potentially curative intervention; rectal cancer—local resection w "pull-through" procedure to avoid colostomy, use transrectal US to determine depth of lesion and nodular metastasis; rx up to 3 solitary liver nodules w resection

Continuous infusion 5-fluorouracil—adjuvant therapy as effective w modulating agents, eg, leucovorin; IL-2 adjuvant rx

Routine f/u: H+P, LFTs, stool guaiac for 2 yr q 3–6 mo, then for 2 yr q 6–12 mo and after yr 4 annually; CEA q 2 mo for 2 yr, then q 4 mo for the next 2 yr, then annually after that; colonoscopy after surgical resection and 1 yr after that, then q 3 yr; chest film q 6–12 mo for 2 yr, then annually (Jama 1989;261:584)

Team Management: For hospice (Table 7-4)

- Bowel obstruction is an oncologic emergency: preventive: liquid or soft diet, stool softeners, antiemetics (metoclopramide); active conventional "conservative" IV fluids, antiemetics, nasogastric suction may cause resolution; if death imminent continue symptomatic rx only with pain relief and antiemetics, eg, Sandostatin (ie, octreotide)—dose is 200–600 μg SC bid (1 mg/mL multi-use vial); surgical treatment justified only in pt with >2–3 mo to live given high morbidity
- Obstructive uropathy common, may present with retention, dysuria, nocturia, frequency, decreased stream; treated with indwelling catheter or surgery
- Widespread pelvic metastases can cause difficult-to-manage neuropathic pain

PROSTATE CANCER

Urol Clin N Am 1999;25:581; Med Clin N Am 1998;83:1423; Am Fam Phys Monograph 1995;191:29; Sci Am Med 1995;12:IXA

Cause: Hormonal, familial (Prostate 1990;17:337), oncogenic viruses, environmental, not associated w BPH (Lancet 1974;2:115) or vasectomy; incidence decreased by selenium, vit E, decreased by soy or tomatoes in diet, increased by rise in fat diet (Cmaj 1998;159:807)

Epidem: 50–70% of men >70 yr old have histologic evidence of prostate cancer on autopsy and <3% of them die from prostate cancer; nevertheless prostate cancer is the 2nd most common cause of

Table 7-4. Pharmacologic Treatment of Pain, Nausea, and Constipation Associated with Bowel Obstruction

Drug	Dose	Comment
Pain		
Morphine or hydromorphone	Titrate to relief po, sl, sc, or IV (Remember, morphine sc dose = 1/3 po dose and hydromorphone sc dose = 1/5 po dose	For cramping pain (colic), may need high dosage or addition or glycopyrrolate (Robinul) 0/4–1/0 mg/d sc or hyoscyamine (Levsin SL) 0.125 mg SL q 4–8 h; if pain unrelieved, consider celiac plexus block
Nausea		
Haloperidol (Haldol)	5–15 mg/d sc, po, or IV	Mix in 5% dextrose for sc infusion
Metoclopramide (Reglan)	60–240 mg/d sc, po, or IV	May cause colic unless combined with a high dose opioid
Hydroxyzine (Vistaril)	100–200 mg/d sc, po, or IV	Add to haloperidol if necessary
Chlorpromazine	25–100 mg/tid po, pr, or IV	Suppositories useful if sc infusion of above agents is unavailable; sedating
Promethazine	12.5–25 mg po or im q 4–6 h, 25 mg pr q 4–6 h	
Methotrimeprazine (Levoprome)	50–300 mg/d sc or IV	Expensive, analgesic, sedating, but very effective; may need daily change of sc site
Scopolamine patch	0.5 mg q 72 h	
Persistent Vomiting of Secretions (despite above measures)		
Octreotide (Sandostatin)	0.1–0.6 mg/d by sc infusion	Expensive, reduces GI secretions
Constipation (in subtotal obstruction)		
Docusate	100 mg po bid–q 4 h	Stimulant laxative like senna or bisacodyl, may cause colic
Dexamethasone	4 mg po or sc bid–qid	May relieve obstruction, but discontinue if ineffective after 5 days
Fecal Incontinence		
Loperamide		Slows motility, augments internal anal sphincter tone

Reproduced by permission from AAHPM publication, Hospice/Palliative Care Training for Physicians, a self-study program, 1996.

cancer death in men; as much as 50% of cancers are clinically advanced at the time of discovery; well-differentiated cancer is least likely to spread (10-yr cancer-specif death rate <10%); most are moderate grade (10-yr cancer-specif death rate 10–20%); poorly differentiated (10-yr cancer-specif death rate 30–60%) (Nejm 1994;330:242)

Incidence 0.8/100,000 in Asians and 100.2/100,000 in black Americans (Ann IM 1994;120:698); prostate is the most common malignancy in black American males and the 2nd leading cause of cancer death among black American men (Med Clin N Am 1998;83:1423; CA 1992;42:7); men w father or brother w prostate cancer before age 65 yr have a 3–5 times risk of developing prostate cancer (Cmaj 1998;159:807); if they have 2 relatives who developed it before age 65 yr, they have 5–8 times risk

Pathophys: 95% adenocarcinoma; remainder are squamous, transitional, sarcomas; adenocarcinoma arises in the peripheral portion of the gland (Med Clin N Am 1998;83:1423), whereas BPH arises from the periurethral area

Crs: PSA >20 ng/mL or poorly differentiated, greater likelihood disease not confined to prostate; clinical pattern of recurrence: local pelvic progression; lymph nodes (obturator, iliac, para-aortic); bony metastases to pelvis, spine, and proximal femur; lung, liver, adrenal gland, supraclavicular nodes, brain

Grading: Gleason

2–4 well differentiated
5–7 moderately differentiated
8–10 poorly differentiated

Staging:

(A or T1) extent of tissue involved incidentally on TURP
(B or T2) detected by digital rectal exam (DRE) confined to prostate
(C or T3) extend thru prostate capsule
(D1 or N1–2) lymph node metastases
(D2 or M) metastases to bone
(D3) progressive after the inanition of hormone therapy or androgen refractory disease

Lab: Age 60–69 yr: nl PSA range 0.0–4.5 ng/mL; 70–79 yr: nl PSA range 0.0–6.5 ng/mL; U.S. Task Force does not recommend screening w PSA because finding prostate cancer early does not decrease mortality (U.S. Preventive Services Task Force. Guide to clinical preventive services. 2nd ed. Baltimore: Williams & Wilkins, 1996); one-third cancers missed w this screening test; false-pos as high as 60%; PSA density >0.15, more likely cancer and not BPH (Mayo Clin Proc 1994;69:59); best used in men w PSAs <9 or 10; PSA velocity >0.75 mg/mL/yr has sensitivity of 72% (Urol Clin N Am 1999;25:581); serial PSA utility unclear (J Urol 1998;158:1243)

Xray: Extraperitoneal lymph node sampling via CT-directed needle bx to determine staging and rx (J Endourol 1992;6:103); bone scan to w/u bony metastases; chest film, CT of abdomen and pelvis

Rx:

Preventive: Large percentage of men w prostate cancer will not die from it; rx causes morbidity, so weigh risks in older people whose life expectancy is limited by other diseases (see 2.2 Cancer, Prostate Cancer)

Therapeutic: Routine f/u after primary prostate cancer treatment:

- H+P (sx of bladder outlet obstruction, pelvic, spine and long-bone pain, neurologic sx from vertebral collapse, sx of renal failure, fixation of prostate to pelvic wall) q 3 mo × 2 yr, q 6 mo next 3 yr and after that annually
- PSA q 3 mo × 2 yr, q 6 mo next 3 yr and annually after that; PSA should fall in 2–3 d after surgery; extremely anaplastic tumors are not differentiated enough to produce PSA, so may not be elevated if recurrent

  Nerve-sparing radical surgery for moderately differentiated localized prostate cancer in 70 yr old instead of expectant management increased survival time by 6 mo (Jama 1993;269:2650); improved survival for patients w locally advanced prostate cancer rx w radiotherapy and goserelin (Zoladex) 79% vs 62% 5 yr survival (Nejm 1997;337:295); hormonal (GNRH agonist: leu leuprolide or goserelin), antiandrogens (flutamide, bicalutamide, nilutamide) (Med Let 2000;42:83) best for locally advanced mets, relief of bone pain, decr serum PSA, decr tumor size, decr obstruction; may partially reverse anemia, improve appetite (Med Clin N Am 1998;83:1231); watch for osteoporosis; radical prostatectomy is associated w significant erectile dysfunction and some decline in urinary dysfunction (Jama 2000;283:354); nodes can be sampled first, then continue procedure only if nodes pos

Team Management: Pts make decisions based on sx previously experienced, eg, choose expectant management if experience dribbling and radical prostatectomy if cannot start stream

(J Am Geriatr Soc 1996;44:934); should refer to literature-based decision making by pt education video (The PSA Decision: What You Need to Know [video]. Hanover NH: Foundation for Informed Medical Decision Making, March 1994); pain due to bone metastases; megestrol acetate effective for hot flashes in 60% pts; pelvic complications: lower extremity edema from lymphadenopathy, urinary dysfunction and neurologic impairment; oncologic emergencies: spinal cord compression, obstructive uropathy, SIADH, disseminated intravascular coagulation

OVARIAN CANCER

Semin Oncol 1998;25:281; Reinke D, American Academy of Family Practice Board Review Course, Seattle, 5/30/95; CA 1995;42:69

Cause: Hereditary (5–10%) w early onset; cosmetic talc to perineum; 80% benign; epithelial: 60%, and 5-yr survival = 20–50%; mucinous: 5 yr survival = 60%; stromal sex cord tumors of which 90% are benign, two-thirds occurring in postmenopausal women; metastatic from stomach, colon, breast, uterus

Epidem: 1/70 women; most common gynecologic cancer causing death in women; 4th most common cause of cancer death in women; mean age 55–61 yr and incidence of ovarian cancer increases w advancing age into 8th decade; industrialized countries; w ovarian cancer have 4 times the risk breast cancer; w breast cancer have 2 times the risk of ovarian cancer; risk factors: low parity, high-fat diet, no bcp use, sedentary lifestyle

Pathophys:
- Unregulated cell division/regeneration of ovarian epithelium
- Pituitary gonadotropin stimulates malignant transformation

Sx: Nausea, dyspepsia, lower abdominal pain; constipation; early satiety w omental metastases; urinary frequency

Si: Ascites; progressive weakness; weight loss; ovarian mass

Crs: 3 hereditary patterns: ovary alone, ovary w breast, ovary w colon (Lynch syndrome) usually detected in advanced stages; mean survival with residual tumor >3 cm = 21 mo; <3 cm = 53 mo; 75% present stage III—5-yr survival rate 10–30%; prognosis: better with young age, good functional status, bcp's, small postop residual tumor

volume, low tumor grade, low tumor ploidy; median time to
recurrence 2–4 mo, first detected by CA125 in asx patients

Staging:
    I = limited to ovary—5-yr survival = 90%
    II = pelvic ext—5-yr survival up to 70%
    III = intraperitoneal metastasis or pos nodes—5-yr survival = 25%
    IV = distant to lung, liver, peritoneal implants occur rapidly—5-yr
      survival = 10%

Lab: Tumor markers: CEA elevated in 60% epithelial tumors; also pos
in cirrhosis, COPD, IBD, smoking; CA125—correlates w disease in
93% pts; also pos in endometriosis, miliary TB, 1% healthy persons

Xray:

Noninvasive: US: solid w papillary projections w involvement adjacent
visceral, distinguish cyst from ascites, bx metastases; transvaginal US
even more effective and should be done if CA125 >2 × nl; CT: for
masses >2 cm, metastases; chest film, IVP, cystoscopy, proctoscopy,
BE, UGI if sx

Rx:

Therapeutic:

  Surgery:
- Laparoscopy discouraged—spill cells
- Debulk primary to <1 cm = 50% cure, >1 cm = 20–25% response
- Bx diaphragm, paracolic gutters, pelvic peritoneum, periaortic,
  pelvic nodes, infra colic omentum
- Peritoneal washings
- TAH/BSO, omentectomy
- Large-bowel resection required in 20–30% cases
- Bladder or ureteral resection required in 5%
- Diaphragm, liver, spleen resection; rarely need
- May have fertility sparing surgery if stage IA

  Chemo rx:
- First-line chemo rx = platinum-based combination, response
  rate = 80%; complete clinical response = 50%
- Paclitaxel (Taxol) most active agent in ovarian and breast cancer
  but risk of anaphylaxis requires dexamethasone as well as H_1- and
  H_2-antagonist antihistamines, decreasing risk of anaphylaxis from
  10% to 1%
- If Cr clearance >45 dL/min and good performance status without
  comorbid disease—age not a factor (CA 1993;71:594)

- Only small portion achieve surgical response documented by 2nd look; even then complete surgical responders progress
- 2nd-line chemo rx = interferon; granulocyte colony-stimulating factor (G-CSF) to prevent neutropenia with chemo rx
- Radiotherapy for small volume tumor, limited by liver and kidney function
- Biological therapy being studied (monoclonal antibodies, gene therapy)

7.3 TREATMENT OF CANCER IN THE ELDERLY

Therapeutic: See Table 7-5 and Table 7-6
- Oldest old tolerate radiotherapy in full doses without serious complications (J Am Geriatr Soc 1995;43:793; CA 1993;72:594; Curr Probl Cancer 1993;17:145)
- Fatigue/weakness: rx depending on etiology
- Hypomagnesemia: magnesium oxide 400 mg 1–2 tab bid–tid
- Adrenal insufficiency: hydrocortisone 5–30 mg bid–qid or dexamethasone 0.03–0.15 mg po/IV/im qd in 2–4 divided doses
- Cord compression: dexamethasone 100 mg IV stat, radiation rx
- Over-sedation by narcotics: methylphenidate 10 mg at 0800 and 5 mg at 1200
- Nausea and vomiting associated w terminal illness: dopamine antagonist such as phenothiazine; benzodiazepine, antihistamine for anxiety (BMJ 1998;316:286; 1997;315:1148)
- Antiemetics for chemo rx: start w prochlorperazine (Compazine), promethazine (Phenergan); serotonin-reuptake antagonists granisetron in combination with dexamethasone more effective than either alone (Nejm 1995;332:1); ondansetron (Zofran) 0.8 mg tid
- Cachexia: megestrol acetate to rx cachexia, inconsistent results w increasing lean body mass; dronabinol, anabolic androgenic steroid, psychostimulants to promote appetite—no systemic studies in frail elderly

Daily pain prevention among NH patients w cancer often untreated in older and minority groups (Jama 1998;279:1877); >33% conscious dying pts have severe pain (Ann IM 1997;126:97); pain management: analgesic dose in a pt who has become tolerant to a narcotic is not lethal because pt also develops tolerance to the

Table 7-5. Specific Causes and Treatments for Dyspnea

B   **Bronchospasm**—If present, consider nebulized albuterol and/or oral steroids: if not, consider lowering doses of theophylline and adrenergic agents to reduce any tremor and anxiety that often exacerbate dyspnea.

R   **Rales**—If volume overload is present, reduce artificial feeding or stop IV fluids; diuretics are occasionally needed; if pneumonia seems likely, decide whether an antibiotic will rehabilitate the patient or just prolong the dying process; patient and family participation in this decision is essential.

E   **Effusions**—Thoracentesis can be effective, but if the effusion recurs and the patient is ambulatory, consider pleurodesis to prevent recurrent lung collapse; if the patient is close to death, palliate the dyspnea with opioids.

A   **Airway obstruction**—Make sure tracheostomy appliances are cleaned regularly; if aspiration of food is likely, puree solids and thicken liquids with cornstarch or "Thick-it," and instruct the family in positioning the patient during feeding and in suctioning if necessary.

T   **Thick secretions**—If the cough reflex is still strong, loosen secretions with nebulized saline; if the cough is weak, dry secretions with hyoscyamine (Levsin) 0.125 mg po or sl q 8 h or Transderm Scop 1–3 patches every 3 days, or add glycopyrrolate (Robinul) 0.4–1.0 mg per day to a sc infusion or by sc or IV bolus 0.2 mg q 3 h pm.

H   **Hemoglobin low**—A blood transfusion may add energy and reduce dyspnea for a few weeks; more often, hemorrhage or marrow failure of the dying process and are best palliated with opioids and living kindness.

A   **Anxiety**—Sitting upright, using a bedside fan, listening to calming music, and practicing relaxation techniques can be extremely effective, as can skillful counseling and the presence of a calming physician; dyspnea exacerbates normal fears and anxiety, so treat with opioids first, then try a benzodiazepine if needed; if the opioid dose is limited by drowsiness, reduce the benzodiazepine and increase the opioid.

I   **Interpersonal issues**—Social and financial problems contribute to dyspnea; counseling and interaction with social workers and other members of the interdisciplinary team may bring relief; when family relationships exacerbate the problem, a few days spent in a peaceful, homelike hospice inpatient unit may help relieve the patient's symptoms.

R   **Religious concerns**—Although faith or an experience of the transcendent can bring profound comfort, some religious beliefs, such as "God is punishing me" or "God will heal me if I have enough faith," can precipitate dyspnea and/or exacerbate its symptoms; take time to listen with full attention and presence; help the patient explore ways to reconnect with God, the cosmos, or the deepest parts of the self; coordinate treatment with the patient's spiritual advisor, chaplain, counselor, other health care professionals, and family members.

Table 7-6. Specific Measure for the Treatment of Nausea

Specific Cause	Possible Remedy

Cortical

- Tumor in CNS or meninges (look for neurologic signs or mental status problems)
- Dexamethasone (consider radiation therapy)

- Increased intracranial pressure (look for projectile vomiting, headache)
- Dexamethasone

- Anxiety and other conditioned responses
- Counseling, tranquilizers

- Uncontrolled pain
- Opioids, other pain medications

Vestibular/Middle Ear

- Vestibular disease (look for vertigo or vomiting after head motion)
- Meclizine and/or ENT consult

- Middle ear infections (look for ear pain or bulging tympanic membrane)
- Antibiotic and/or decongestant

- Motion sickness (travel-related nausea)
- Transderm Scop, meclizine

Chemoreceptor Trigger Zone

The most common causes of nausea are mediated by this area in the brain, which senses changes in the blood.

- Drugs, eg, opioids, digoxin, chemotherapy, carbamazepine, antibiotics, theophylline
- Decrease drug dose or discontinue drug if possible

- Metabolic, eg, renal or liver failure
- Haloperidol po or sc or ondansetron (Zofran) po or sc

- Hyponatremia
- Salt tablets, demeclocycline

- Hypercalcemia
- Diphosphonate or other therapy

Gastrointestinal Tract

- Irritation by drugs (eg, NSAIDs, iron, alcohol, antibiotics)
- Stop drug if possible, add H_2 blocker or misoprostol

- Tumor infiltration, radiation therapy to the GI tract, or infection (eg, candida esophagitis, colitis)
- Haloperidol sc, possibly with hydroxyzine sc or Transderm Scop

- Distention from constipation or impaction
- Laxative, manual disimpaction

- Obstruction by tumor or poor motility
- Metoclopramide (Reglan)

- Tube feedings
- Reduce feeding volume

- Gag reflex from feeding tube
- Remove it

- Nasopharyngeal bleeding
- Packing, vitamin K, sedation

- Thick secretions (cough-induced vomiting)
- Nebulized saline if good cough reflex, anticholinergic if poor cough reflex

Reproduced by permission from Drugs of choice for cancer chemotherapy. Med Lett Drugs Ther 1997;14;39:21–8.

life-threatening side effects of respiratory depression (McCaffery M, Phoenix, AZ, 1997 AMDA Annual Meeting); World Health Guidelines for stepwise approach to cancer pain:

1. Acetaminophen, ASA, OTC NSAID as well as nonpharmacologic interventions (radiation, relaxation, psychotherapy)
2. Weak opiate (codeine)
3. Graduated dose of strong narcotic (morphine)
   - Equianalgesic doses: morphine 10 mg im or sc = 30 mg po = meperidine (Demerol) 75 mg im = 300 mg po = acetaminophen-oxycodone HCl (Percocet) 2 mg po = codeine 200 mg po = fentanyl 0.1 mg im or IV (Prim Care 1992;19:793); may need up to 1800 mg po morphine sulfate (Nejm 1996;335:1124); bone metastasis: 4 mCi strontium chloride 89 IV q 3 mo; neuropathic: 150–300 mg mexiletine tid; formal pt education about pain helpful (CA 1994;74:2139); fentanyl patch 21.5 mg q 3 d; avoid meperidine-accumulation of toxic metabolite normeperidine resulting in dysphoria, myoclonic jerks, sz (see Tables 1-3 and 1-4)
   - Biofeedback, hypnosis, behavior modification for chronic pain (Ann IM 1980;93:588)

Terminal hydration leads to untoward effects such as pulmonary edema (Cancer Nurs 1990;13:62)

Hypercalcemia: IV saline and loop diuretics; pamidronate 60–90 mg IV over 4 h, repeat q 2 wk; or calcitonin 4 units/kg IM or sc q 12 h; or plicamycin 25 µg/kg IV q 4–6 h (Drugs 1993;46:594)

Team Management: Ethical dilemmas in feeding the terminally ill (Nejm 1988;318:25; J Am Geriatr Soc 1984;32:237; 1984;32:525); Chapter 13, Ethics

Psychological issues: isolation, lack of understanding of dx/px, role changes in family, guilt, financial difficulties, loss of intimacy, anticipatory grief, anger at loss of independence

Family meeting w dying pt (simple nonjudgmental listening):

1. Have pt tell the story of how he/she became ill and the course of the illness; the pt may ask spouse to tell the story but it is important that the pt do so, regaining confidence and connection w the family this way
2. Have pt talk about his/her worries and fears; first, fears for the family
   A. Spouse—describe how met spouse, evaluate the marriage, voice disillusionments, resentments so they may be let go

B. Children—speak to each, reframe crying not as "breaking down" but as "breaking through"; important for pt to realize that he/she does not have control over how the children will live the rest of their lives and that he/she must let this go; can now only simply give the "gift of love"; grandchildren may have separation and individuation issues (Kubler-Ross E, Children facing death, Presented at the 4th international seminar on terminal care, Montreal, Canada, 1982)

C. Self—his/her worries for him/herself: suffering, loneliness, fear, loss of control

3. Concerning roots: have the pts recount stories about parents and siblings, unmourned deaths

4. Family tells of the pt: spouse evaluates marriage; secrets may emerge (alcohol, incest) not to inflame guilt but to keep secrets from being buried only to reappear in future generations (Murphy M, Hospice Conference, New York, 1992)

Transportation for radiation rx

Caregivers (informal and formal) need to care for themselves (BMJ 1998;316:208)

8 Cardiology

8.1 HYPERTENSION

Clin Ger Med 1999;15:663; NIH Pub No. 98-4080 (www.nhlbi. nih.gov/guidelines/hypertension/jncintro.htm); Ger Rev Syllabus 1996:219; Arch IM 1995;155:563; 1993;153:177; Hypertension 1994;23:275–285; NIH Pub. No. 93–1088

Cause: Consider meds, eg cough and cold preparations, NSAIDs

Epidem: 50% of pts >65–74 yr old have HT; 60–70% black, Hispanic, Native American have HT; >1/3 have BP >160 (Hypertension 1995;25:305); diastolic BP rises until age 55, when it begins to level off; thus rise in isolated systolic BP accounts for the overall increase in age-related HT: 10% at 70 yrs, and 20% at 80 yrs independent of race; elevated systolic BP or elevated pulse pressure is the single greatest risk for cardiovascular disease in persons >65 yrs; even isolated systolic hypertension 140–159 (Nejm 1993;329:1912); LVH in hypertensives may confer increased risk for ventricular arrhythmias; ~90% HT primary (essential) associated w family hx, DM, obesity, diet, ETOH use, drug/med use; ~10% HT secondary: primary renal disease, renovascular causes, pheochromocytoma, Cushing, Conn syndrome (Nejm 1992;327:543)

Sleep apnea associated with HT even when adjustment for weight, ETOH, smoking made; treatment of obstructive sleep apnea w BiPAP has been shown to lower BP (Jama 2000;283:1829)

Pathophys:

- Increased vascular resistance results from age-related decrease in elastic tissue and development of atherosclerosis; also decrease in vasodilatory response to alpha adrenergic stimulation, while adrenergic response remains the same

- Decreased baroreflex secondary to decreases in arterial distensibility; requires larger change in BP to activate and then responds w large effects in sympathetic nervous system outflow
- Renally secreted prostaglandins protect from HT; renin/aldosterone/angiotensin worsen HT, although not a major cause in the development of HT in the elderly; basal and stimulated levels of renin and aldosterone decline with age; however, older pts respond well to smooth-muscle relaxants and ACE inhibitors
- Calcium and sodium intakes modulate BP via PTH and the renin-angiotensin system (Ann IM 1987;107:919)
- "Salt-sensitive" HT depends on Na and Cl together; BP decreases w Na citrate (Nejm 1987;317:1043)

Sx: Usually asymptomatic but long-standing HT may first present with end-organ damage, ie, retinal hemorrhage, decreases renal function

Sudden onset (see Table 8-1) or recalcitrant HT suggests secondary HT, particularly occlusive renovascular disease, rarely hyperaldosteronism, hypokalemia, pheochromocytoma

Si: Systolic BP >140 on three occasions or average DP >90 (but see pseudo-HT)

Systolic BP >160 mmHg more significant risk factor than diastolic BP >95 mmHg (Lancet 2000;355:865); ambulatory BP better predictor of risk in elderly (Jama 1999;282:539)

Auscultate for peripheral arterial bruits, 4th heart sound, displaced PMI, retinal changes

Si of secondary HT: abdominal bruit (renovascular disease); hyperglycemia, fat distribution (Cushing); headache, palpitations, diaphoresis, paroxysmal elevations of BP (pheochromocytoma); worsening of BP control or BP that remains uncontrolled on trip therapy; malignant HT: abrupt development of diastolic HT (unusual in light of general decrease in diastolic BP in pt >60 yrs)

Pseudo-HT w rigid arteries that cannot be compressed by sphygmomanometer cuff, giving falsely high readings, but can still palpate radial pulse (Osler sign, may be unreliable); however, pt often exhibits BP out of proportion to end-organ damage (Hypertension 1994;23:275)

Crs: Older pts w HT at higher risk for orthostatic hypotension; pressures should be measured in both sitting and standing position; rx of systolic and diastolic HT up to age 85 yr (Lancet 1991;338:1281); LVH decreases over 6 mo and function improves in

elderly when rx with verapamil or atenolol (Nejm 1990;322:1350);
ACE inhibitors best preserve renal function (see Rx)

Isolated moderate systolic HT also associated w 1.5 times increased
cardiovascular risks (Nejm 1993;329:1912)

Rx of isolated systolic HT (>160) in elderly reduces CVAs by one-
third (NNT − 5 = 33) (Jama 1991;265:3255), stroke mortality
by 36%, and cardiac mortality by 25% (Ann IM 1994;121:355),
NNT − 5 = 18 to prevent MI/CVA (Jama 1994;272:1932)

Cmplc: CVA, hypertensive crisis; chronic renal failure; cardiovascular
including afib and LVH, which increases risk of MI, CVA, vtach,
death, and sudden death 3−4 times more than HT alone (Nejm
1992;327:998; 1987;317:787; Ann IM 1986;105:173)

Lab: Routine initial w/u:
- Family hx, DM II high likelihood of essential HT; r/o sleep apnea
  (30%) (Ann IM 1985;103:190; 1994;120:382)
- Alcohol, sodium (water softeners?), diet (r/o hyperparathyroid, Ca,
  Mg, K deficiency) and other drug/med use, primary renal disease
- Urinalysis w micro exam, K, BUN/Cr, EKG (3−8% sens) or
  echocardiography (100% sens, ?specif) for LVH

For recalcitrant HT or HT emergency:
- Renovascular causes (40% have bruits), hypo/hyperthyroidism,
  pheochromocytoma, Cushing, Conn syndrome (Nejm 1992;
  327:543)

See specific topics in Chapter 3, Endocrinology

Xray: For renovascular HT: renal scan before and after captopril 50 mg
po shows decreased flow in affected kidney (90% sens and specif)
(Ann IM 1992;117:845; Jama 1992;268:3353)

Rx:

Assessment: focused PE for neuro, cardiovascular, renal, ocular si/sx

Major Trials:

Non-pharmacologic: The Trials of Hypertension Prevention, DASH,
Modification of Diet in Renal Dis, TONE

Pharmacologic: SHEP, NHANES III, TOMHS, INDANA, Syst-EUR,
SAVE, ELITE, MRFIT, ALLHAT, SOLVD, AASK, MRC, etc.

Non-Drug Regimens: (BMJ 1994;309:436); reduced sodium intake and
weight loss (Jama 1998;279:839); decrease ischemic stroke with
leisure time physical activity (Stroke 1998;29:380); reduce ETOH
(Hypertension 1992;20:533); avoid or stop NSAIDs (Jama 1994;
272:781; Ann IM 1994;121:289)

Pharmacologic Strategies: (Ann IM 1994;121:35; Hypertension 1994;23:275; www.nhlbi.nih.gov/guidelines/hypertension/jncintro.htm)

- Titrate med according to standing BP to avoid hypotension
- Treatment goal: Gradual reduction of BP as cerebral blood flow to mean arterial pressure curve is shifted rightward; too rapid decline in BP may precipitate stroke or hypotension, as well as reflex tachycardia/sympathetic activation (especially w β-blockers)
- No more than 10 mmHg decrease per dose increment (over 1 mo) with end goal of 120–140 systolic/<90 diastolic (lower BP confers added protection for DM); do not lower below 140/85 mmHg (Swedish trial in old persons w HT, STOP-HT; Lancet 1991;338:1281); Finnish cohort study: lowering BP 5 mmHg from 90 to 86 associated w decreased 5-yr survival (J Hypertens 1994;7:1183); vs lowering diastolic BP <85 did not cause cardiovascular compromise (Lancet 1998;351:1755); BP <70 a danger (Arch IM 1999;159:2004); when withdraw pts from chronic antihypertensives, 40% of pts require restarting them within 1 yr (J Intern Med 1994;235:581)
- Treat according to risk stratification: treat mild HT (140–159/90–99) w 12-mo lifestyle modification unless risk factors, then treat w 6-mo lifestyle modification, if target organ damage or clinical cardiovascular disease treat w drugs; treat BP >160/100 w drugs (>140 if w DM) (Clin Ger Med 1999;15:663)
- Guiding principles for drug rx: Start 1/2 usual adult dose; simple dosing regimens; alternative routes such as patches when needed; lower doses of two different agents sometimes better than larger dose of single agent; 1/2 of elderly controlled w single drug (Jama 1996;277:1577); keep cost in mind
- Monitor for hypotension, hypovolemia, kidney function, potassium especially w diuretics or ACE I or on Digoxin
- Diuretics better than β-blockers in decreasing BP and preventing cardiovascular morbidity and mortality (Stroke 1998;29:380); β-blockers relatively ineffective as monotherapy for older hypertensives (Jama 1998;279:1303); diuretics actually help prevent cardiovascular mortality in hyperlipidemic pts (Jama 1991;265:3255); reduce LV mass (Jama 1998;279:778)
- Dyazide (hydrochlorothiazide 12.5–25.0 mg + triamterene 50 mg) avoids all the MRFIT mortality risks (Ann IM 1995;122:223; Nejm 1994;330:1852)

CARDIOLOGY

- Chlorthalidone 2.5 mg qd for isolated systolic HT results in 80% risk reduction of CHF in pts w prior MI (Jama 1997;378:212)
- β-blockers w diuretic also reduce mortality (Jama 1991;265:3255); atenolol reduced lipid solubility (less depression, lethargy)
- Calcium channel blocker: second choice in elderly after diuretics (Arch IM 1991;151:1954), eg, diltiazem SR 60–180 mg bid; but some studies suggest produces more cognitive impairment than atenolol (Ann IM 1992;116:615); mortality controversy (J Am Geriatr Soc 1995;43:1309); black men do best with diltiazem: 85% success rate compared w 33% w captopril (Am J Hypertens 1995;8:189); long-acting dihydropyridine resulted in 42% reduction in stroke in pts w ISH (Lancet 1997;350:757)
- ACE inhibitor may best preserve renal function even w early renal failure, eg, enalapril 5 mg po qd–qid (NNT = 4) (BMJ 1994;309:833); age better predictor of renin response than renin profile (Jama 1998;280:1160); ACE inhibitors more effective than calcium channel blockers in preventing vascular outcomes in hypertensive type 2 diabetes (Diabetes Care 1998;21:597; Nejm 1998;338:645)
- Effects on lipids (Geriatrics 1995;50:13): diuretics increase total cholesterol and triglycerides; sympatholytics decrease total cholesterol and HDL; ACE inhibitors decrease triglycerides; calcium antagonists have no effect on lipids; β-blockers decrease total cholesterol, LDL, triglycerides, and increase HDL; vasodilators decrease total cholesterol, LDL, and increase HDL

HT Crisis: Rise in BP with imminent risk of organ damage (Table 8-1) predicated less by BP rise than by the potential vital organ damage; BP must be lowered immediately but not too low (target BP ~160–170/100–110); make sure pt is euvolemic

Lab: CBC, lytes, BUN/CREAT, UA, CXR, EKG; consider renal US and head CT/MRI if indicated; BP

Table 8-1. Hypertensive Emergencies and Treatment

Type	Drugs of Choice	Second-Line Drug	Relative Contraindications
Hypertensive Emergency			
General	Best given IVI for accurate titration then PO as IVI weaned	—	Caution: in pt w chronic HT lower BP slowly to avoid cerebral ischemia clonidine
Hypertensive encephalopathy (some form of following sx in 20–60%: HA, emesis, vision changes, MS changes)	Nitroprusside (see contraindications) 0.5–10 µg/kg/min onset 1–2 min duration 2–3 min	Labetalol 0.5–2 mg/min onset 5–30 min duration 5–6 hrs	Trimethaphan (monitor thiocyanate level in renal insuf or when given over 72 h or at dose >3 µg/kg/min)
Intracranial hemorrhage (~5%)	Labetalol	Nitroprusside	Vasodilators*
Left ventricular failure and pulmonary edema (11%)	Nitroprusside ± loop diuretic	Labetalol	Verapamil
Acute myocardial infarction, unstable angina (~8%)	± enalapril (ACE I) 0.625–25 mg q6h onset 10–60 min duration 2–6 hrs Nitroglycerin 5–100 µg/min onset 2–5 min duration 5–10	Nitroprusside, Labetalol	Vasodilators*
Dissecting aortic aneurysm	± labetalol		
Adrenergic crisis	Propranolol 0.5 mg q 5 min to max 6 mg total onset 1–2 min duration 4–12 hrs +/– Nitroprusside Nitroprusside ± β-blockers	Labetalol	Monotherapy with β-blockers

Table 8-1. (cont'd)

Type	Drugs of Choice	Second-Line Drug	Relative Contraindications
Hypertensive Urgency (potential for end-organ damage; requires lowering of BP over hours)			
Uncomplicated malignant HT (papilledema present without above conditions)	Labetalol, Captopril	Nifedipine, Clonidine	
Acute renal failure	Labetalol, Minoxidil +/– β-blocker	Diuretics (in volume overload only) Hemofiltration (in oliguria)	Nitroprusside (renally cleared)
Perioperative HT	NTG, Nitroprusside	Labetalol, Nicardipine	

Note: Pt should have intra-arterial BP monitoring. ACEI = angiotensin-converting enzyme inhibitor.
* Vasodilators with reflex sympathetic stimulation, eg, hydralazine, minoxidil, diazoxide, and short-acting nifedipine.
Reproduced by permission from Kitiyakara C, Guzman NJ. Malignant hypertension and hypertensive emergencies. J Am Soc Nephrol 1998;9:133–42.

8.2 CORONARY ARTERY DISEASE

J Am Geriatr Soc 1998;46:1157; Ger Rev Syllabus 1996:222

ATHEROSCLEROSIS

Nejm 1996;344:1311; J Am Coll Cardiol 1995;25:1000 (women)

Cause: Cholesterol (Nejm 1981;304:65); >300 independent risk factor in elderly (Ann IM 1993;153:1065; J Am Geriatr Soc 1988;36:103);

smoking; HT; lack of estrogen (Ann IM 1976;85:447); genetic (especially in women); not increased by triglyceride elevations alone, although they are markers for other risk factors (Nejm 1993;328:1220); decreased B_6 (Circ 1998;97:437)

Epidem: By age 70 yr, 15% M, 9% F have symptomatic CAD; most common cause of death, >50% of deaths among people >65 yr (DHHS Pub. No. 97-1789); risk of CHD death from hypercholesterolemia 2.2 times at 60 yr to 11.3 times at 75 yr (Ann IM 1990;113:916)

Increased in diabetes, HT, obesity (Nejm 1990;322:882), homocystinuria (Jama 1992;268:877)

Low HDL predicts cardiac mortality in pts >70 yr old; elevated total cholesterol not associated w mortality in men but may be in women (Jama 1995;274:539); decreased in women who take postmenopausal estrogens (Nejm 1991;325:756)

Pathophys: (Nejm 1992;326:242,310) Earliest change: lipid-laden cells or fatty streak in intimal layer of artery (Am Heart J 1994;128:1300); age-related changes: decreases in LDL receptors, cholesterol clearance, bile acid production and estrogen; insulin resistance syndrome: hyperlipidemia, hyperglycemia, and hyperinsulinemia

Wall stress causes fibrous plaques which later infiltrate with cholesterol; impaired fibrinolysis may also play a role in genesis; IL-1, cytokines suggest immunologic mechanism (Basic Res Cardiol 1994;89:41); HDL protective because it stabilizes vasodilator prostaglandin I (Circ 1994;90:1033); HT may induce endothelial dysfunction (Hypertension 1995;25:155); hemorrhage into plaque causes sudden occlusions

Sx: Claudication, angina, MI, sudden death, TIA/CVA, abdominal angina

Si: Renal HT; bruits, absent peripheral pulses; CVAs; retinal fundal vessel plaques

Crs: Reversible with rx (Ann IM 1994;121:348)

Rx: (J Am Geriatr Soc 1999;47:1458) NHANES III study (DHHS Pub No. 97-1789) 50% elderly would benefit from dietary changes, 10–25% qualify for medication (NCEP II guidelines in JAMA 1993;269:3009)

See Table 8-2

• Rx of elevated cholesterol, LDL >130 mg/dL (NH Med 1997; Supplement D:ID), if two other cardiac risk factors (Ger Rev Syllabus 1996:84), which helps by both decreasing plaques and

Table 8-2. Treatments for Elevated Cholesterol

	First Choice	Alternative
ISOLATED ELEVATED LDL	STATIN (in order of most effect on serum lipids):	STATIN + BAS
	Atorvastatin 10–80 mg qd Simvastatin 5–40 mg qd Pravastatin 10–40 mg qd Lovastatin 10–40 mg qd bid Cerivastatin 0.2–0.3 mg qhs Fluvastatin 20–40 mg qd bid	
	BILE ACID SEQUESTRANT (BAS) (eg, Cholestyramine)	BAS + NA
	NICOTINIC ACID (NA)	STATIN + NA*
ELEVATED LDL + LOW HDL	STATIN	STATIN + NA*
ELEVATED LDL + TRIGLYCERIDES (200–400 mg dL)	STATIN	STATIN + GEMFIBROZIL/FENOFIBRATE* STATIN + NA*

* Increased risk of myopathy and hepatitis.

preventing coronary artery spasm (Nejm 1995;332:481,488; Circ 1994;90:1056; 1994;89:1329; Lancet 1994;334:1383); reducing cholesterol may be hazardous (BMJ 1994;308:373)
- Exercise (Jama 1995;273:402) decreases hospitalizations (J Am Geriatr Soc 1996;44:113); maximum heart rate: M = 220 − Age, F = 224 − 0.6 × Age; because maximal inotropic and chronotropic response to catecholamine and sympathetic nervous system is markedly impaired w age
- ASA: 85–325 mg qd (Med Let Drugs Ther 1995;37:14; Arch IM 1995;155:1386)
- Diet that produces LDL <100 induces plaque regression (Lancet 1994;344:1383); "Mediterranean diet" helps (Lancet 1994; 343:1454); Ornish program leads to disease regression, 8% improvement angiogram vs 28% worsening without diet (Jama

1998;280:2001); however, low fat diet may reduce HDL; diet and exercise combined with weight loss may increase HDL; caution dietary changes in pts at risk for malnutrition
- Diet <30% fat, <7% saturated fat, <200 mg chol/d; then HMG-CoA reductase inhibitor; nicotinic acid 1.5–3.0 gm/d (lowers triglycerides, increases HDL) (Am Fam Phys 1997;55:2250); estrogen replacement decreases ASHD incidents in women by up to 50% (Jama 1995;273:199); alcohol at 2–3 drinks qd decreases mortality by 25% (Am J Pub Hlth 1993;83:805); perhaps vit E, an antioxidant, prevents LDL oxidation and decreases ASHD 40% (Nejm 1993;328:1444,1450; Am Heart J 1994;128:1333)
- Folate 400 mg/d, B_6 3 mg/d to treat increased homocystinemia which leads to atherosclerosis (Jama 1998;279:359)
- Estrogen/progesterone reduces risk by 50% (Jama 1995;273:199,240); perhaps medroxyprogesterone to increase HDL cholesterol in postmenopausal females (Nejm 1981;304:560); in a blinded multicenter trial estrogen did not decrease coronary events in women w preexisting CAD (Jama 1998;280:605)
- Raloxifene 60 mg/d (selective estrogen receptor modulator w estrogen agonist) many have good effects on bone and antagonist effects of breast and uterus and bad effects on LDL-C, fibrinogen, and HDL-C2 (Jama 1998;278:1445)
- Preop assessment of cardiac risks:
Clinical variables: <6 mo s/p MI, advanced age, h/o angina, non-Q-wave MI, DM, HT, ventricular ectopy requiring rx; asx pts w bradycardia or chronic bifascicular block do not need prophylactic pacing
Preop angioplasty in pts w >3 clinical variables and dipyridamole thallium test that demonstrates either redistribution or EKG changes associated w dipyridamole infusion; if 1–2 clinical variables and pos thallium, risk of having cardiac event (unstable angina, MI, pulmonary edema, cardiac death) increased from 3.0% to 30% (Nejm 1996;344:1311)
61% of MIs in 1st wk postop are silent

ANGINA

Am Fam Phys 1994;49:1459; Mod Concepts Cardiovasc Dis
1988;57:19; Nejm 1984;310:1712

Cause: Atherosclerotic heart disease; myopathic disorders; mitral valve
prolapse; reduced vasodilator reserve in coronary arteries (Nejm
1993;328:1659,1706); mental stress is as good an inducer of angina
as exercise (Nejm 1988;318:1005)

Epidem: Silent ischemia: coexistent w angina; potential benefit of
β-blockers, calcium channel blockers, coronary revascularization
(J Am Geriatr Soc 1996;44:83)

Pathophys: Spasm may occur even when there is no fixed lesion;
unstable angina usually due to a platelet thrombus (Nejm
1992;326:287)

Sx: Onset with first exercise after rest; more frequently in unfamiliar
settings; worse supine; relieved by TNG (r/o esophageal spasm)

Si: S_4; mitral regurgitant murmur during pain

Crs: Prognosis depends on extent of coronary involvement evidenced by
angiography and LV function (Circ 1994;90:2645); C-reactive protein
may predict early mortality from acute ischemia (J Am Coll Cardiol
1998;31:4160)

Cmplc: MI

R/o esophageal reflux (which can mimic) (Ann IM 1992;117:824),
PUD, biliary colic, pleurisy, pancreatitis, pulmonary infarct,
pneumothorax (Geriatrics 1995;50:33); consider carbon monoxide
induction if onset at home in winter (Nejm 1995;322:48)

Lab:

Chemistry: CPK-MB may elevate mildly

Noninvasive: ETT contraindicated in CHF, aortic stenosis, IHSS,
unstable angina; cannot interpret ST changes in face of LBBB, WPW,
digoxin, LVH; submaximal test (<85% maximal pulse achieved)

- Depressions (from 0.5 mm to >2 mm and start in first 3 min or last
≥8 min) (Nejm 1979;301:230) and/or hypotension during ETT; this
scoring system predicts 5-yr survival and annual mortality (Nejm
1991;325:849)
- Thallium scan at peak exercise and 2–4 h later a better predictor
of long-term outcome than ETT or Holter (Ann IM 1990;113:575);
dipyridamole (Persantin) used when pt cannot walk on treadmill

- Echocardiogram w dobutamine stress (Am J Cardiol 1993;72:605); about same sens and specif as dipyridamole thallium

Rx:
- ASA 75–325 mg po qd prevents MIs

Antianginal Meds: (Med Let Drugs Ther 1994;36:111)

Nitrates to dilate, reduce spasms, increase collaterals and decrease platelet adhesion; po, sl, buccal patch or paste; tolerance develops so avoid hs or 24-h rx

β-Blockers decrease pulse, block action of sympathetic nervous system caused by mental stress (Circ 1994;89:762), lower BP, decrease platelet adhesion; avoid in Prinzmetal type because can increase spasm

Calcium channel blockers dilate, reduce spasm

Imipramine 50-mg po hs helps microvascular

Surgical:

Angioplasty (Nejm 1994;331:1037,1044; 1994;330:981) preferred in severely symptomatic pt w 1- or 2-vessel CAD and nl LV EF w multiple medical problems; increased risk for stroke w CABG because of cerebrovascular disease or diffuse aortic disease; increased risk for developing postop cognitive dysfunction or frail physical condition; more complications than medical rx (Nejm 1992;326:10); angioplasty long term requires more antianginal med and surgical interventions than CABG (Nejm 1994;331:1037)

CABG increases survival significantly (Circ 1994;89:2015; Lancet 1994;344:563); preferred in high-risk symptomatic elderly (even age >80 yr; Ann IM 1990;113:423) w left main artery disease, in pts w significant 3-vessel disease with EF >30% (Nejm 1988;319:332; 1987;316:981), in pts w significant 2-vessel disease, decreased LV EF and proximal left anterior descending artery disease, in pts w clinical evidence of heart failure during ischemic episodes w ischemic but viable myocardium w few other medical problems, younger physiologic age and in pts who are prepared for 3–4 mo convalescence; diabetic pts do better w CABG than angioplasty (Nejm 1996;335:1290)

If unstable angina: ASA 75–325 po qd (Nejm 1992;327:175) in men (Nejm 1983;309:396); heparin alone or better with TNG (Nejm 1988;319:1105) (see tirofiban (Aggrastat))

If silent ischemia: Angioplasty (J Am Coll Cardiol 1994;24:11), atenolol (Circ 1994;90:762)

CARDIOLOGY

MYOCARDIAL INFARCTION

J Am Geriatr Soc 1998;46:1157,1302; Am J Med 1992;43:315

Cause: Atherosclerotic (85%) including spasm; emboli 15% (Ann IM 1978;88:155)

Epidem: Increased incidence with h/o:

- Surgical menopause pts not placed on estrogen; but no sharp increase if natural menopause or put on estrogen (Nejm 1987;316:1105)
- Smoking increases risk 3 times, but risk decreases to normal over 2 yr after stopping (Nejm 1985;313:1511); increases risk 5 times if >1 ppd, 2 times if 1–4 cigarettes qd in women (Nejm 1987;317:1303)
- Elevations of total and/or LDL cholesterol (often with cholecystitis hx) (Nejm 1981;304:1396)
- Diabetic, hypertensive women at higher risk for MI (F = 23%, M = 15%) and mortality rate as high as 46%
- HT
- Myocardium at more risk secondary to comorbidities: decreased HR variability, reduced vagal tone makes elderly pt more at risk for sudden death w MI
- Decreased incidence with exercise >6 METS >2 h/wk divided 3–4 × wk (Nejm 1994;330:1549); 2–3 alcoholic drinks qd (Nejm 1993;329:1829; Ann IM 1991;114:967)
- Elderly under-treated and lidocaine overused (Arch IM 1996; 156:805)

Pathophys: Platelet aggregations and thrombi (Nejm 1990;322:1549); early morning increase in catecholamine-induced platelet aggregation and decrease in plasminogen activator inhibitor type 1 contribute to thrombogenesis (J Am Coll Cardiol 1993;22:1228); myocardial damage severe because of long-standing HT, DM, valvular disease associated w LV damage, ongoing electrical instability, multivessel CAD and ischemia, reduced diastolic compliance, increased vascular resistance increasing cardiac workload

Sx: Chest pain, substernal, in "distribution of a tree," worse supine; diaphoresis, dyspnea; associated with heavy exertion

50% >60 yr present with CNS sx especially confusion; silent MI more common in the elderly, 15–20% of MIs; DM often the cause; might also be due to increased myocardial collateral circulation from gradual coronary artery narrowing (J Am Geriatr Soc 1994;42:732)

Si: Elderly may present w flash pulmonary edema, arrhythmia, sudden drop in BP, delirium, sudden weakness; in pts who have dementia or language barrier any pain in torso could be MI; can present w abdominal pain and vertigo as well; toothache

Pericardial rub on day 2+, usually without ST changes (Nejm 1984;311:1211); S_4 gallop; fever <103°F (39.4°C); transient S_2 paradoxical split (Geriatrics 1995;50:2)

RV infarct syndrome (Nejm 1994;330:1211) more common in elderly, mortality 75% (Circ 1997;96:436); acute inferior MI, high CVP with low PAPs and PCWPs

Rectal exam important for guaiac and detection of BPH so do not omit on admission physical

Crs: 42% are "silent" and unrecognized (Ann IM 1995;122:96); non-Q-wave MI 10% hospital mortality, 36% 1-yr mortality, 23% develop afib, 53% develop CHF (Am J Cardiol 1995;75:187); TIMI III registry: most severe CAD, least likely to get angiography and most likely to have the most adverse outcomes from disease both in hospital and at 6 wk (Jama 1996;275:1104)

Cmplc: Mortality 4+ times higher in elderly because do not go to the ER as quickly (J Am Geriatr Soc 1999;47:151; Ann IM 1997;126:593; Circ 1995;92:1133)

- Shock (7.5%) (Nejm 1991;325:1117)
- Arrhythmias
- Rupture of septal wall more frequent in elderly than younger pts
- Pericardial tamponade (r/o RV infarct)
- Aneurysm, occurs in 40% with anterior MI, develops in first 48 h, leads to emboli, CHF, and PVCs
- Mural thrombi without aneurysm in 11% of anterior MIs, 2% of others (J Am Coll Cardiol 1993;22:1004)
- Dressler syndrome
- Papillary muscle rupture causes CHF
- Heart block (Mod Concepts Cardiovasc Dis 1976;45:129) occurs in 5% of inferior MIs, 3% of anterior MIs, and in 100% with anterior MI w RBBB causing 75% mortality
- Excessive adrenergic tone: analgesia and sedation appropriate, β-blockers should be considered (Am Heart J 1994;9:1)
- Atrial flutter: if electrical cardioversion unsuccessful, use procainamide; can use sotalol (β-blocker) with no arrhythmic effect

- CHF: rx systolic dysfunction with dobutamine for positive inotropic effect

Lab:

Chemistry: Enzymes (Ann IM 1986;105:221):

- Troponin released into circulation after all death, elevated within 4–6 h 10–15 d; total CPK and/or fractions up in 12 h, peak at 2 d, last 4 d; CPK-MB rise during 1st 6 h after onset of pain has 95% sens and specif and may be used for early r/o MI in ER (Nejm 1994;331:561,607); total CPK correlates with MI size, but may not be as elevated in the elderly (Mayo Clin Proc 1996;71:184)
- LDH and fractions (isoenzymes 4 and 5) increased; r/o renal and red cell source
- AST (SGOT) up in 24 h, peaks at 2–4 d, lasts up to 7 d
- Cardiac troponin I elevation is specific to myocardium, useful perioperatively when surgery may increase CPK (Nejm 1994; 330:670)

EKG: See Table 8-3; non-Q-wave MI more common in the elderly (Mayo Clin Proc 1996;71:184); T-inversions: r/o acute cholecystitis (Ann IM 1992;116:218); in RV infarct, these changes are present in V_3–V_6R, especially V_4R w 80+% sens and specif (Nejm 1993; 328:981); new RBBB indicates occlusion of anterior descending proximal to 1st septal branch (Nejm 1993;328:1036); >10 PVCs/h associated with a 10+% 1-yr mortality (Nejm 1983;309:331)

ETT: (Nejm 1999;340:340) contraindicated in CHF, aortic stenosis, IHSS, unstable angina; cannot interpret ST changes in face of LBBB, WPW, digoxin, LVH, or lack of changes w submaximal test (<85% maximal pulse achieved)

Nuclear (Sestamibi or thallium) scan at peak exercise and 2–4 h later better predictor of long-term outcome than ETT or Holter (Jama 1966;277:318)

Non-exertional testing w dipyridamole (Persantine), dobutamine, arbutamine (Med Let 1998;40:19) as good as ETT; may need in elderly w arthritis, COPD, who may not be able to accomplish ETT

Angiography Indications: CHF, LV dysfunction (EF <50%); high-risk noninvasive test results; persistent sx, failure of medical rx; previous angioplasty, CABG, or MI; malignant ventricular arrhythmia; contraindications: very elderly; significant risk of bleeding; coexisting medical problems, eg, liver disease, terminal condition; do not need in uncomplicated non-Q-wave MI (Nejm 1999;388:785)

Table 8-3. EKG Changes in MI

Area	Leads	Findings	Artery
Anterior	V_3, V_4	Q, ST elevation, T inversion	Left anterior descending
Anterior septal	V_1, V_2	Q, ST elevation, T inversion	"Watershed"
Anterior lateral	V_4–V_6	Q, ST elevation, T inversion	"Watershed"
Lateral	I, aVL, V_5, V_6	Q, ST elevation, T inversion	L coronary
Inferior	II, III, aVF	Q, ST elevation, T inversion	R coronary
Posterior	V_1, V_2	Tall broad R, ST depression, tall T	Associated w inferior
RV	V_1, V_2	ST elevation	Associated w inferior

Rx:

Prophylactic Interventions: ASA (see 8.2 Coronary Artery Disease); stopping smoking decreases risk to baseline in 3 yr (Nejm 1990;322:213); lowering cholesterol helps (meta-analysis) (Nejm 1990;323:1112); atorvastatin best (J Am Coll Cardiol 1998;32:665), as does American Heart Association diet (BMJ 1992;304:1015)

- 60–70% of coronary deaths due to acute MI before arrival hospital; pre-hospital thrombolysis important (Am Heart J 1992;123:181); aggressive rx of acute MI w angiography, angioplasty
- CABG of minimal benefit (J Am Coll Cardiol 1995;25:47A; Jama 1994;272:859) vs CABG beneficial (J Am Coll Cardiol 1994;24:425)

Coronary Care unit (CCU):

- Oxygen only when objective evidence of desaturation (AHCPR Pub. No. 94-0602); ASA 325 mg po stat
- β-Blockers help older post-MI pt (J Am Geriatr Soc 1995;43:751; Am J Cardiol 1994;4:674); adverse outcome of underuse of β-blockers in elderly survivors of MI (Nejm 1998;339:489,551; Jama 1997;227:115)
- β-Blocker rx (metoprolol 5 mg IV q 5 min × 3, then 50 mg po bid × 1 d, then 100 mg bid or atenolol 50–100 mg po qd) if no

CARDIOLOGY

contraindications helps prevent recurrent MIs (Circ 1994;90:762); mortality reduction 40% in elderly (Am J Med 1992;93:315)

- Diltiazem for non-Q-wave MI (60–90 mg po qid)
- Captopril 50 mg tid, if ETT is impaired to <40% (Ann IM 1994;21:750; Nejm 1992;327:669) or acutely × 6 wk for all (Lancet 1994;343:1115) or at least for anterior MI (Nejm 1995;332:80), ages 55–74 yr (Circ 1998;97:2202)
- TNG rx (IV if volume ok) goal to decrease systolic BP by 10%; excessive reduction in BP may result in extension of infarct (Mayo Clin Proc 1996;71:184)
- Heparin does not reduce mortality in old AMI pts (J Am Coll Cardiol 1998;31:964) except if large AMI, where can reduce risk of mural thrombus, emboli, severe CHF, afib, recurrent ischemia in first few days (J Am Geriatr Soc 1999;47:271; J Am Coll Cardiol 1996;28:328; Lancet 1994;343:311)
- Lovenox better than Lopurin for non-Q-wave MI (Nejm 1997; 337:447)
- Thrombolytics: several studies support the efficacy in pts >65 yr (ISIS-2, GISSI, ASSET, AIMS), but age distribution skewed in these studies (<20% in pts >75 yr) (J Am Geriatr Soc 1994;42:127); contraindications: active internal bleeding, aortic dissection within 10 d, prolonged traumatic CPR, hemorrhagic CVA within last 2 mo, head trauma, intracranial neoplasia, retinopathy, persistent uncontrollable HT; relative contraindications: diabetic retinopathy, prolonged need for CPR; streptokinase preferred over TPA (60% increase risk of cerebral bleeds); ASA+ thrombolytic rx better for survival (ISIS-2), ischemia × 30 min within 6–12 h w 1–2 mm ST elevation in >2 leads or presence of LBBB, also w >12 h if BP decreased or cardiogenic shock, particularly in elderly who present late; risk/benefit high in IMI (J Am Geriatr Soc 1998;46:1157; Circulation 2000;101:2239); primary angioplasty comparable if not superior results compared to thrombolytic rx if not delayed (Nejm 1999;341:1413)
- Intravenous monoclonal antibody and peptide and nonapeptide antagonists of GPIIb/IIIa receptor (the final common pathway in platelet aggregation) (Jama 1999;281:1407): use in pts w non-ST-elevation acute coronary syndromes w positive troponin (Jama 2000;284:876); IIb/IIIa inhibitors: coronary stenting plus IIb/IIIa (abciximab ReoPro) leads to a greater degree of myocardial salvage and a better clinical outcome than do fibrinolytics w IIb/IIIa

inhibitors (abciximab) but antithrombin rx is still required (Am J Cardiol 2000;85:32C); PURSUIT Trial showed that bleeding more common in IIb/IIIa (eptifibatide (Integrilin)) group but no increase in incidence of hemorrhagic stroke (Nejm 1998;339:436); tirofiban (Aggrastat) as part of triple drug rx of unstable angina (Nejm 1998;338:1488,1498,1539)

- ACE inhibitor (Jama 1995;273:1450; Nejm 1995;332:80) beginning 3 d after MI w EF <40%, captopril 6.25 q 6–8 h, stop if hypotensive; diltiazem for non-Q-wave MI if no LVH or CHF

Rehab: Depression in CCU s/p MI: 10%, 3–4 times increase in mortality rate in 6 mo if persists; return to work part-time in 4–6 wk (Barker LR, et al., eds. Principles of ambulatory medicine. Baltimore: Williams & Wilkins, 1995:712); if can walk 100 m without angina or dyspnea, can do air travel 10 d after MI (Dardick K. Travel medicine—what the family physician should know. 16th Annual family practice review. St. Petersburg, FL: Bayfront Medical Center, 1994); lifestyle changes, then thiazides, then β-blockers? (Jama 1994;272:842; Hypertension 1994;23:275)

Post-MI: (J Am Geriatr Soc 1998;46:1459)

- β-blocker indefinitely regardless of whether HT present
- Cholesterol reduction after MI benefits elderly of both sexes (Circ 1997;96:4211); keep LDL <100 w simvastatin (Circ 1997;95:1683)
- ASA 160–325 mg indefinitely (Circ 1996;94:2341)
- Warfarin INR 2.0–3.0 for persistent afib, LV thrombus
- Calcium channel blockers if persistent angina despite nitrates, β-blockers
- Nitrates: increase gradually, isosorbide dinitrate po to 30–40 mg tid or 60 mg dose isosorbide-mononitrate qd, nitrate-free period = 12 h (Nejm 1987;316:1440); β-blocker can be given during nitrate-free period
- No antiarrhythmics except β-blocker
- Implantable cardioverter-defibrillator for VF, VT, high risk sudden cardiac death (Nejm 1996;335:1933)
- Hormone replacement: debatable as secondary prevention (Jama 1998;280:605; Nejm 1996;335:453; Jama 1995;273:119; Circ 1994;89:2545)
- CABG 73% success rate vs PTCA 89% success rate
- Dipyridamole thallium after MI independent predictor of outcome (J Am Geriatr Soc 1999;47:295)

CARDIOLOGY

8.3 CONGESTIVE HEART FAILURE

Clin Ger Med 2000;16:407; Am J Cardiol 1999;83:9A; Cardiol Clin 1999;17:123; J Am Geriatr Soc 1998;46:525; 1995;43:1035; www.acc.org/clinical/guidelines/failure

Cause:

Systolic: Dilated cardiomyopathy (10% >65 yr old, due to ischemia, infarction, HT, MR, chronic ethanol abuse, idiopathic); high output failure (chronic anemia, hyperthyroidism, thiamine deficiency, AV shunting) (J Am Geriatr Soc 1997;45:972)

Diastolic: Hypertrophic cardiomyopathy (CAD and HT account for >70% of all heart failure cases; also consider calcific AS, DM, and hypertensive hypertrophic cardiomyopathy, which is more common in elderly women); restrictive cardiomyopathy, especially due to senile amyloid deposition (J Am Geriatr Soc 1997;45:972)

Precipitating Factors: Noncompliance with meds and/or diet most common cause; also excessive fluid intake, arrhythmias; iatrogenic: β-blockers, calcium channel blockers, NSAIDs, estrogen, corticosteroids, clonidine (J Am Geriatr Soc 1997;45:972)

Epidem: Prevalence increases 2 times every decade after 45 yrs so that prevalence in adults >80 yr old approaches 10% (J Am Geriatr Soc 1997;45:968); fewer than 30% elderly survive 6 yrs after first hospitalization for CHF (Clin Ger Med 2000;16:407); diastolic dysfunction much more prevalent in elders, accounting for up to 47% of elder pts with heart failure (J Am Geriatr Soc 1997;45:1132)

The nl EF in elderly = 50–60% (Cur Probl Cardiol 1987;12:1); at autopsy, 50% pts with CHF did not have CAD (Mayo Clin Proc 1988;63:552); diastolic CHF in absence of CAD has low mortality; single marital status correlated w death from CHF (Am J Cardiol 1997;78:1640); atrial natriuretic hormone level predictive of mortality (J Am Geriatr Soc 1998;46:453)

Pathophys: In general, four principal changes in cardiovascular system with aging diminish heart's ability to respond to stress:

1. Reduced responsiveness to β-adrenergic stimulation limit heart rate, contractility, $β_2$-mediated vasodilation
2. Increased vascular stiffness, increased afterload
3. Increased heart stiffness, impaired diastolic filling, increased resting atrial, and ventricular pressures increase preload

4. Decreased mitochondrial ability to respond to increased demand for ATP (J Am Geriatr Soc 1997;45:969)

Systolic (EF <40–45%): inadequately contracting ventricle resulting from and contributing to several factors, often additive in vicious cycle:

1. Increased afterload: increased arterial tone due to increased sympathetic tone and increased activation of renin-angiotensin-aldosterone system (RAAS)
2. Increased preload: increased venous tone which shifts blood from periphery to central circulation, increasing venous return to heart; also, failing ventricle has decreased cardiac output, decreased renal blood flow, increased sodium absorption by proximal tubule, and increased activation of RAAS
3. Hypertrophy and dilatation of heart: response to chronic pressure and volume overload or to post-MI remodeling of infarcted area; hypertrophied muscle operates at lower inotropic state than normal muscle; postulated that angiotensin II, aldosterone, and catecholamines may all directly promote deterioration of the heart
4. Atrial natriuretic peptide (ANP): released in response to atrial stretch, ANP increases GFR, natriuresis, and diuresis, while suppressing release of aldosterone, vasopressin, renin; levels of ANP may be depressed in some pts with heart failure

Diastolic (EF ≥45%): impaired capacity of ventricle to fill is much more common in older pts due to impaired ventricular relaxation, increased myocardial stiffness, increased end-diastolic pressures

Sx: Must distinguish systolic from diastolic dysfunction, as this will determine rx:
- Systolic: fatigue, sx of prerenal azotemia, cool skin, mental obtundation, anxiety, insomnia, nightmares, anorexia, nausea; orthopnea, PND may not occur due to compensatory pulmonary vasculature changes; pts may present initially with only dry cough (J Am Geriatr Soc 1997;45:1129)
- Diastolic: increased filling pressures cause congestion, exercise intolerance

Si: JVD more reliable than peripheral edema in the elderly; classic sx such as pulmonary and peripheral edema occur late in disease and are neither sens nor specif in elderly (J Am Geriatr Soc 1997;45:1129); rales lower half of lung not always CHF; need echocardiography (Jama 1994;271:1277); tachypnea; resting tachycardia uncommon; murmurs and gallops may be difficult to detect; S_4 very nonspecif in

Table 8-4. New York Heart Association Functional Classification of Cardiovascular Disability

Class	Characteristics	Annual Mortality
I	Asymptomatic LV dysfunction	<5%
II	Slight limitation of physical activity	10–20%
III	Marked limitation of physical activity	10–20%
IV	Inability to carry on any physical activity without discomfort	>40%

Source: New York Heart Association.

elderly and may simply reflect age-related diastolic dysfunction; pulse contour abnormalities obscure due to stiff vessels (J Am Geriatr Soc 1997;45:1129)

Crs: Elderly pts with systolic dysfunction have higher mortality at 16 and 23 mo than pts with diastolic dysfunction (J Am Geriatr Soc 1995;43:1038); 28% mortality elderly men; 6-min walk test provides independent prognostic data in pts w LV dysfunction (Jama 1993;270:1702); new LVH new CHF (J Am Geriatr Soc 1998;46:1280); wide pulse pressure >67 mmHg 55% increased risk of CHF (Jama 1999;281:634); shift in differential WBC (decreased lymphocytes) poor px CHF (activation of sympathetic nervous system) (Circ 1998;97:19)

Px most closely related to extent of impairment in ejection fraction, degree of ventricular dilatation, and decrease in LV sphericity

See Table 8-4

Lab: CBC, U/A, lytes, BUN, Cr, glu, calcium, magnesium, phosphorus, albumin, TSH in pts with afib and unexplained heart failure (J Am Coll Cardiol 1995;26:1376)

Noninvasive Studies: Systolic and Diastolic: echocardiography in all cases to assess ventricle size and function, atrial size, valvular function, pericardium; EKG evidence of LV dysfunction due to CAD, eg, Q waves, LVH; CXR, though cardiomegaly need not be present and pulmonary congestion may be subtle or absent in elderly pts (Cardiol Clin 1999;17:125); noninvasive stress testing to detect ischemic myocardium for pts without angina but with high probability of CAD who would be candidates for revascularization (J Am Coll Cardiol 1995;26:1376); also must assess functional capacity, including physical capacity, emotional status, social function, cognitive factors (J Am Coll Cardiol 1995;26:1376)

Table 8-5. Initial and Maintenance Doses of ACE Inhibitors and Other Drugs for CHF in Older Persons

Drug	Initial Dose	Maintenance Dose
Captopril	6.25 mg tid	50 mg tid
Enalapril	2.5 mg qd	20 mg qd
Lisinopril	2.5 mg qd	20 mg qd
Quinapril	5 mg qd	5 mg bid
Ramipril	2.5 mg qd	5 mg bid
Losartan		50 mg qd
Hydralazine		300 mg qd
Isosorbide Dinitrate		120–160 mg qd
Carvedilol	3.125 mg bid	25–50 mg bid

Note: Contraindications to ACE Inhibitors: Symptomatic hypotension, progressive azotemia, intolerable cough, angioneurotic edema, hyperkalemia; cautious use of ACE inhibitor if BP <90, K >5.5, Cr >3.0 (Jags 1998;46:545).
Adapted from Cardiol Clin 1999;17:123 and J Am Geriatr Soc 1997;45:1252.

Invasive Studies: Coronary revascularization shown to be beneficial in pts with both ischemia and LV systolic dysfunction; consider arteriography in pts with angina and CHF to assess suitability for revascularization (J Am Coll Cardiol 1995;26:1376)

Rx: Major trials include: VHeFTI (Nejm 1986;314:1547); CONSENSUS I (Nejm 1987;316:1429); The SAVE Trial (Nejm 1992;327:669); The SOLVD Prevention Trial (Nejm 1992;327:685); CONSENSUS II (Nejm 1992;327:678); VHeFT II (Nejm 1991;325:303); CONSENSUS Trial (Nejm 1987;316:1429; AIRE (Lancet 1993; 342:821); ELITE (Lancet 1997;349:747); DIG (Nejm 1997;336: 525); CIBIS II (Lancet 1999;353:9); MERiT-HF (Lancet 1999;353: 2001); HOPE (Nejm 2000;342:145); PRAISE (Nejm 1996;335: 1107)

See Table 8-5 for recommended doses

Systolic:

Asymptomatic = Class I

- ACE-inhibitors attenuate progressive LV dysfunction post MI by inhibiting remodeling; 19% mortality reduction w captopril in post-MI pts with EF <40% but without overt heart failure (Nejm 1992;327:685); use of IV enalapril directly after MI not recommended (Nejm 1992;327:678)

- Use diuretic only if pt has peripheral edema or mild jugular venous distention despite sodium restriction; thiazide should suffice (J Am Coll Cardiol 1995;26:10)
- Dietary Na^+ 2–3 gm/d (J Am Geriatr Soc 1998;46:525)
- Prolonged bed rest dangerous; exercise helps: 4 h/wk at 75% maximum heart rate in home walking program (Ann IM 1996;124:1051; Jama 1994;272:1389)
- Oxygen rx helps

Mild = Class II

- ACE inhibitors help all pts with symptomatic heart failure (Lancet 1993;342:821; Nejm 1991;325:303; Nejm 1987;316:1429)
- Diuretics 1st line rx to decrease venous return and filling pressures, reduce congestion and edema (may need thiazide + loop, or potassium-sparing thiazide + loop; may even have to try metolazone + loop; if BUN is increased, then must curtail diuretic rx)
- Carvedilol (nonselective β-blocker, also blocks receptors) + ACE inhibitor reduced clinical progression of mildly symptomatic heart failure, but start at low dose (Circ 1996;94:2800)

Mild–moderate = Class II–III

- Continue diuretics as above
- Enalapril decreases mortality by 28% in Class II–III pts; reduces afterload, enhances myocardial shortening, increase stroke volume (Nejm 1991;325:303)
- Angiotensin II receptor blockers: if unable to tolerate ACE because of cough, rash, altered taste try angiotensin II type I receptor antagonist such as losartan (J Am Geriatr Soc 1996;46:545); losartan shown to have fewer adverse effects than captopril (Lancet 1997;349:747), though may have decreased efficacy; thus use only as alternative to ACE
- Nitrates and hydralazine: isosorbide dinitrate (reduces preload) and hydralazine (reduces afterload) also recommended for pts with Class II–III failure who cannot tolerate ACE due to cough or increased creatinine (Nejm 1991;325:303); if pt has low cardiac output and pre-renal azotemia, try hydralazine only (Sci Am 1998;2:12); hydralazine protects against tolerance of the hemodynamic effects of TNG, so use in combination in CHF (Cardiology 1995;26:1575)
- Digoxin decreases hospitalizations and deaths due to heart failure, but not overall mortality, with greatest effect in pts with EF <25% and in Class III (Nejm 1997;336:525); appropriate serum levels in elderly range from 0.5–1.3 ng/mL

- β-Blockers: in addition to ACE, diuretic, ± dig, bisoprolol (selective $β_1$-blocker) decreased all-cause mortality, with greatest effect in Class III heart failure pts (Lancet 1999;353:9); metoprolol also reduced all-cause mortality by 38% (Lancet 1999:353–2001

- Calcium channel blockers: short-acting such as nifedipine, diltiazem, and verapamil not used in CHF pts with abnormal EF because may exacerbate CHF (Circ 1990;82:1954); recent trials of amlodipine indicated decreased mortality in pts with non-ischemic cardiomyopathy (Nejm 1996;335:1107); use only in pts with abnormal EF if needed to control HT or angina and then use only amlodipine or felodipine (Cardiol Clin 1999;17:128)

Severe = Class IV

- Diuretics, ACE-inhibitors, angiotensin II receptor blockers, digoxin, nitrates, and hydralazine as above

- Spironolactone in low doses decreases hospitalization and mortality in pts with severe heart failure already taking ACE inhibitor, loop diuretic, and in most cases digoxin (Med Let 1999;41:81; Nejm 1999;341:709)

- β-Blockers not recommended in pts with Class IV heart failure (Am J Cardiol 1999;83:20A); carvedidol of benefit (Nejm 2001;344:1651)

Diastolic:

- Paucity of large-scale randomized controlled trials in pharmacologic rx of diastolic dysfunction (Nejm 2001;344:17,56)

- Diuretics, nitrates: goal is to enhance effective ventricular filling; very sensitive to preload reduction, eg, nitrates, diuretics can make worse, so start with small doses (J Am Geriatr Soc 1997;45:1252)

- ACE inhibitors: rx HT with ACE and it will decrease LVH by 15%; ACE promotes filling by reduction of venous and arterial tone, regression LVH and interstitial fibrosis, attenuation coronary vasoconstriction (J Am Geriatr Soc 1995;42:1040); ramipril reduces mortality in pts without low EF or heart failure, but who are at high risk due to DM, HT, elevated cholesterol, tobacco use (Nejm 2000;342:151)

- Direct-acting angiotensin II receptor antagonist (ATA) losartan improves exercise capacity and quality of life in pts w diastolic dysfunction perhaps by blocking the increase of circulating angiotensin II during exercise (J Am Coll Cardiol 1999;33:567)

- Calcium channel blocker verapamil helps to decrease afterload, regress LVH, enhances ventricular relaxation, and gives improved exercise tolerance in pts with hypertrophic cardiomyopathy (J Am Geriatr Soc 1995;43:1039; Am J Cardiol 1990;66:981)
- β-Blockers slow rate and promote ventricular filling, thereby increasing stroke volume and reducing symptoms (Cardiol Clin 1999;17:129); β-blockers also effective anti-ischemic agents and reduce LVH (Am J Cardiol 1997;80:207); propranolol + ACE + diuretics decreased mortality and increased LVEF in pts >80 yr with CHF, normal systolic function, and prior MI (Am J Cardiol 1997;80:207)
- Digoxin in pts with EF >45% had no effect on overall mortality, but did reduce hospitalizations and deaths due to heart failure (Nejm 1997;336:525)

Miscellaneous:

- Warfarin indicated in pts with afib, rheumatic mitral valve disease, mechanical prosthetic valves, or prior thromboembolic events (Chest 1995;108(suppl):225S); older pts are at risk for increased bleeding complications
- Revascularize if absence of comorbid disease (renal failure, pulmonary disease, CVD, EF <20%, life expectancy <1 yr); potential benefit highest w severe limiting angina or angina equivalent (J Am Geriatr Soc 1998;46:545)
- Triple-drug rx (ACE, diuretics, digoxin) instead of initial stepped care (J Am Coll Cardiol 1998;32:686)

Nonpharmacologic Rx: Interdisciplinary team to address issues of pt education, prognosis, diet consultation, lipid lowering agent if hyperlipidemic; dietary supplementation in elderly heart failure patients (Clin Ger Med 2000;16:480); med review, social services, daily weight chart, support stockings, activity prescription and follow-up reduces hospitalization, improves quality of life, and decreases costs; cardiac rehab activity should emphasize duration and not intensity of activity; supervision of activity initially recommended for those with Class III–IV failure (Cardiol Clin 1999;17:130)

8.4 SYNCOPE

Cardiol Clin 1997;15:295; Ger Rev Syllabus 1996:221; Geriatrics 1995;50:24; Sci Am Med 1995:1; Clin Ger Med 2001;7:9–12

Cause: Unlike in younger pts, syncope is usually multifactorial: occurs usually in the setting of multiple medical problems, medications and age-related physiologic impairments
1. Cardiac: (associated w 20–30% 1 yr mortality rates vs 5% for noncardiac syncope)
   • Electrical: vtach, afib, tachy or bradyarrhythmias (Stokes-Adams-Morgagni)
   • Mechanical: aortic stenosis (most common) with decreased preload or arrhythmia, pulmonary HT
   • MI: ~6% present as syncope
   • Hypertrophic obstructive cardiomyopathy: pts >60 represent 33% of cases
2. Medications: antihypertensives, nitrates, diuretics, phenothiazines, tricyclics; particularly fluoxetine, acepromazine, haloperidol, L-dopa (J Clin Epidemiol 1999;50:313)
3. Hypotension:
   • Orthostatic: decreased baroreceptor sens, volume depletion, venous pooling
   • Postprandial: pts w HT more at risk for postprandial hypotension (Ann IM 1995;122:286; Circ 1993;89:391)
4. Reflex-mediated:
   • Vasovagal: pain, fatigue, fear
   • Situational: cough, defecation, micturition: 3+ voidings per night in men associated with 1.9 times mortality rate over 54 months (BJU Int 1999;84:297)
   • Carotid sinus hypersensitivity R > L; commonly in males >60
5. Endocrine:
   • Diabetes: autonomic instability, hypoglycemic crisis, osmotic diuresis with dehydration
   • Addison disease, chronic adrenal suppression
6. Other:
   • Cerebrovascular (arteriosclerotic vascular disease, carotid-basilar artery steal, subclavian steal) (J Cardiovasc Surg 1994;35:11); subarachnoid hemorrhage

CARDIOLOGY

- Psychiatric (rare): panic, MDD
- Shy-Drager
- Pulmonary embolism
- Billowing mitral valve
- CNS tumor
- Pheochromocytoma
- Carcinoid
- Sepsis
- Deconditioning, starvation
- Positional

Epidem: Annual incidence 6% in the elderly

Sx:

- Cardiac: premonitory symptoms are usually absent; possible palpitations, dyspnea, angina
- Vasovagal: nausea, fatigue, dimming vision, diaphoresis, dizziness upon wakening
- TIA: diplopia, dysphagia, confusion after episode
- Symptoms are not useful for risk stratifying pts w unexplained syncope (Arch IM 1999;159:375)

Si: Orthostatic BP from lying or sitting to standing after 1 min; positive if P increased >30, and/or systolic BP decreased >20 mmHg (Jama 1999;281:1022)

Carotid sinus massage w EKG only if no carotid bruits—if after 5 sec, produces 3-sec asystole or drop in systolic BP of 50 mmHg, then carotid sinus hypersensitivity likely etiology; massage should be done in the head-up tilt position if initial supine test neg (Heart 2000;83:22)

Aortic stenosis: murmur (see Table 8-6); delay of carotid artery impulse; observe for signs of trauma

Cmplc: R/o seizures (bowel/bladder incontinence, aura, tongue biting) Fall-related injuries and fx

Lab: History and physical reveal 56–85% of ultimately identifiable causes (Ann IM 1992;268:2553); lab tests generally low yield although CBC w diff, electrolytes, blood glucose, BUN, Cr, drug levels helpful; EKG is indicated in all pts presenting with syncopes; dx infection with CXR, UA

Noninvasive: (Cardiol Clin 1997;15:195)

- Cardiogenic (arrhythmic): monitor 24–48 h (Arch IM 1990; 150:1073); Holter monitoring not helpful because complex ventricular arrhythmias recur despite rx; 50% of pts without significant findings on Holter have recurrence of arrhythmias; poor correlation of symptoms with Holter recorded arrhythmias (Chest 1980;78:456); telemetry rarely diagnostic as most arrhythmias brief, not associated with symptoms (Ann IM 1990;113:53)

- Pt-activated memory loop recorders: useful and cost effective in pts with infrequent episodic syncope with previously negative w/u; records several min before event; implantable loop recorders also available
- Ambulatory BP monitoring: may help detect orthostatic, postprandial, or medication-induced hypotension
- Electrophysiologic studies (EPS): 3–4 yr mortality = 60% w abnormal EPS vs 15% w normal EPS; EF >40% correlates highly w neg EPS (Jama 1992;268:2553)
- Cardiogenic (nonarrhythmic): echocardiogram indicated to w/u aortic stenosis
- Cerebrovascular: carotid US, cerebral angiography in pts who are good surgical candidates; CT not indicated unless focal findings or symptoms of neurologic disease
- Electroencephalogram: minimal value unless pt exhibits focal neurological abnormalities or sx/si of seizures
- Tilt table: helpful for evaluation of recurrent, unexplained syncope in pts without underlying heart disease; positive endpoints are vasovagal symptoms; common protocol is 60 degrees for 45 min; sens 67–83%, specif 75–100% for vasovagal mechanism of syncope (Am J Med Sci 1999;317:110); variable reproducibility (Am J Cardiol 1997;80:1492); can be used to assess therapeutic efficacy

Neurally mediated hypotension (Jama 1995;274:961): strong ventricular contractions may cause via C-fiber induced peripheral dilatation (Ann IM 1991;115:871); brought out w tilt table and isoproterenol infusion; if bradycardia and hypotension occur quickly on tilt alone, may be more sure of dx (Nejm 1993;328:1117)

Rx:
Therapeutic:
- Although most syncope in the elderly is multifactorial, rx should be aimed at reducing specific contributory diseases and processes
- Cardiac (see 8.6 Arrhythmias)
- Cardiac (nonarrhythmic): valve replacement for aortic stenosis
- Neurocardiogenic: rx by avoiding diuretics, vasodilators, and tricyclics; increase salt intake; try fludrocortisone (Florinef),

β-blockers, and anticholinergics like disopyramide (Norpace)
(Jama 1995;274:961) or SSRI like paroxetine 20 mg qd
(J Am Coll Cardiol 1999;33:1227); caffeine no help
- Orthostatic hypotension: elastic stockings, fludrocortisone
0.1 mg/d increasing to as much as 1.0 mg/d
- Medication-induced: document and review pt medications;
consider alternatives or discontinuation

Team Management: Education on physical activities/movements that
bring on syncope and careful discussion of drugs that cause syncope
as side effects

8.5 VALVULAR DISEASE

Ger Rev Syllabus 1991, 1994, 1996
See Table 8-6

8.6 ARRHYTHMIAS

SUPRAVENTRICULAR TACHYARRHYTHMIAS

J Am Geriatr Soc 2000;48:224; Clin Ger Med 1999;15:645; Ger Rev
Syllabus 1996:222; Nejm 1995;332:162; Am Fam Phys
1994;50:959; 1994;49:823,1805; J Am Coll Cardiol 1994;23:916

Cause:
- Afib: associated w HT in 70% of pts; associated w mitral stenosis,
atrial septal defect; also associated with hyperthyroidism or
subclinical hyperthyroidism especially in the elderly (Nejm
1994;331:1252); toxic multinodular goiter present in 20% of
the elderly with afib associated w hyperthyroidism (Med Aud
Dig 1983;30:18); alcoholic myocardiopathy; COPD; CAD; fever;
pericarditis; aflutter and multifocal atrial tachycardia often
(60%) from pulmonary disease including pulmonary emboli
- Supraventricular arrhythmias: hypokalemia, low serum magnesium;
concomitant administration of digoxin and quinidine has 6.5%
complication rate in older population

Table 8-6. Valvular Heart Disease

	Aortic Stenosis	Aortic Insufficiency	Mitral Stenosis	Mitral Regurgitation
Cause	Degenerative valve disease > rheumatic disease; associated w DM, hyperlipidemia; calcific AS age 50–60 yr (50% associated w CAD)	Rheumatic heart disease (mitral disease may also be present); cystic medial necrosis of the aortic root associated w aneurysm of the ascending aorta; HT and renal disease can lead to fenestrations of the valve	Rheumatic heart disease, 1/3 of mitral valve disease in the elderly	Rheumatic fever rare; CAD w papillary muscle dysfunction, ventricular dilatation, prolapse mitral valve, rupture chordae tendineae, CHF may be presenting sx
Pathophys	Leaflet calcification in the elderly rather than fusion of the commissures as w younger pts	—	Commissural fusion fibrosis and calcification of leaflets and chordae	Calcium posterior cusp leaflets lifting them toward L atrium resulting in MR
Sx	Exertional chest pain, dyspnea, syncope; sedentary elderly: low-output state: weight loss, pleural effusions, hepatic and renal failure; afib can lead to CHF in low-output state	CHF; more problems at rest than when they maintain exercise	Afib precipitates clinical deterioration	If dyspnea, orthopnea, edema, or fatigue present, valve replacement indicated; associated w afib
Si	Low-output state: murmur not very loud; late peaking systolic ejection murmur as opposed to early peaking in AS; may be confused w MR; S₄ decreased carotid upstroke, associated AI murmur w calcific AS	W aortic root dilatation high-pitched blowing diastolic murmur heard best at the right rather than the left sternal border; wide pulse pressure; LVH	In older pts calcified leaflets less mobile, therefore first heart sound at apex is diminished, no opening snap; diastolic murmur heard best w bell at apex w pt in left lateral position; often associated murmur of mitral insufficiency	May be difficult to differentiate from AS in elderly because increased AP diameter results in diminished AS m. MR if not cres-cendo–decrescendo, and radiates axilla or left sternal border

CARDIOLOGY

Table 8-6. (cont'd)

	Aortic Stenosis	Aortic Insufficiency	Mitral Stenosis	Mitral Regurgitation
Test	Doppler gradient >40; hemodynamic studies needed for low-output state; aortic valve area <0.75 cm^2 or peak systolic valve gradient of 70 mmHg	Pts where end-systolic dimension exceeds 5 cm^2 may be approaching LV dysfunction—indication for valve replacement before irreversible damage takes place	LAE on EKG; echo for severity	End-diastolic valve dimension >4.5 cm^2, refer cardiologist
Prognosis	W onset sx: mortality rate = 30–50%; aortic valve surgery (Circ 1993;8:17): encouraging results w human homographs; treat porcine and human homographs w warfarin for 3 mo at INR of 2–3, then D/C warfarin; mechanical heart valves: use warfarin long-term (INR at 2.5–3.5); ASA 160 mg/d may provide added protection; favorable results of CABG +/- valve replacement in pts >80 yr old (Cardiovasc Surg 1993;1:68); malfunction of aortic bioprosthesis if aortic diastolic murmur (Nejm 1996;335:407); surgery for asx pts if LVH dysfunction at rest, hypertrophic cardiomyopathy, ventricular ectopy, pts may be denying their sx	Nifedipine delays need for valve replacement (Nejm 1994;331:689); replace valve w exercise intolerance and before LV dysfunction (Ann Thorac Surg 1992;53:191); presence of coronary disease worsens postop outcome; may see associated rheumatic MS although less common in older people but when seen is more often accompanied by afib worsens sx of fatigue and CHF, and embolization may occur resulting in stroke	Anticoagulate if afib present, valve replacement for progressive, severe sx; malfunction of bioprosthesis if high-frequency holosystolic murmur (Nejm 1996;335:407); good outcome w valvotomy if class I or II (New York Heart Association) or class III, IV in octogenarians (J Am Ger Soc 2000;48:971)	If CAD present, operative mortality = 25% (Ann Thorac Surg 1993;55:333), then manage medically w diuresis, afterload reduction; afib: rx w anticoagulation, embolus less likely w MR than MS; good prognosis w repair of mitral valve prolapse

D/C = discontinue; LAE = left atrial enlargement.

Pathophys: Afib: age-associated loss of sinoatrial node fibers, atrial myocardial fibers; amyloid deposition; atrial dilatation from decreased ventricular compliance; SVT reentrant pathways

Epidem: Afib: 6% of pts >65 yrs; 50% of pts w afib >75 yrs

Sx: Polyuria, palpitations, faintness, neck pounding in AV reentrant types but not accessory pathway SVT (Nejm 1992;327:772); CHF and stoke in afib

Crs: Afib: unfavorable markers for successful conversion: >1-yr duration or markedly dilated LA (5 cm) or recurrent after previous conversion

Cmplc: Elderly more dependent on atrial kick, thus afib may lead to CHF; 7-fold risk of stroke in nonrheumatic afib and a 17% risk in mitral stenosis; post-PAT T-wave inversions may last days to weeks (Nejm 1995;332:161); chronic afib causes embolic CVA in 20% if recent CHF, chronic HT, or previous embolus (Ann IM 1992;116:1); increased cognitive disorders (J Am Geriatr Soc 2000;48:387)

Lab:

Chemistry: TSH

Noninvasive: EKG; sick sinus syndrome dx by SVTs alternating w some heart block; suggested by P <90 after 1–2 mg atropine or asystole >3 sec after carotid sinus massage; supraventricular arrhythmias: normal QRS, regular tachycardia without visible P waves = AV nodal reentrant arrhythmia: controlled w digoxin or verapamil

Multifocal atrial tachycardia: P >100 and 3 or more different PR intervals and P-wave morphologies; looks superficially like afib but digoxin will not help

Rx:

Therapeutic: Overall goal is ventricular rate control to protect cardiac output; all but β-blockers may prolong or cause ventricular arrhythmias (Ann IM 1992;117:141); need to lower digoxin dose by one-half in the presence of quinidine to avoid digitalis toxicity
Afib (Nejm 1992;326:1264):

Acutely: IV verapamil, diltiazem, β-blocker like esmolol, metoprolol, sotalol (Ann Emerg Med 2000;36:1) which is a non-selective β-adrenergic blocker, also helps decrease CHF, sudden cardiac death (J Am Coll Cardiol 1999;34:1522); for VT, implantable cardioverter-defibrillator (J Am Coll Cardiol 1999;34:1090)

Digoxin to slow; conversion with digoxin alone no better than placebo (Ann IM 1987;106:503): rate easily overridden by catechol/exercise stimulation (Ann IM 1991;114:573); if recalcitrant may need quinidine po (holds in NSR better but death rate 3 times placebo) (Circ 1990;82:1106) or procainamide or ibutilide or amiodarone (Ann IM 1992;116:1017) or clonidine (0.075 mg po, repeat in 2 h, decreases sympathetic tone) (Ann IM 1992;116:388); if LA size is <50 mm, use cardioversion (J Am Geriatr Soc 1999;47:740); if onset within 48 hours consider transesophageal echocardiogram to rule out left atrial clot; pt may need long-term agent to keep in normal sinus rhythm (eg, amiodarone, procainamide, quinidine) but these drugs are not benign (systemic adverse effects 40% with amiodarone—routinely screen with CXR, liver, and thyroid 94 mo; dysrhythmias, pulmonary fibrosis, sudden death, drug interactions) (Lancet 1997;350:1417); intermediate: heparin, coumadin for 2 wks, then convert, then 2 wks of coumadin and as above (Nejm 1993;328:750,803)

Chronic/paroxysmal (failed conversion): With coumadin, 50–70% reduction of stroke risk (Nejm 1995;332:238); valvular: if no contraindications, heparinize and coumadinize, rate control; non-valvular: controversial, depends on risk of bleeding versus risk of embolic disease in particular pt; increased risk of stroke if: age >65, diabetes, high BP, history of stroke/TIA, CHF, LV dysfunction; increased risk of bleeding if: stroke, GI bleed, severe recent illness, afib, high INR, age >80 (debated); special case: "lone afib," meaning no comorbidities and age <65, then no rx or ASA; unless contraindication exists, adjusted-dose coumadin with INR of 2–3 (J Am Geriatr Soc 2000;48:224; Nejm 1995;333:5) yields 64% risk reduction vs placebo and 40% vs ASA (Nejm 1995;332:238); similar guidelines found in Clinics in Geriatric Medicine November 1999

"Clinical Practice Guidelines": coumadin for pts older than 65 years (J Am Geriatr Soc 2000;48:224); use in high-risk individuals, including age >75 yr, TIA/stroke, DM, HT, CHF, LV dysfunction (Clin Ger Med 1999;15:645) vs only ASA in pts >75 yrs (Lancet 1994;243:687)

ASA for those who can't take coumadin

Warfarin is underused in at-risk populations with afib (Ann IM 1999;131:927; J Am Geriatr Soc 1998;46:1423; Arch IM 1998;158:2093; Lancet 1998;352:1167)

Bleeding risk cited among reasons not to anticoagulate (J Am Geriatr Soc 1997;45:1060); 9 studies show no age-related risk of bleeding, 10 studies show age-related risk of bleeding

(Ann IM 1996;124:970); appears that risk is balanced best with effectiveness if INR maintained at 2–3 (Lancet 1996;348:633)
One-third in NH under-treated (Circ 1995;92:2178)

PAT and Aflutter: Carotid sinus pressure; then, for PAT only, adenosine 6–12 mg IV, metabolized in 10 sec, potentiated by dipyridamole and carbamazepine, inhibited by theophyllines (Med Let Drugs Ther 1990;32:63); or verapamil 5–10 mg IV; perhaps propranolol 1–5 mg IV; then either digoxin + quinidine or electrical cardioversion with syncope; OK to do even if digoxin on board as long as levels therapeutic and not toxic and K^+ OK (Ann IM 1981;95:676)

Multifocal Atrial Tachycardia: Verapamil IV with pretreatment with IV $CaCl_2$ (Ann IM 1987;107:623) or po for chronic; MgH IV, especially if low; β-blockers if no COPD

BRADYARRHYTHMIAS AND HEART BLOCKS

Cause: ASHD, digoxin
Epidem: Idiopathic 3rd-degree heart block fairly common in the elderly
Sx:
   1st-degree heart block usually causes no sx
   2nd-degree may cause dizziness or dyspnea
   3rd-degree may cause syncope, especially during standing
Si:
   1st-degree heart block = PR >0.22 sec
   2nd-degree = some unconducted P waves
   3rd-degree = no relationship between P waves and QRS intervals
   Sick sinus syndrome (sinoatrial node dysfunction due to CAD or sclero-degenerative process) presenting w chest pain, palpitations, or sinus pause; treat brady part of the bradycardia-tachycardia syndrome w permanent pacer; see Table 8-7
Crs: 5-yr mortality 50%; not significantly reduced by pacing, but pacer improves sx
Lab:
Noninvasive: EKG; Holter monitor may still miss a majority of intermittent heart blocks (Nejm 1989;321:1703); event monitor

Table 8-7. Indications for Pacemaker

A. Acquired Atrioventricular Block in Adults

1. Third-degree AV block at any anatomic level association with any one of the following conditions:
   a. Bradycardia with symptoms presumed to be due to AV block.
   b. Arrhythmias and other medical conditions that require drugs that result in symptomatic bradycardia.
   c. Documented periods of asystole ≥3.0 seconds or any escape rate <40 beats per minute (bpm) in awake symptom-free patients.
   d. After catheter ablation of the AV junction. There are not trials to assess outcome without pacing, and pacing is virtually always planned in this situation unless the operative procedure is AV junction modification.
   e. Postoperative AV block that is not expected to resolve.
   f. Neuromuscular disease with AV block such as myotonic muscular dystrophy, Kearns-Sayre syndrome, Erb dystrophy (limb-girdle), and peroneal muscular atrophy.
2. Second-degree AV block regardless of type or site of block, with associated symptomatic bradycardia.
3. Asymptomatic third-degree AV block at any anatomic site with average awake ventricular rates of 40 bpm or faster.
4. Asymptomatic type II second-degree AV block.
5. Asymptomatic type I second-degree AV block at intra- or intra-His levels found incidentally at electrophysiological study for other indications.
6. First-degree AV block with symptoms of pacemaker syndrome and documented alleviation of symptoms with temporary AV pacing.

B. Chronic Bifascicular and Trifascicular Block

1. Intermittent third-degree AV block.
2. Type II second-degree AV block.
3. Syncope not proved to be due to AV block when other likely causes have been excluded, specifically ventricular tachycardia (VT).
4. Incidental finding at electrophysiological study of markedly prolonged HV interval (≥100 milliseconds) in asymptomatic patients.
5. Incidental finding at electrophysiological study of pacing-induced infra-His block that is not physiological.

C. Sinus Node Dysfunction

1. Sinus node dysfunction with documented symptomatic bradycardia, including frequent sinus pauses that produce symptoms. In some patients, bradycardia is iatrogenic and will occur as a consequence of essential long-term drug therapy of type and dose for which there are no acceptable alternatives.
2. Symptomatic chronotropic incompetence.
3. Sinus node dysfunction occurring spontaneously or as a result of necessary drug therapy with heart rate <40 bpm when a clear association between significant symptoms consistent with bradycardia and the actual presence of bradycardia has not been documented.

Table 8-7. (cont'd)

D. To Prevent Tachycardia
1. Sustained pause-dependent VT, with or without prolonged QT, in which the efficacy of pacing is thoroughly documented.
2. High-risk patients with congenital long QT syndrome.

E. Hypersensitive Carotid Sinus Syndrome and Neurally Mediated Syncope
1. Recurrent syncope caused by carotid sinus stimulation; minimal carotid sinus pressure induces ventricular asystole of >3 seconds' duration in the absence of any medication that depresses the sinus node or AV conduction.
2. Recurrent syncope without clear, provocative events and with a hypersensitive cardioinhibitory response.
3. Syncope of unexplained origin when major abnormalities of sinus node function or AV conduction are discovered or provoked in electrophysiological studies.

F. After the Acute Phase of Myocardial Infarction
1. Persistent second-degree AV block in the His-Purkinje system with bilateral bundle branch block or third-degree AV block within or below the His-Purkinje system after AMI.
2. Transient advanced (second- or third-degree) infranodal AV block and associated bundle branch block. If the site of block is uncertain, an electrophysiological study may be necessary.
3. Persistent and symptomatic second- or third-degree AV block.

Source: Based on evidence and favorable opinion about efficiency by American College of Cardiology/American Heart Association practice guidelines (ACC/AHA).

CARDIOLOGY

Rx:

- 2nd- and 3rd-degree: isoproterenol IV or sl, atropine IV, or external pacer until can get transvenous pacer; symptomatic pts w sinus pause >3 sec with sx or pause >2 sec with sx as well as Mobitz type II block should be considered for pacemaker; pts w Mobitz type I should avoid digitalis, β-blockers, calcium channel blockers, and antidepressants
- Sick sinus syndrome: lower incidence of afib w dual-chamber pacing (Nejm 1998;338:1097; Lancet 1994;344:1523)
- Transvenous pacemaker: temporary first, then permanent, unless inferior MI, when block will usually reverse spontaneously
- Permanent pacemaker (RV in Nejm 1996;344:89; Mod Concepts Cardiovasc Dis 1991;60:31): dual-chamber types more expensive; use only when need atrial kick (Ann IM 1986;105:264); see Table 8-8

Table 8-8. The North American Society of Pacing and Electrophysiology/British Pacing and Electrophysiology Group Generic Pacemaker Code

Position I (Chamber Paced)	Position II (Chamber Sensed)	Position II (Response to Sensing)	Position IV (Programmable Functions: Rate Modulation)	Position V (Antitachyarrhythmia Functions)
V—ventricle	V—ventricle	T—triggered	P—programmable rate and/or output	P—pacing (antitachyarrhythmia)
A—atrium	A—atrium	I—inhibited	M—multiprogrammability of rate, output, sensitivity, etc.	S—shock
D—dual (A & V)	D—dual (A & V)	D—dual (T & I)	C—communicating (telemetry)	D—dual (P + S)

Reproduced by permission from Gregoratos G. Permanent pacemakers in older persons. J Am Geriatr Soc 1999;47:1125–35.

8.7 DEEP VENOUS THROMBOSIS

Cause: Venous stasis from incompetent valves; increased hct leads to greater blood viscosity and clotting

Epidem: Occult cancers; extended sedentary periods (illness, travel); obesity; hip fx; estrogen

Pathophys: Decreased levels of antithrombin III can lead to venous dilatation and stasis

Sx: None or calf pain; unilateral edema

Si: None or increased calf diameter/tenderness/elevated skin temperature; Homan sign not sens/specif

Cmplc: Chronic postphlebitic syndrome: occurring after thrombosis involving destruction of the deep and communicating valves of the leg and obliteration of thrombosed veins; rarely painful; chronic edema (enlarged and hard leg because of trapped fluid from lymphedema due to scarring); hypopigmentation; stasis dermatitis; hyperemic ulcers; varicose veins; rx w 30 mmHg pressure stocking toe to knee; legs 3–4 inches above heart level at night if significant swelling persists; elevate legs intermittently, but ambulation should not be limited

Lab:

Noninvasive: Duplex US: in pts w sx, better than IPG (Nejm 1993;329:1365); in high-risk asx pts only 38% sens (Lancet 1994;343:1142); in pts w sx of recurrence it is difficult to distinguish on US up to 1 yr after initial DVT (Acta Radiol 1992;33:297); use serial IPG if had normal IPG before; venograms may be indeterminate, so use degree of clinical suspicion in deciding anticoagulation (Geriatrics 1995;50:29)

Rx:

Preventive: In hip replacement initiating low-molecular-weight heparin rx 1 mo prior to elective surgery results in fewer DVTs (Nejm 1996;335:696; 1993;329:1370)

Therapeutic: Heparin IV × 5 d + coumadin started on d 1 (Nejm 1992;327:1485); continue coumadin × 6 mo (Nejm 1995;332:1661); 1–2 mo only if transient specific cause; lifelong if recurrent idiopathic (Nejm 1995;332:1710); low-molecular-weight heparin as good as heparin for DVT (Arch IM 1995;155:601); see 10.2 Hip Fracture for hiradin

CARDIOLOGY

8.8 ANTICOAGULATION

Anticoagulants
- ASA (Nejm 1994;330:1287): 75–325 mg po qd (Med Let Drugs Ther 1995;37:14) inhibits platelet aggregation; can be used safely w coumadin (Nejm 1993;329:530); adverse effects: gastric intolerance (Ann IM 1994;120:184), asthma, increased bleeding time for 2 d, platelet dysfunction for 7–10 d; low cost
- Enoxaparin (Lovenox): 30 mg sc bid, low-molecular-weight heparin (Med Let Drugs Ther 1993;35:75) are clearly better with less bleeding (Ann IM 1994;121:81) and better DVT/PE prevention over 6 d (Nejm 1992;326:975); $23/d as rx for DVT (Nejm 1996;334:677,682; 1996;335:1816); after 24 h Lovenox may start warfarin and may discontinue heparin after 4 d if INR 2.0 for 2 consecutive days (Arch IM 1998;158:1809; Nejm 1997;337:657, 663,688; 1996;335:1821); not for massive PE (Clinics in Ger Med 2001;17:15)
- Heparin: also inhibits activated prothrombin-platelet interaction; renal excretion, half-life = 105 min (Nejm 1991;324:1565); prophylactic regimen = 5000 units IV q 12 h; therapeutic regimen = 5000-unit load, then 1200 units IV/h; measuring q 6 h PTT until stable at 1.5–2.0 × control
- Ticlopidine (Ticlid): stoke prevention after cardiac stenting, may cause neutropenia, thrombocytopenia, cholestasis, TTP, so only use 2–4 wks (Ann IM 1998;128:541)

Prophylaxis of thromboembolism for surgical or orthopedic procedure where short-term need (<1 mo): once-daily evening doses of 5.0–7.5 mg; lower doses should be used in elderly pts; during initiation of rx, PT INR should be monitored daily, response to a given dose may not be accurately measured for up to 36 h, doses should not be changed for 3–5 d; 3 wk before procedure: hct, PT, APTT, and platelet count; overlap prolonged PT 2–5 d with heparin as switch over (Nejm 1984;311:645) because it inhibits liver synthesis of factors X (3-d half-life), IX (1.25 d), VII (7 h), and II (4 d); INR of 2–3 for routine anticoagulation, 3.0–4.5 for artificial valves (ACP J Club 1994;120(suppl 2):52)

Preop and on coumadin: withhold 4 d prior to surgery and use heparin; discontinue antiplatelet rx 5 d prior to surgery and restart 48–72 h after surgery (Chest 1995;108:312S)

Coumadin Protocol: If INR <1.5, increase total dose/wk by 10%; INR >3.4, decrease total weekly dose by 10% after one dose is held; INR 5.0–9.0 w increased risk of bleeding, coumadin may be omitted and vit K (1.0–2.5 mg) given po w additional dose in 24 h if INR remains high; >9.0 without serious risk of bleeding may give vit K 3–5 mg po; significant elevation of INR w severe bleeding, give vit K (10 mg) slow IV infusion q 12 h prn w FFP and transfusion if needed

For minor surgery w pts at low risk for thromboembolic event, stop coumadin several days preoperatively and perform surgery when INR <1.5; for pts w significant risk for thrombolic event, admit for heparin infusion when INR reaches 2.0; stop infusion 4 h prior to surgery, resuming as soon as possible postoperatively (J Am Geriatr Soc 2000;48:226)

Adverse effects: bleeding, especially when given with probenecid or if renal failure; risk of serious bleeding >10%/yr in therapeutic range; correlates w higher PTs and first 3 mo of rx, not age or gender (Ann IM 1993;118:511); risk of intracranial bleed = 2%/yr w PT 2 × control, risk much higher if PT higher (Ann IM 1994;120:897); blue toe syndrome (cholesterol emboli) rare complication (South Med J 1992;85:210; Surgery 1989;105:737)

Potentiated by foods and drugs (Ann IM 1994;121:676) that either displace from carrier protein or compete for degradation enzyme; includes allopurinol (Nejm 1970;283:1484), amiodarone, Antabuse, ASA, cimetidine (Ann IM 1979;90:993); or by decreased warfarin metabolism (cimetidine, erythromycin, tricyclics, TMP/SMZ); vit K deficiency (inadequate diet, fat malabsorption, mineral oil, broad-spectrum antibiotics); unknown mechanisms: clofibrate, quinine, phenothiazines, acetaminophen (J Am Geriatr Soc 1998;279:657)

Decreased w increased coumadin metabolism (barbiturates, carbamazepine); excess vit K (dietary supplements); impaired coumadin absorption (malabsorption syndromes, mineral oil, cholestyramine)

CARDIOLOGY

9 Pulmonology

9.1 CHRONIC OBSTRUCTIVE PULMONARY DISEASE

Geriatrics 1995;50:24; Ger Rev Syllabus 1996:278 (asthma, bronchitis, emphysema)

Cause: Smoking in overwhelming majority of pts; asthma may "reappear" late in life

Epidem: Asthma (increased bronchial and bronchiolar responsiveness to various stimuli resulting in airway narrowing): 1–3% of new cases in the elderly; prevalence 3.8% M, 7.1% F; increased mortality in the elderly

Pathophys: Normal changes in lung w aging: decreased elastic recoil resulting in collapsed airways during respiratory cycle, especially in lower part of lung leading to V/Q mismatch; chest wall compliance, number of alveoli, vital capacity, maximum voluntary ventilation, FEV_1, maximum expiratory flow rate all decreased

Increase in residual volume and functional residual capacity; all changes accentuated by pulmonary disease

Limitation of expiratory flow, usually combination of emphysema and chronic bronchitis

Emphysema: destruction of air spaces distal to terminal bronchioles

Chronic bronchitis: daily production of sputum for 3 mo during 2 consecutive yr

Asthma: relatively few new cases in elderly and may have collagen-vascular etiology

Sx: Fear of shortness of breath may lead to blunting of emotional response in interpersonal interactions (Heart Lung 1973;2:389)

Si: Final stages: cor pulmonale—barrel chest, prolongation of expiration, wheezing, pulmonary HT, elevated jugular venous pressure, pronounced pulmonic closure sound (P_2), hepatic congestion, peripheral edema, cyanosis

    Asthma: indicators of acuity: difficulty walking 100 feet or more; speech fragmented by rapid breath; syncope; pulsus paradoxus >12 mmHg; inability to lie supine; accessory muscle use; respiratory rate >30; heart rate >120; FEV_1 or peak expiratory flow rate <30% predicted value

Cmplc: R/o lung cancer, CHF, GE reflux, recurrent aspiration, thromboembolic disease (pleuritic pain, hemoptysis, unexplained right-sided heart failure, hypoxemia), cough secondary to β-blockers, ACE inhibitors

Lab: Normal Pao_2 for patient >65 yr old = 80–85 mmHg (Eur Respir J 1994;7:856); Pao_2 decreased approximately 3 mmHg/decade; FEV_1/FVC <0.70; FEV_1 falls 30 mL/yr and 75–80 mL/yr in smokers

    Asthma: reversible w bronchodilators; FEV_1 improves by 15% or 200 mL

Xray: Chronic bronchitis: increased bronchiolar markings, increased heart size; emphysema: elongated heart, hyperinflation of lungs, bullae

Rx:

Therapeutic:

    Bronchodilator therapy: symptomatic improvement, but does not change survival; 40% patients use metered-dose inhalers (MDIs) inappropriately; spacers help (correct use: National Heart, Lung, and Blood Institute, National Asthma Education Program. Guidelines for the diagnosis and management of asthma. Bethesda, MD: National Institutes of Health, U.S. Dept. of Health and Human Services, Public Health Service, 1991:57); reasons for noncompliance include expense, memory lapse, denial, anxiety; all pts need instruction

    β2-Adrenergic agonists most effective for acute episodes of asthma and prevention of exercise-induced asthma; long-acting β2-adrenergic agonists prevent nocturnal asthma and should be prescribed only at regular intervals (never prn); elderly asthmatics have diminished receptor response and may not respond as well to β-adrenergic agonists (Geriatrics 1995;50:24); salmeterol not approved for COPD, just asthma (Nejm 1995;333:499)

    Anticholinergic: ipratropium bromide best as chronic therapy in addition to β2-adrenergic receptor agonists; not advantageous to

Table 9-1. Theophylline Levels

Increased Levels	Decreased Levels
Caffeine	β-Blockers
Erythromycin	Barbiturates
Clarithromycin (Biaxin)	Phenytoin
Ciprofloxacin (Cipro)	Rifampin
Pentoxifylline (Trental)	Felodipine (Plendil)
Cimetidine	High protein
Ranitidine (Zantac)	Low carbohydrate
Enoxacin (Penetrex)	Carbamazepine (Tegretol)
Disulfiram (Antabuse)	Smoking
Mexiletine (Mexitil)	
Ticlopidine (Ticlid)	
Estrogen/progestin	
Isoproterenol (Isuprel)	
Propranolol	
Flu shot	
Untreated hypothyroid, CHF	
Thiabendazole (Mintezol)	

use both in the acute setting (Ann Pharmacother 1994;28:1379); precipitates glaucoma if sprayed in eye

Corticosteroids: first-line therapy for asthma; loss of bone density if given systemically; rinsing mouth after inhaler avoids oral candidiasis, cataracts cromolyn anti-inflammatory blocks mast cell degranulation, 1–2 puffs qid; nedocromil anti-inflammatory w sometimes unpleasant taste, nausea, vomiting, rhinitis occasionally

Theophylline (Chest 1995;107:206S) (Table 9-1): in older pts w emphysema may be of value initially for airflow obstruction that is irreversible; may reduce the work of breathing, augmenting diaphragmatic breathing and acting centrally to increase respiratory drive; may also work as a mild diuretic; high serum levels may be more helpful to pts w asthma, but toxicity (nausea, cardiac arrhythmias, confusion, seizures) 17 times more frequent in the elderly, thus has limited role in COPD (Nurs Home Pract 1995;3:17); erythromycin and cimetidine inhibit cytochrome P450 metabolism of theophylline; liver disease and CHF reduce clearance; decrease theophylline by 50% if giving ciprofloxacin at the same time; measure levels after 2–5 d of therapy; therapeutic trough = 5–15 μgm/mL

Indication for long-term oxygen therapy at home: $O_2:Pao_2$ <55 mmHg or cor pulmonale or polycythemia w Po_2 <60 mmHg; goal is to increase Po_2 >60 mmHg; after 1, 6, 12 mo, ABGs should be measured to determine ongoing need for and appropriate dose of oxygen; long-term oxygen therapy: increased survival (Nejm 1995;333:710)

Team Management:

- Avoid irritants: smoking, dust, air pollution, humidity; pts >65 yr gain 4 yr of life expectancy if they quit smoking; MAO inhibitors may help w the addiction, counteracting nicotine stimulation of dopamine release (Jama 1995;275:1217)

- For substantial sputum production: percussion and postural drainage given by a family member; flutter valve device pts can use alone

- Severe dyspnea: conscious slowing of respirations, purse-lipped breathing, relaxation techniques

- Arm movement exercise controversial

- Daily 15-min periods of exercise-induced hyperpnea increase ventilatory capacity in pts 65–75 yr old; 8-wk training program produces significant reduction in breathlessness (Geriatrics 1993;48:59); pulmonary rehabilitation program improves exercise capacity in older pts w COPD (Chest 1995;107:730)

- Nutrition: high ratio of fat to carbohydrate; fat metabolism generates the least amount of carbon dioxide, carbohydrates the most; very hot and very cold foods stimulate coughing

- Psychosocial support: family education, eg, care and crisis

- Asthma: color-coded peak expiratory flow meters may make it easier for older pts to monitor asthma in outpatient setting (Am Fam Phys Monograph 1995:2); stepwise approach to asthma management (Med Let Drugs Ther 1999;41:5; Reuben DB, et al. Geriatrics at your fingertips 2000. Dubuque, IA: Kendall-Hunt: 2000:125):

  1. Intermittent: prn inhaled β_2-agonist less than twice a week; inhaled β_2-agonist or cromolyn or nedocromil before exposure to trigger

  2. Mildly persistent: daily inhaled corticosteroid (200–500 μg) w β_2-agonist prn less than once a week

  3. Moderately persistent: daily inhaled corticosteroid (800–2000) plus long-acting β_2-agonist plus prn β_2-agonist not exceeding 3–4 d/wk

4. Severely persistent: inhaled corticosteroid (800–2000 µg) plus long-acting β_2-agonist plus sustained-release theophylline and or ipratropium plus prn β_2-agonist (Reuben et al. 2000:125; National Institutes of Health Pub No. 95–3659, 1995)

- Always heed "subjective" responses to empiric rx trials as well as "objective" (eg, peak flow responses) since perception of breathlessness important to pt, reducing anxiety component

Preop Assessment: Only absolute indication for preop PFTs, even in COPD pts, is to measure lung volume before lung resection; consider local vs general anesthesia to avoid a 30–50% fall in tidal volume; preop postural drainage w chest percussion to avoid complications postop; bronchial secretions increase for 6 wk after cessation of smoking, increasing risk for postop infection (Ger Rev Syllabus 1996:65)

9.2 PULMONARY EMBOLUS

Epidem: 15% of cancer patients will have one within 2 yr (Ann IM 1982;303:1509)

Pathophys: Thrombophlebitis causes thrombus migrating to lungs; recurrent small emboli more common than single large one; mostly thigh and pelvis veins (Ann IM 1981;94:439); no si or sx in 50%

Sx: Dyspnea may be sudden, intermittent, or chronic; pleuritic chest pain w infarct; hemoptysis; fever; syncope w large emboli; common to have minimal sx

Si: 33% pleural effusion of which 67% bloody (rbc >100,000/dL); unexplained arrhythmias; resistant heart failure; tachycardia

Crs: Resolves over 10–30 d (Nejm 1969;280:1194); 60% survival without rx, 90% w rx 3 d heparin

Cmplc: Chronic leg edema, chronic pulmonary HT

Lab: nl a-a = <10–15 mmHg and is abnormal if there is intrinsic lung problem

Neg D-dimer rules out PE w near certainty; false-pos results appear to be less likely in nonsurgical patients or without underlying cancer or liver disease (Am J Respir Crit Care Med 1999; 159:1445)

EKG: partial right bundle branch block ($S_1S_2S_3$), right axis deviation 20%, $S_1Q_3T_3$

Xray: V/Q scan mismatch (PIO-PED in Jama 1990;262:2753); B-mode duplex US; arteriogram false-neg rate w 1–5% complication rate, 1–4/1000 mortality rate; spiral CT

Rx:

Preventive: Mild to moderate alcohol consumption decreases risk of DVT and pulmonary embolus (J Am Geriatr Soc 1996;44:1030)

Therapeutic: Heparin PTT 1.5–2.5 times control for 5–10 d; overlap coumadin 5 d and continue 6 mo at INR 2–3 (Nejm 1995;332:166)

If major bleeding, stop heparin and allow anticoagulation effect to dissipate over hours; if cannot tolerate coumadin long term, give heparin sc 10,000 units q 12 h; vena cava filter for pts w persistent contraindication to anticoagulation; adverse effects include chronic leg edema, thrombus formation above the filter, recurrent embolization through collateral veins, perforation of vena cava, migration of filter

Aim of prophylaxis is to prolong quality of life; if pt terminally ill, eg, w cancer, anticoagulation may only prolong suffering

9.3 PULMONARY HYPERTENSION

Cause: LVH, valvular heart disease, COPD, chronic recurrent thromboembolic disease

Epidem: F > M

Pathophys: Excess platelet thromboxane A, deficient endothelial cell prostaglandin (Nejm 1993;328:1732)

Sx: Dyspnea, chest pain, pedal edema, fatigue

Si: Right-sided S_3, pulmonary systolic and diastolic murmurs, tricuspid insufficiency, enlarged RV

Crs: If PA pressure >85 mmHg, then median survival time 2.8 yr

Lab: ABG: low P_{CO_2}

Rx:

Therapeutic: Selective use of oxygen; low-dose diuretics; phlebotomy for hct exceeding 50%; calcium channel blockers; coumadin anticoagulation (Nejm 1992;327:76); epoprostenol (prostacyclin) infused or inhaled has some hemodynamic and sx benefit (Ann IM 2000;132:425); may be no long-term benefit (Nejm 2000;342:1866)

10 Orthopedics/ Rheumatology

10.1 OSTEOPOROSIS

Jama 2000;283:1318; 2001;285:785; Ann IM 1995;123:452; Nejm 1992;327:620; Bull Rheum Dis 1988;38:1

Cause: See Table 10-1.

Epidem: More common in female smokers from changes in estrogen metabolism (Nejm 1985;313:973; 1994;330:387); less frequent in blacks and Polynesians because they start with higher adolescent bone densities (Nejm 1991;325:1597)

Pathophys: Simple estrogen deficiency postmenopausally (Nejm 1980;303:1571)

Sx: Fx usually of vertebrae, distal forearm bones, proximal femur; bone pain, especially vertebral, although many w/o sx

Si: Decreased height/kyphosis from vertebral compression fx; if incidental vertebral fx of T7 or 8, patient has osteoporosis by definition (Cummings, 2000); hip fx imparts prescriptive dx osteoporosis

Crs: Chronic, slowly progressive

Cmplc: Rib and vertebral fx (Nejm 1983;309:265), hip fx

Lab:

Chemistry: PTH, serum and urine calcium to r/o hyperparathyroid and renal calcium leak; bone turnover markers: bone-specific alkaline phosphatase, osteocalcin (Geriatrics 1996;51:24); osteoclast-mediated procollagen carboxyl-terminal peptide (N-telopeptide) turnover in urine (Osteomark) (J Clin Endocrinol Metab 1995;80:3)

Xray: Osteopenic bones and fx; densitometry screening controversial, much debated (Nejm 1991;324:1105; Ann IM 1990;113:565;

Table 10-1. Causes of Osteoporosis

Acromegaly

Alcoholism

Anorexia (AIM 2000;133:790)

Cushing disease/syndrome (even 10 mg prednisone qd enough), including chronic steroid use in asthmatics (Nejm 1983;309:265) and rheumatoid arthritis (Ann IM 1993;119:963)

Diabetes, type I

Estrogen deficiency in postmenopausal women or amenorrheic athletes (Nejm 1984;311:277); hypogonadotrophic hypogonadism in men

Homocystinuria

Hyperparathyroidism

Hyperthyroidism

Idiopathic, at least some of which is genetic in structure of bone matrix protein (Nejm 1998;338:1016)

Malabsorption

Myeloma

Renal calcium leak (rx w thiazides)

Soda intake, excessive

Vitamin A, chronic excessive intake (Ann IM 1998;129:770)

Vitamin D, winter deficiency (Jama 1995;274:1683)

Vitamin D antagonist meds like phenytoin

1990;112:516; Nejm 1987;316:212); might consider w pts indecisive re ERT or in high-risk pts (chronic steroid use, renal disease, hyperparathyroidism, Graves disease, malabsorption); dual-energy xray absorptiometry (DEXA) most precise and lowest cost (Am Fam Phys Monograph 1996;1:1; Med Let Drugs Ther 1996;38:103); T scores (SD from mean density of 20-yr-old F) >2.5 has a 5-times increased risk of fx; Z score is SD from same age group, scores may take 2 years to change w rx (Jama 2000;283:1318); at cost of $5 per scan, femoral neck measurement most accurate because does not pick up calcification of aorta that a spine measurement would; vs FIT trial data suggesting that yr to yr variation makes it difficult to use DEXA to follow therapy; MXA better because less radiation and gives information on density as well as morphology (Cummings, 2000)

Rx:

- All rx is preventive or instituted to slow progression (Med Let 2000;42:97) including progression of steroid-induced type (Nejm 1993;329:1406); weight-bearing exercise (Ann IM 1988;108:824); smoking cessation (Ann IM 1992;116:716); posture and balance exercise (fall prevention)

- Calcium replacement therapy (Med Let Drugs Ther 2000;42:29) w $CaCO_3$ 1.5 gm of elemental Ca^{+2}/d (milk has 300 mg Ca^{+2}/cup; chewable Tums, 200–500 mg/tab; Os-Cal, 500 mg/tab) (Med Let Drugs Ther 1989;31:101); first 800 mg qd as calcium citrate (Citracal), higher cost but absorbed better, especially in achlorhydrics/elderly (Nejm 1985;313:70), then add $CaCO_3$ (Nejm 1990;323:878); substantial effect even without estrogen (Ann IM 1994;120:97), eg, 50% less loss/yr (Nejm 1993;328:460); calcium content in supplements and foods (Med Let Drugs Ther 2000;42:29; 1996;38:108); increased protein in diet may exert calciuretic effect (Am J Clin Nutr 1988;48:880); no association of decreased fx w increased dietary calcium (Am J Publ Hlth 1997;87:992)
- Vit D as 225–400 IU qd (400 IU in multivitamins, or as high as 600–800 IU) or calcitriol (D3) 0.25 μg po bid markedly decreases fx without producing stones by preventing increased PTH of winter at least (Nejm 1998;338:828; 1993;327:1637; 1992;326:357; Ann IM 1991;115:505); 400 IU × 2 yr preserves femoral neck bone density in F >70 yr (1995;80:1052); sunscreen prevents vit D absorption—difficult trade-off w rising skin cancer rates
- ERT (decreases responsiveness of bone to PTH, preventing bone resorption) 0.625 mg decreases fx rates by two-thirds (wrist, hip, other); even smaller estrogen doses help (Obgyn 1996;27:163), start soon after menopause and continue (Ann IM 1995;122:9) as late as age 75 yr; may also start as late as age 60 yr (Jama 1997;277:543) vs estrogen not fx preventive unless on it for 10 yrs (HERS study: Med Let Drugs Ther 2000;42:97); unknown long-term effects of even selective estrogen receptor modulators (raloxifene [Evista]) on breast (Cummings, 2000; Jama 2000;283:534)
- Testosterone in men, especially if hypogonadism, watch cancer of prostate and rx pts
- Bisphosphonates (Am Fam Phys 2000;61:2732)
    - Alendronate (Fosamax) (Am Fam Phys 1996;54:2053; Med Let 2001;43:26–38:965; Nejm 1995;33:1437), 10 mg po qd or 70 mg qwk clearly helps prevent progression over 3 yr; prevents nonvertebral fx over 3 yrs (Jama 1997;277:1159; Lancet 1996;348:1535) or 5–10 qd for prevention in high-risk F, eg, on steroids (J Bone Miner Res 2000;15:993) or F who cannot take ERT (Ann IM 1998;128:253,313; Nejm 1998;339:292,338,485); in men (Nejm 2000;343:604) give where life expectancy 2–3 yrs at least and pt walking; analgesic

effect (Bone Miner 1991;15:237); adverse effects: various GI sx, eg, esophagitis, diarrhea (Nejm 1996;335:1216); give w caution in pts w renal insufficiency; can give once a week 70 mg (Cummings, 2000); for M too (Nejm 2000;343:604); high cost

- Risedronate (Actonel) (Jama 1999;282:1344) 5 mg po qd (Med Let Drugs Ther 2000;7:26) reduces vertebral and hip fx (Med Let Drugs Ther 2000;42:100); etidronate disodium (Didronel) 400 mg po qd × 14 d, then 13 wk off in cycles (Nejm 1997;337:382) to avoid osteomalacia (Ger Rev Syllabus 1996:157)

- Pamidronate (Aredia) 150 mg po qd (Med Let Drugs Ther 1992;34:1); 2 h infusion 40–80 mg IV q 4 mo (Ann IM 2000;132:734; Am Fam Phys 2000;61:2732); unknown: long-term value, when to stop, micro fx after 5 yrs therapy (Cummings, 2000)

- Calcitonin interferes w osteoclasts and inhibits bone resorption; 100 IU salmon calcitonin sc qd, may also relieve acute fx pain, possibly via opiate effect (J Fam Pract 1992;35:93); 200 IU qd alternating nostrils (Med Let Drugs Ther 1996;38:965; Am J Med 1995;98:452); nausea from calcitonin self-limited and <10% of pts discontinue med; other side effects include flushing, diarrhea, and pain at injection site; human calcitonin has more side effects than salmon calcitonin; recrudescence when rx discontinued, even after a year of rx; PROOF trial supporting calcitonin flawed because 1/2 patients lost to f/u (Am J Med 2000;109:330); alendronate maintains bone density more effectively than intranasal calcitonin (J Clin Endocrinol Metab 2000;85:1783)

- STATINS for increased cholesterol Rx, also slows osteoporosis (Jama 2000;283:3205,3211,3255 v.s. Jama 2001;285:1850)

- Thiazides may help bone density and fx rate (Ann IM 1996;129:187; 1993;118:657,666; Nejm 1990;322:286); others report increased fx rate (Nejm 1991;325:1)

- Vertebral plasty reinforces collapsing vertebrae w polymethyl-methacrylate alleviating pain and increasing mobility; best for in-pts w 1–2 new fx (Am J Neuroradiol 1997;18:1897)

10.2 HIP FRACTURE

Nejm 1966;334:1519

Cause: Falls and osteoporosis

Epidem: 90% pts >50 yr old; rates lower in blacks; increased w low BMI, maternal h/o hip fx, alcohol use, CVA hx (Nejm 1994;330:1555), smoking (Nejm 1987;316:404), hyperthyroidism, visual impairment (Nejm 1991;324:1326), and drugs like long-acting benzodiazepines, tricyclics, SSRIs (Lancet 1998;351:1303), phenothiazines (Nejm 1987;316:363), as well as other psychoactive drugs, especially in NHs (Nejm 1992;327:168); paradoxically also may be increased by restraints (Ann IM 1992;116:369); associated w being on feet <4 h/d, higher resting pulse rate (Nejm 1995;332:767)

Pathophys: Falls and fx occur in the elderly because:
- Slow gait results in more sideways and backward falls on hips rather than on other body parts
- Diminished protective responses; less fat and muscle protection
- Diminished strength (J Gerontol 1989;44:M107)

Subcapital fx (45%) disrupts blood supply to femoral head; higher incidence nonunion and necrosis of femoral head

Intertrochanteric fx (10%) and subtrochanteric fx (45%) leaves blood supply to femoral head intact

Sx: H/o fall; hip pain (may be vague in the elderly)

Si: External rotation of the leg w shortening; pain w motion; persistent immobility in demented

Crs: 25% of fall-induced hip fx associated w death within 6 mo; 25% have subsequent functional dependence; 50% of pts walking independently 1 yr after fx (Am J Pub Hlth 1987;79:279); pre-fx mental status and physical functional level best predictors of eventual outcome (J Am Geriatr Soc 1992;40:861)

Cmplc: After fx, frequently develop confusion (49%), UTI (33%), arrhythmia (26%), pneumonia (19%), depression (15%), CHF (7%), DVT; femoral neck fx: avascular necrosis in 20%, nonunion 30%; intertrochanteric: failure of fixation devices (tremendous muscle forces on bone) (J Gen IM 1987;2:78; Ger Rev Syllabus 1996:245)

Xray: Fx, often subtle, especially if impacted; best view: anteroposterior w internal rotation 15–20 degrees; delayed repeat films may be necessary; after 72 h, bone scan or MRI if dx still in doubt

Rx:
Prevention:

- Positive relationship between physical activity and lower risk of hip fx (Intern Med 1998;129:81)
- W ERT (see 10.1 Osteoporosis)
- In elderly NH women, by 1.2 gm calcium + 800 IU vit D (calcitriol) qd (Nejm 1992;327:1637) (see 10.1 Osteoporosis)
- W hip protectors in NH (Lancet 1993;341:11; Nejm 2000;343:1506)
- Statins (HMG-CoA reductase inhibitors) prevent hip fx (Jama 2000;283:3205,3211,3255; Lancet 2000;355:2185,2218)
- Avoid use of throw rugs in home, restraints (Ann IM 1992;116:369)

Surgical:

- Subcapital fx: Austin-Moore prosthesis, early weight bearing; if nondisplaced: pin, weight bearing in 12 wk
- Intertrochanteric fx: screw w early ambulation
- Subtrochanteric fx: nail and rod, no weight bearing till healed

Delay surgery if pt must be on anticoagulation; delay is associated w more postop risk (J Bone Joint Surg Am 1995;77:1551); recombinant hirudin (desirudin) a specific inhibitor of thrombin administered 30 min before total hip replacement—more effective than enoxaparin in preventing DVT (Nejm 1997;337:1329)

After surgery, consider heparin and/or coumadin DVT prophylaxis if pt not able to be up quickly, or at least compression stockings (Arch IM 1994;154:67); low-molecular-weight heparin q 12 h for 1 mo post-op (Nejm 1996;335:696); ASA reduces risk PE, DVT even w those receiving other prophylaxsis (Lancet 2000;355:1295)

- Austin-Moore prosthesis: weight bearing in 1–2 d
- Compression screw internal fixation: in 2–3 d
- Pinned: not for 6–8 wk but can be discharged from hospital within 2–5 d, sooner if advanced dementia

Loosening of prosthesis: groin pain w acetabular component and upper thigh pain w femoral component

Selected patients (advanced Alzheimer, Parkinson, CHF, CVA, near terminal illness) for no repair if high surgical risk or nearing end of ambulatory life; pain management often no worse or prolonged than w postop course

Early rehab (Jama 1998;279:847) as good in NH as in rehabilitation unit (Jama 1997;277:396)

- Anterior approach hip repair: rehab limited to flexion, adduction, internal rotation
- Posterior approach: should have less than 90 degrees in relation to sitting surface and no internal rotation
- Walker use s/p hip fx (advance 20–30 cm, then move weak leg first)
- Cane use s/p hip fx only if ipsilateral upper extremity and contralateral lower extremity are strong; <25% of pt weight should be placed on cane; when going up or down stairs, keep good leg up higher (ie, "up with good, down with bad"); although ipsilateral cane use can reduce the force acting on the hip, placing the cane in the contralateral hand useful in relieving hip pain; watch for development of new shoulder problem with added stress (J Am Geriatr Soc 1996;44:434); cane height should allow 30 degrees of flexion at pt elbow w top of cane parallel to greater trochanter

Rx osteoporosis in walking NH patients (Jama 2000;284:972)

10.3 OSTEOARTHRITIS

Jama 1996;276:486; Klippel JH, Dieppe PA, eds., Rheumatology. St. Louis: Mosby-Year Book, 1994; see Tables 10-2 to Table 10-4, and Figure 10-1

Cause: Aging: decreased proteoglycan aggregation, decreased resistance of cartilage to procollagen (Lancet 1989;1:924); obesity; postural defects (genu valgum/varum); excessive repetitive stress; crystalline deposit disease; previous inflammatory joint disease; hemochromatosis; Wilson disease; acromegaly; in familial may be ank gene (Science 2000;289:265,289)

Epidem: Uncommon <35 yr old, more common >65 yr old (30–40% population >65 having sx); F/M = 1.5:1.0 (Arth Rheum 1987;30:914)

Pathophys: Injury to articular cartilage leads to destruction of proteoglycan matrix, which in turn leads to cellular proliferation in attempted repair, release of enzymes with increased destruction of all cartilage elements and proliferation of subchondral bone

Sx: Aching worse with activity; relieved by rest; morning stiffness; hip arthritis begins in groin and radiates to thigh (getting up from chair)

Table 10-2. Does the Clinical Presentation Meet ACR Criteria for the Diagnosis of Osteoarthritis?

Hand OA	Knee OA	Hip OA
Hand pain, aching, or stiffness *And* Hard tissue enlargement of 2 select joints *And* Radiographic femoral or Fewer than 3 swollen MCP joints *And* 2 or more DIP hard tissue enlargement *Or* Deformity in 2 or more select joints	Knee pain *And* Radiographic osteophytes *And* 1 or more of the following: • Age ≥50 • Morning stiffness <30 minutes • Crepitus on motion	Hip pain *And* 2 or more of the following: • ESR <10 mm/hour • Acetabular osteophytes • Radiographic joint space narrowing

Select Joints = DIP, PIP, 1st CMC.
Reproduced by permission from Ling SM, Bathon JM. Osteoarthritis in older adults. J Am Geriatr Soc 1998;46:216–25.

Table 10-3. Potential Markers of Osteoarthritis

Cartilage Staining	Synovial Fluid or Serum	Urine
Denatured type II collagen	Type II procollagen peptide	Pyridinoline crosslinks

Chondroitin sulfate 846 pitope	Cartilage oligomeric protein
	Hyaluronic acid
	Stromelysin (metalloproteinase 3)
	IGF-1
	Osteocalcin
	Chondroitin sulfate 846 pitope
	  Synovial/serum ratio
	Keratan sulfate
	  Synovial/serum ratio
		Deoxypyridonline crosslinks

Reproduced by permission from Ling SM, Bathon JM. Osteoarthritis in older adults. J Am Geriatr Soc 1998;46:216–25.

Si: Knee > hip > spine, ankles, elbows, shoulders; wrist not involved; involvement of base of thumb; joint crepitus; decreased ROM, minimal soft tissue swelling + bony enlargement, minimal warmth or erythema; rare effusions; Bouchard, Heberden nodes

Table 10-4. Functional Assessment Measures

Osteoarthritis specific indices
- Lequesne algofunctional index
- Western Ontario McMaster University (WOMAC) osteoarthritis index

General measures of function
- Self report
  Katz Activities of Daily Living
  Instrumental Activities of Daily Living
  Geriatric Arthritis Impact Scale

• Objective performance upper body	
Grip Strength	Squeeze the examiner's fingers or maximum pressure squeezed with a rolled sphygmomanometer cuff inflated to 30 mmHg
Pinch Strength	Patient firmly holds a piece of paper between the thumb and index finger while the examiner tries to pull the paper out
Dexterity	Patient picks up a coin or small object from a table top or floor
• Objective performance lower body	
Balance	Tandem gait and stance
	Functional reach
	"Get up and go" test Tinetti Balance and Gait evaluation
Speed & Mobility	Walk speed
Gait evaluation	Time to rise from a chair
	Antalgic gait due to pain from weight bearing joint (knee or hip)
	Trendelenburg lurch indicates gluteus medius weakness: often accompanies hip arthritis
	Tinetti Balance and Gait evaluation

Reproduced by permission from Ling SM, Bathon JM. Osteoarthritis in older adults. J Am Geriatr Soc 1998;46:221.

Crs: Insidious onset; slowly progressive

Cmplc: Joint pain and instability; contractures, tendonitis, bursitis; r/o osteoporosis, malignancy, Paget, osteomyelitis, neuropathy, parkinsonism, avascular necrosis of hip, trochanteric bursitis (lateral bone pain instead of groin/hip pain seen w arthritis, also still have ROM and no radicular signs), reflex sympathetic dystrophy (RSD:

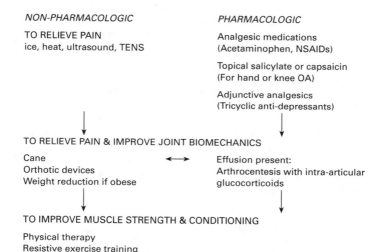

NON-PHARMACOLOGIC	PHARMACOLOGIC

NON-PHARMACOLOGIC

TO RELIEVE PAIN
ice, heat, ultrasound, TENS

PHARMACOLOGIC

Analgesic medications
(Acetaminophen, NSAIDs)

Topical salicylate or capsaicin
(For hand or knee OA)

Adjunctive analgesics
(Tricyclic anti-depressants)

TO RELIEVE PAIN & IMPROVE JOINT BIOMECHANICS

Cane ⟷ Effusion present:
Orthotic devices Arthrocentesis with intra-articular
Weight reduction if obese glucocorticoids

TO IMPROVE MUSCLE STRENGTH & CONDITIONING

Physical therapy
Resistive exercise training
Aerobic conditioning

PAIN IS LIMITING FUNCTION IN SPITE OF MAXIMAL THERAPY

IS THE PATIENT A SURGICAL CANDIDATE?

NO YES

Chronic pain management *SURGICAL EVALUATION*
Trials ongoing using alternative Total joint replacement
forms of medicine, e.g., acupuncture Osteotomy

Figure 10-1. Management of osteoarthritis. Medicinal and nonmedicinal modalities may be initiated concurrently. Reproduced by permission from Ling SM, Balton JM. Osteoarthritis in older adults. J Am Geriatr Soc 1998;46:216

precipitated by trauma, stroke, MI, skin of hand hyperesthetic, warm vasodilation proceeding to cold vasoconstriction w edema on dorsum of fingers; after 6 mo skin becomes atrophied, proceeding in 6 mo to diffuse osteopenia; 3-phase bone scan to make dx early in disease, rx w steroids, stellate ganglion block)

Of hand: r/o hypertrophic pulmonary osteoarthropathy (clubbing fingers, swollen wrists); de Quervain (pain in base of thumb elicited by gripping thumb under fingers and flexing wrist in ulnar direction, rx w splinting and steroid injection, surgery); Dupuytren contracture (fibrous contraction of palmar fascia causing flexion of fingers, rx w stretching, steroid injection, and surgery)

Of knee: r/o anserine bursitis (medial aspect of knee), Baker cyst (rx w steroid injection into joint helps because of direct communication w joint and cyst)

Lab: ESR, CRP nl; synovial fluid WBC <200/dL, protein <4 gm/dL, glucose < serum glucose

Xray:

Early: slight loss of cartilage thickness with narrowing of joint space

Middle: marginal osteophyte formation

Late: loss of joint space, sclerosis of subchondral bone, subchondral cysts, loose bodies, subluxation deformity

Hip films correlate w sx more than hand, knee films

Rx:

Therapeutic:

Tylenol, ASA, NSAIDs (Nejm 1991;325:87) (see Table 10-5); topical salicylates, other topicals worth trials (low risk); capsaicin cream not prn because takes several d to establish effects (see 1.3 Geriatric Pharmacology); ice, cooling packs, corticosteroid injection

Glucosamine sulfate 500 mg tid (Med Let Drugs Ther 1997;39:91), most side effects GI; other agents under investigation: insulin-like growth factor 1, degradative enzyme inhibitors (J Am Geriatr Soc 1997;45:850)

COX-2 inhibitors: (see 10.4 Rheumatoid Arthritis)

Joint irrigation through arthroscope

Joint replacement good option in elderly without other medical problems; consider when major instability in weight-bearing joint, loose bodies in joint, intractable pain

Team Management:

F/u frequently inadequate in clinical practice

Exercise improves function (Jama 1997;277:1863), preserves ROM and increases muscle strength and stability of joint; may reduce med requirements (Ann IM 1992;116:529); water exercises

Emotional, social support; early education for long duration of disease

Common splints: first carpometacarpal joints

Assist knee and quad strength with appropriately fitted chairs and toilets, wall support handles

Support proximal tarsal joint with lacing corset footwear

Hallux valgus: rocker shoe helps reduce stress on joint
Cervical pillow
US deep heat increases tolerance, not cost-effective (Ann IM
    1994;121:133); TENS for knee pain
Assistive devices: jar holder, key holders
Decrease weight (Ann IM 1992;116:535)

10.4 RHEUMATOID ARTHRITIS

Geriatrics 2000;55:30; J Am Geriatr Soc 1991;39:284

Cause: Humoral immune response (rheumatoid factor, IgM, IgG or
  IgA complexed w antigens producing immune complexes w fixed
  complement) resulting in an inflammatory process; cellular immunity
  involving lymphocytes and macrophages; viral

Epidem: 20% new onset after age 60 yr, elderly-onset RA (EORA)

Sx: Pain; inflammation small joints accompanied by constitutional sx
  such as malaise, anorexia, weight loss; prolonged morning stiffness
  lasting >1 h

Si: Criteria for diagnosis (at least four of which must be present for
  6 mo): morning stiffness; arthritis of three or more joint areas;
  hand-joint arthritis (symmetric involvement); rheumatoid nodules;
  rheumatoid factor; radiologic features

  Extra-articular manifestations of RA occur more in young-onset RA
    (YORA): anemia, thrombocytosis, eosinophilia, Felty syndrome,
    splenomegaly, neutropenia, diffuse lymphadenopathy, osteoporosis,
    vasculitis, pericarditis w effusion, conduction abnormalities,
    valvular incompetence, Raynaud phenomenon, pleuritis w
    effusion, interstitial fibrosis, bronchiolitis, entrapment syndromes
    (eg, carpal tunnel), atlantoaxial subluxation, monoarthritis
    multiplex, distal sensory abnormalities, autonomic changes, disuse
    atrophy, keratoconjunctivitis, scleritis, corneal ulceration,
    xerostomia, amyloidosis, cryoglobulinemia, hyperviscosity

Crs: Possibilities include:
  • Few months of sx followed by complete remission
  • Intermittent periods of active disease alternate w relative or
    complete remission
  • Unrelenting progressive disease

Indicators of good prognosis: monoarticular, unilateral, proximal, more abrupt onset, brief duration of initial sx, M sex, absence of IgM and rheumatoid factor, absence of high ESR or CRP, no extra-articular involvement, no erosions on xray; milder course has 50% chance remission vs 30% for YORA; only 6% w EORA have subcutaneous nodules vs 20% with YORA

Cmplc: Late articular complications: deformities of knees and hips result in decreased ambulation; subluxation of cervical vertebrae may lead to neurologic deficits; septic arthritis of knees, elbows, wrists (*Staphylococcus* most common)—19% mortality if not treated early

R/o:

- Osteoarthritis: improves after rest and worsens w activity; weight-bearing joints; distal interphalangeal (Heberden nodes); proximal interphalangeal
- Polymyalgia rheumatica (see 10.5)
- Gout (see 10.6)
- Pseudogout: common in knees, but may also be seen in the wrists, carpal joints; calcium pyrophosphate crystals in joint fluid
- Primary Sjögren syndrome in elderly: milder; less positive ANA, fewer antibodies to SS-A, SS-B (more in RA)
- Fibromyalgia: multiple tender points; disturbed sleep; no synovitis
- Scleroderma: may present w diffuse swelling of digits, but will also see skin changes and anti–Sci-70 antibodies; Raynaud phenomenon
- SLE: 15% of pts present after age 50 yr; less F predominance in elderly; milder course w fewer renal changes and more serositis and joint manifestations; rheumatoid factor occurs more frequently while hypocomplementemia and anti–double-stranded DNA antibodies occur less frequently in elderly SLE patients; r/o rx-induced SLE with mitochondrial and histone antibodies
- Polymyositis/dermatomyositis
- Carcinomatous polyarthritis: direct invasion of bones or joints by lung or breast malignancy; asymmetric; spares small joints; mild inflammatory joint fluid; xrays nl

Lab: Rheumatoid factor pos in 70% of pts; ESR >40 mm/h (elderly run high); mild normochromic, normocytic anemia

Xray: Periarticular osteopenia; periarticular soft tissue swelling; symmetric joint involvement; loss of cartilage; deformities (usually in late disease)

Rx:

Therapeutic (Nejm 1994;330:1368)

- ASA 650–1000 mg qid (elderly more susceptible to salicylism and possible development of pulmonary edema and high risk for GI irritation and bleeding); ASA + NSAIDs may decrease institutionalization rate (J Am Geriatr Soc 1996;44:216)
- Gold (toxic in elderly, causes diarrhea, rash, ulcers, nephropathy, marrow depression, colitis; check CBC, UA, q 2 wk then q mo) 3 mg bid
- D-penicillamine 250 mg qd–tid (toxic in elderly; skin rash and taste abnormalities more common in elderly)
- Hydroxychloroquine 200 mg qd–bid (maculopathy more frequent in elderly)
- Azathioprine 50 mg qd–tid (beneficial effects within 2–6 mo)
- Methotrexate 5–15 mg once a week (oral ulcers, liver abnormalities, marrow suppression, pneumonitis)—more early use recommended
- Sulfasalazine 1–3 gm/d in divided doses (nausea and vomiting more common in the elderly), check lytes, BP, blood sugar, CBC, fecal occult blood test q 1–3 mo
- Steroid injections no more frequently than q 3 mo; use systemic steroids for short courses in conjunction w other agents; steroid side effects in 2–4 wk; low-dose steroids 15 mg prednisone well tolerated during first 2 yrs (BMJ 1998;316:811); >7.5 mg/d glucocorticoid (prednisone) × 6 mo results in rapid loss of trabecular bone in hip, spine, forearm, thus measure BMD and begin preventive measures w calcium, vit D, HRT, weight-bearing exercise; if deterioration BMD give thiazide, sodium restriction, biphosphonate or calcitonin (Arth Rheum 1996;39:179); caution with >3–5 steroid injections in joint pending replacement

Early intervention w disease-modifying antirheumatic drugs (DMARDS) to control disease activity, alleviate pain, maintain function and slow progression of joint damage:

- Hydroxychloroquine is recommended for patients w mild arthritis, methotrexate for moderate to severe disease; sulfasalazine an alternative to either drug (Med Let Drugs Ther 2000;42:57)
- Etanercept (Enbrel) inhibits tumor necrosis factor (TNF, a pro-inflammatory cytokine produced by synovial cells); can be used in combination w methotrexate, glucocorticoids, ASA, NSAIDs; or analgesics; response in 1–2 weeks, lose effect after 1 mo discontinuation; 25 mg twice weekly sc; side effects: more frequent infections, long-term effects unknown

- Leflunomide (Arava) inhibits clonal expansion of T cells by inhibiting cell cycle progression; inhibits cytochrome P450; effect evident by 1 mo; 100 mg tab for 3 days then 20 mg qd; side effects include diarrhea, elevated ALT/AST, alopecia, rash; potential for immunosuppression; watch for renal insufficiency
- Infliximab (Remicade) a monoclonal antibody that blocks TNF; (Lancet 1999;354:1932) can give w methotrexate; 3 mg/kg IV q 8 wks; watch immunosuppression
- COX-2 inhibitors selectively inhibit cyclooxygenase that is involved in inflammation and not prostaglandins that protect gastrointestinal lining: watch clinical liver function and dehydration; reduces effects of ACE inhibitors, furosemide and thiazide; celecoxib (Celebrex) (Med Let Drugs Ther 1999;41:11) 200 mg bid: can be used w methotrexate, timing of meals does not effect absorption, no platelet aggregation so can be given w low-dose ASA, monitor INR w coumadin; rofecoxib (Vioxx): increased gastric ulcer incidence from normals but better than NSAIDs; unknown long-term effects (Gastroenterology 1999;117:776); nephrotoxicity same (Ann IM 2000;133:1)

Opioids have definite role in treating pain (Arth Rheum 1998;41: 1603)

Obtain neck films of pts w long-standing RA and limited ROM of neck to detect subluxation

Team Management:
- Physical and occupational therapy
- Acute episodes: avoid pillows under knees, prevents contractures
- Knee, ankle, wrist splints part of the day to stabilize painful joint while still allowing function
- Isometric maximal contraction of muscle groups in mid-joint range
- Raised soft heel protector for Achilles tendonitis
- Molded insoles to maintain longitudinal arch of shoe
- Hot soaks 20 min tid
- If other associated joints functioning, can consider joint replacement
- Swimming, water exercise if available
- Establish long-term relationships w occupational/physical therapists

10.5 POLYMYALGIA RHEUMATICA AND TEMPORAL ARTERITIS

Am Fam Phys 2000;61:2061; J Am Geriatr Soc 1992;40:515

Cause: HLA-D4 genetic susceptibility; inappropriate immune response
Epidem: 0.1–1.0% of people over 70 yr; F/M = 2:1, white/black = 6:1
Pathophys: Medium and large arteries segmentally; smaller arteries may also be involved, eg, lung
Sx: May be sudden onset:
- Most w muscle pain which is relieved w activity
- Fever
- Jaw claudication
- Transient blindness or blurred vision (occlusion of ciliary artery causing infarction of optic nerve head or, more commonly, central retinal artery causing normal-appearing disk with the remainder of the retina pale w segmented vessels)
- Diplopia
- Headache, usually unilateral
- Thickening of temporal artery

Also slower onset:
- Malaise
- Anorexia
- Weight loss
- Anemia

Less common sx:
- Leg/arm claudication
- CHF
- Aortic arch syndrome
- Facial swelling
- Delirium/dementia
- Peripheral neuropathy

Si: Criteria for dx of PMR: pain and stiffness in two of the following areas: shoulders and upper arms, or pelvic girdle (hip and thighs), or neck and torso; morning: stiffness >1-h duration; duration at least 4 wk; no muscle weakness on exam; no other collagen-vascular disease; elevated ESR (>40 mm/h); relief of symptoms within a few days of starting low-dose steroids (Clin Ger Med 1998;14:455)

Criteria for dx of giant cell arteritis (3 of the following 5): >50 yrs old, new onset of localized headache, temporal artery tenderness or decreased temporal artery pulse, ESR >50 mm/h, abnormal temporal artery biopsy

Crs: Average duration 3 yr

Cmplc: Most PMR resolves uneventfully; 5% have synovitis in sternoclavicular joints; occasionally death from giant cell arteritis (cerebrovascular infarct, MI, aortic aneurysm) (Clin Ger Med 1998;14:455)

R/o RA, which responds to NSAIDs where as PMR does not

Other causes of polymyalgia: SLE; dermatomyositis; periarteritis nodosa; neoplastic diseases, eg, carcinoma, multiple myeloma; Waldenström macroglobulinemia; sarcoidosis; infective endocarditis; osteomalacia; HMG-CoA reductase inhibitors

Xray: Color duplex US for dx temporal arteritis (Nejm 1997;337:1336)

Lab:

Chemistry: ESR >30 mm/h (80–95%), often >100 mm/h; elevated plasma viscosity and CRP (80–95%); normochromic, normocytic anemia (50–80%); elevated globulin fraction in serum electrophoresis (50%); elevated alkaline liver function (50%); neg rheumatoid factor (85%); negative ANA (85%)

Invasive: Temporal artery bx: not necessary in PMR without objective signs of temporal arteritis because clinical outcomes for giant cell arteritis same as pts who only have PMR (Drugs Aging 1998;13:109; J Am Geriatr Soc 1992;40:515); excise 3–5 cm because shorter segment may miss involved segment; if bx neg, still a 5–10% chance that dx has been missed; bx rarely causes scalp necrosis, but more likely when both arteries are removed; 2 wks of steroid will not change characteristic pathologic findings on temporal artery bx

Rx:

Therapeutic:

- PMR: Prednisone 10–20 mg/d until ESR nl, asx; ↓ 1 mg/d q 4 wk; monitor ESR q 4 wk × 3 mo, then q 2–3 mo until 1 yr, then q yr (Am Fam Phys 2000;61:2000)

- Temporal arteritis patients need higher doses of steroids during infections, surgeries, increased physiologic stress; calcium, vit D supplementation and Fosamax; lose 20% BMD within 1 mo on high-dose chronic steroids; alternate-day steroid therapy not recommended; after corticosteroids discontinued, monitor pt for at least 6 mo, checking ESR

- Prednisone 40–60 mg/d until ESR nl; ↓ 10% q 2 wk to 10 mg/d, then ↓ 1 mg/d q 4 wk; monitor ESR q 4 wk × 3 mo then q 2–3 mo until 1.0–1.5 yr after cessation rx (Am Fam Phys 2000;61:2000)

10.6 HYPERURICEMIA AND GOUT

Ann IM 1979;90:812

Cause: Hyperuricemia defined as plasma urate >420 mol/L (7.0 mg/dL); consequence of increased total body urate due to overproduction and/or underexcretion of uric acid; plasma and extracellular fluid saturation with urate leads to crystal formation and deposition; uric acid is the final breakdown product of purine metabolism; 66–75% excreted in kidney and the rest is excreted in the small intestine

Epidem: More common in women

Pathophys:

Gout characterized by:
1. Hyperuricemia
2. Attacks of acute, monoarticular inflammatory arthritis
3. Tophaceous deposition of urate crystals in and around joints (calculi)
4. Interstitial deposition of urate crystals in the renal parenchyma

Si: Extraordinarily painful joint, exquisitely sensitive to touch/pressure; patients do not tolerate any but gentle exam; may be subacute or chronic pain; tophi likely to occur in and around Heberden nodes

Complc: R/o pseudogout calcium pyrophosphate deposition (more common in elderly, in larger joints, often following trauma, surgery or ischemic heart disease); gout associated w hyperthyroidism; pos birefringent rhomboid crystals under polarized light; xray reveals chondrocalcinosis in wrists, knees, pubis symphysis

Crs: Attacks less frequent in the elderly

Lab:

- Evaluation of hyperuricemia: >800 mg/24 h in urine indicates overproduction
- Aspiration of involved joint or tissue key to dx with demonstration of intracellular mono-urate crystals in synovial fluid, PMNLs or tophaceous aggregates; needle-shaped crystals show strong neg birefringence

Rx:

Preventive: Most hyperuricemic individuals never develop gout, so routine screening for asx hyperuricemia is not indicated; for diet, avoid high-purine foods (shellfish, wild game, organ meats); alcohol, dehydration can precipitate attack; if pt has diseases w increased cell breakdown, watch for increased production

Therapeutic: Asx hyperuricemia: treatment is not beneficial or cost-effective except for chemotherapy pts (overproduction) who are at risk for acute uric acid nephropathy

Acute Gouty Arthritis

- NSAIDs: better tolerated than colchicine (former first-line treatment); indomethacin-most widely used in younger age groups but more toxicity in elderly; continue rx 3–4 d after all signs of inflammation have disappeared; use with caution in patients w PUD, heart failure, HT because of problems with salt retention; may precipitate hyperkalemia and renal insufficiency; anemia, check CBC early and during use

- Colchicine: can be useful if NSAIDs not tolerated; inhibits the release of leukocyte-derived crystal-induced chemotactic factor; oral doses of 0.6 tid; cannot be tolerated in up to 80% pts because of abdominal pain, diarrhea, and nausea; increased toxicity when given w other drugs that are P450 enzyme inhibitors, eg, cimetidine, erythromycin, tolbutamide (Nejm 1996;334:445); can also be given IV but w significant toxicity risks; in pts with renal insufficiency, colchicine may produce a reversible neuromuscular toxicity that leads to a subacute myopathy, axonal neuropathy, and increased serum creatinine kinase

- Intra-articular injection of corticosteroids: use when pt cannot take po and when colchicine and NSAIDs are contraindicated or ineffective; po steroids (60–80 mg w quick taper), IM steroids (methyl prednisone acetate [Depo-Medrol] 50 mg), IM ACTH can also be effective (but unavailable at most pharmacies)

Chronic Gout

Patients with recurrent attacks, chronic sx, evidence of tophi, gouty arthritis, or nephrolithiasis

- Biggest issue in elderly is toxicity of long-term med use for chronic gout; all use worth evaluating periodically; stop drugs if possible

- Before starting a urate-lowering agent, pt should be free of inflammation and have started colchicine for prophylaxis (0.6 mg tid is 90% effective in preventing further attacks); treatment goal is urate concentration <300 μmol/L (<5.0 mg/dL); diet modification plays a helpful role but pharmacotherapy is also effective; roles of hyperlipidemia, obesity, DM, HT, and ETOH abuse should be addressed

- Colchicine at 0.6 mg/d for long-term suppression if only sx is joint pain/low-risk regimen
- Allopurinol (for overproducers only): potent competitive inhibitor of xanthine oxidase; absorbed from the GI tract; half-life = 3 h; for pts with evidence of urate overproduction, nephrolithiasis, renal insufficiency (creatinine clearance <80 mL/min), tophaceous deposits, pts at risk for acute uric acid nephropathy; maximum reduction in urate seen at 2 wk; initiation may induce gout attack so concomitant colchicine is usually prescribed; minor side effects: skin rash, GI, diarrhea, headache; serious side effects: alopecia, fever, lymphadenopathy, bone marrow suppression, hepatic toxicity, interstitial nephritis, renal failure, hypersensitivity vasculitis; death can occur in pts with renal insufficiency and pts taking diuretics

  Drug interactions: Allopurinol prolongs the half-life of 6-mercaptopurine, cyclophosphamide, and azathioprine, all of which are degraded by xanthine oxidase; pts taking ampicillin or amoxicillin have a threefold increase in skin rashes; more toxic in the elderly, therefore reduce doses to 100 mg qod
- Uricosuric agents (for underexcretion, most common cause): Decrease serum urate by inhibition of proximal tubule reabsorption; use carefully w renal monitoring in pts >60 yr old, creatinine clearance <80; most commonly used agents:
  1. Probenecid 250 mg po bid up to 1.5 gm/d
  2. Sulfinpyrazone 50 mg po bid (maintenance dose 300–400 mg po tid/qid)

10.7 CERVICAL AND LUMBAR STENOSIS (SPINAL STENOSIS)

Jama 1995;274:1949; Clin Ger Med 1994;10:557

Cause: Congenital size of spinal canal and progression of degenerative spinal disease (soft and bony tissue) lead to vascular compromise of nerve roots (claudication sx) caused by a 50% reduction in one segment relative to normal segments above and below as seen on CT

Pathophys: Most common at L3/L4 or L4/L5 where there is disk degeneration leading to anterior, posterior disk height reduction and longitudinal ligament laxity and subluxation of facet joints; posterior ligamentum flavum hypertrophies in effort to keep segments from falling off each other, resulting in spinal stenosis

Sx:

Cervical: upper extremity radiculopathy; loss bowel, bladder functions; lower extremity spasticity, Babinski, sensory changes; cervical spondylotic myelopathy: neck stiffness, unilateral or bilateral deep aching neck, arm, shoulder pain; numbness, tingling hands; clumsiness while walking; weakness, stiffness legs; electric shock down back w flexion (Lhermitte sign); cervical spondylosis C5–6 no biceps reflex but hyperreflexic triceps; Hoffmann sign reflex contraction of the thumb and index finger after nipping the middle finger (Am Fam Phys 2000;62:1064)

Lumbar: calf, leg, quad, hip pain after walking a discrete distance; back pain less common; lumbar spinal canal increases in size w flexion and decreases w extension; thus increased pain on standing, walking on flat surface, or downhill, which extends the spine

Si: Neurologic exam usually neg w earliest sx but can progress to asymmetric ankle jerk, knee jerk; decreased quad, anterior tibial, extensor hallucis longus strength (check heel and toe walking, hip abduction); bicycle test (can bike farther than can walk, for in sitting position lumbar spine is flexed, which opens up spinal canal and the foramen at each level); straight-leg raising neg; repeating exam after pt walks downhill may bring out subtle neurologic signs (Jama 1995;274:1949)

Cmplc: R/o:

- Acute and chronic disk pain increased by sitting forward; pts often roll to one side and sit up sideways; plantar flexion = L4, dorsiflexion and hip adductors = L5; clearer dermatome pain distribution; chronic disk herniation pain may closely mimic spinal stenosis pain

- Acute central disk: saddle anesthesia; sphincter tone loss (can be common finding in elderly); crossover leg pain (Bull Rheum Dis 1983;33:1)

- Peripheral vascular claudication: pulses absent

- Tumor or infection: rapidly increasing pain or dysfunction, night pain

Xray: LS spine film helpful; MRI

Rx:

Preventive: General conditioning, particularly walking

Therapeutic:

- Conservative: bicycling program, follow pt over long enough time to get careful reading on trend of sx before costly therapy; walker, wheelchair for exercise (NH patients)
- Acupuncture, acupressure, stress reduction, pain treatment programs (Semin Spine Surg 1994;6:156)
- Spinal manipulation not recommended (BMJ 1995;311:349; Ann IM 1992;117:590)
- Epidural steroids (Anesthesiology 1994;81:923)
- Surgical: posterior decompression helps calf pain (2–8 wk to normal activities); fusion (4–6 mo return to normal activities); 85% of pts helped, 12% of pts no better, 3% of pts worse (J Neurosurg 1994;81:699; Spine 1992;17:1); no randomized trial has compared efficacy of surgical vs conservative rx (J Am Geriatr Soc 1996;44:285); rapid increase in surgical intervention w high regional variation suggests need for more research on pt selection (American Hospital Association, Center for Health Care Leadership. The Dartmouth atlas of health care. Chicago, IL: American Hospital Publishing, 1996)

10.8 PAGET DISEASE OF THE BONE

Clin Ger Med 1994;10:719; J Am Geriatr Soc 1998;46:1025; see Figure 10-2

Cause: Autosomal dominant characteristics; seven times greater risk if 1st-degree relative afflicted; may result from viral infection

Epidem: Second most common bone disease (after osteoporosis) affecting older population; although severe disease much less common

Pathophys: Localized increased rate of bone turnover and blood flow; pelvis, axial skeleton, skull and weight-bearing bones affected most frequently; large increase in number and size of osteoclasts and increase in number of nucleoli; irregular resorption of bone produces "mosaic pattern"; reactive osteoblasts produce less organized "woven" bone

Diagnosis:

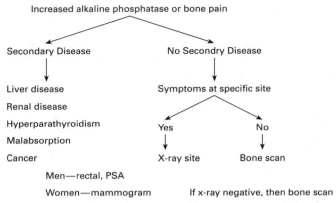

Increased alkaline phosphatase or bone pain

Secondary Disease → Liver disease, Renal disease, Hyperparathyroidism, Malabsorption, Cancer

No Secondary Disease → Symptoms at specific site

Yes → X-ray site

No → Bone scan

Men—rectal, PSA

Women—mammogram   If x-ray negative, then bone scan

Treatment: If alkaline phosphatase 2–3× normal

OR

Pain unrelieved by NSAIDs

OR

Present or potential neurologic sequelae
Surgical intervention (ie, joint replacement)
Or fracture risk (ie, involvement of femur)

First-line therapy: bisphosphonates, calcitonin for patients unable to tolerate

Baseline labwork: alkaline phosphatase and either free pyridinoline crosslinks or N-telopeptides

Follow-up: 3 months, repeat baseline exam and assays
6 months, treatment failure if no remission of symptoms or alkaline phosphatase remains abnormal

Referral: Neurologic symptoms, treatment failure, or uncertainty of diagnosis.

Figure 10-2. Proposed algorithm for Paget disease of bone (osteitis deformans). Reproduced by permission from Ankrom MA, Shapiro JR. Paget's disease of bone (osteitis deformans). J Am Geriatr Soc 1998;46:1010.

Sx: 5% experience pain, especially at night in warm bed secondary to vasodilation in vascular bone; fx, hip arthritis; 1% develop osteosarcoma which presents w excruciating pain unrelieved by analgesics; when pt skull affected, may become apathetic and lethargic (South Med J 1993;10:1097); mental status changes could result from shunting of blood from internal to external carotid system through anastomotic channels; bone compression of CNs II, V, VII, VIII produces monocular visual loss, atypical trigeminal neuralgia, facial paresis or paralysis, hearing loss; middle ear ossicles may be affected as well

Si:

- Deformities: anterior tibial bowing along lines of least resistance; anterolateral femoral bowing; weight of skull causes it to sink into spine, producing short neck and compression of cranial nerves at the base of the skull, spinal neuropathy, hydrocephalus from distortion of the sylvian aqueduct and obstruction of CSF
- Vertebrae: kyphosis, nerve entrapment, spinal stenosis, vascular steal syndrome which may be mistaken for direct cord compression (Aus NZ J Surg 1992;62:24)

Crs: Variable

Cmplc: Osteosarcomatous changes (Clin Orthop 1991;265:306); high-output CHF; heart block due to bundle calcifications; renal stones, especially w immobilization; r/o viral, traumatic causes of bone pain

Lab:

- Alkaline phosphatase reflects activity of the osteoblasts (Horm Metab Res 1991;23:559); common minor alkaline phosphatase elevations nl in elderly—need elevations 1.5–2.0 times nl to pursue dx
- Urinary hydroxyproline levels reflect activity of osteoclasts and bone resorption; both lab values used to monitor active disease and response to rx; free pyridinoline crosslinks, N-telopeptides-specific (J Am Geriatr Soc 1998;46:1025)
- Urine and serum calcium nl unless suddenly immobilized; secondary hyperparathyroidism not uncommon

Xray: Trabecular and cortical bone irregularly thickened; sclerosis and deformity of periarticular bone; fissure fx perpendicular to long axis of bone; inner and outer table of skull bones indistinguishable; thus entire thickness consists of spongiosa, producing "cotton wool" appearance; w osteosarcomas (most commonly in pelvis, femur, humerus) technetium uptake reduced and gallium uptake increased

Rx:
Therapeutic:
- Treat asymptomatic Paget disease of the skull or vertebrae; otherwise only rx disability, pain (not relieved by analgesics), increased bone deformity, frequent fx, vertebral compression, rapid decline in hearing, high-output CHF
- Early intervention w CN decompression results in better prognosis
- Biphosphonates: etidronate 200–300 mg/d in frail elderly for 6 mo; alendronate (Fosamax): reduces the rate of bone turnover and decreases bone blood flow; newly formed bone is lamellar; effects long lasting and persist after treatment stopped and more effective than etidronate and calcitonin (Nejm 1997;336:558); tiludronate (Skelid) 200 mg might be tolerated better than other bisphosphonates (Med Let Drugs Ther 1997;39:65); risedronate, zoledronate 3rd generation
- Calcitonin: 200 IU/dose, alternate nostrils qod; nausea from calcitonin self-limited and <10% of patients discontinue med; other side effects include flushing, diarrhea, and pain at injection site; human calcitonin has more side effects than salmon calcitonin; recrudescence when therapy discontinued even after 1 yr therapy
- Plicamycin: cytotoxic antibiotic reserved for nerve compression; 15–20 µg/kg over 5–10 d period; give w calcium and vit D
- Surgical hip replacement (J Bone Joint Surg Am 1987;69:760); total knee replacement (J Bone Joint Surg Am 1991;73:739)

10.9 LOW BACK PAIN

J Am Geriatr Soc 1993;41:167; Ger Rev Syllabus 2001:213

Cause: Major and minor soft tissue trauma and overuse injuries; UTI; cancer; spontaneous vertebral compression fx (osteoporosis)
Epidem: Very common in elderly; frequently chronic or recurrent
Sx: Nonspecific limb sx (pseudoclaudication), loss of continence
Si: Decreased lower extremity muscle strength; decreased lower extremity muscle circumference; altered lower extremity reflexes; altered lower extremity sensory exam; pos straight-leg raising; check sitting knee extension; palpate for lower abdominal masses; pelvic and rectal exam if pain severe or long-standing

Palpate point and general tenderness—spinous processes of lumbar vertebrae, iliolumbar ligaments, lumbar paravertebral muscles, sacroiliac joints, gluteal muscles; evaluate landmark asymmetries —leg length discrepancies, tibial tuberosities, iliac crest heights; pelvic compression—osteopathic maneuver to detect sacroiliac joint instability; pelvic roll—osteopathic maneuver to detect mobility of LS spine; standing and seated flexion; sacral motion

Cmplc: R/o fx, spinal stenosis, infection, tumor, cauda equina syndrome

Lab: CBC, alkaline phosphatase, Ca^{2+}, ESR, UA, serum immunoelectrophoresis later if multiple myeloma suspected

Xray: LS plain films can be useful if fx or neoplasm suspected; prior film(s) always helpful for comparison; bone scan if malignancy or osteomyelitis suspected

Rx: Brief bed rest periods only (if at all); encourage frequent brief walks; discourage sitting (particularly in auto) for any lengths of time; maintain regular f/u (frequency depends on pain); firm bed, lumbar pillow, abdominal muscle-strengthening exercises (after acute phase)

Osteopathic:

Principles of Treatment
- Use shorter, less frequent treatments
- Avoid thrust techniques in people with severe osteoporosis or osteoarthritis
- Reestablish motion as quickly as possible
- Use steady, gentle techniques

Specific Manipulative Treatments
- Muscle and fascial stretching
- Muscle energy technique: improve muscle-resting length by having pt actively engage the muscle group and then passively stretch it during relaxation
- Counterstrain: reduction of inappropriate neuromuscular reflexes by placing joint into a position of comfort for 90 sec
- Soft tissue release: massage of muscle to improve fluid mobilization

Team Management: Establish physical therapy or osteopathic relationship early if musculoskeletal origin of pain

10.10 ADHESIVE CAPSULITIS OF SHOULDER (BURSITIS, TENDONITIS)

J Am Geriatr Soc 1998;46:1144; Ger Rev Syllabus 1996:237

Cause: Adhesive capsulitis: often secondary to impingement syndromes

Sx: Long head biceps tendonitis: arm motions w fixed flexed elbow, eg, screwing caps on jars; working overhead forcefully turns plantar surface of hand upward against resistance with elbow fixed; tennis serve motion

Adhesive capsulitis: contraction glenohumeral capsule

Si:

- Long head biceps tendonitis: tender bicipital groove, pain on resisted supination forearm w elbow adjacent to side and flexed 90 degrees
- Rotator cuff tendonitis (age >45 yr): 60–120 degrees extension with painful arc; pain at anterolateral aspect shoulder at greater tuberosity of humerus may lead to complication of subdeltoid bursitis, giving pain at tip acromion and over humeral head; supraspinatus: pain on resistance in abduction; infraspinatus: pain on resistance in external rotation; no pain on resisted movement w subacromial bursitis; rotator cuff tears: weakness w elevation of arm in abduction and external rotation; impingement sign: putting hand behind head cannot hold hand in 90 degree position, infra- and supraspinatus atrophy (J Am Geriatr Soc 2000;48:1633)
- Subacromial bursitis: swelling, warm, tender
- Adhesive capsulitis: decreased movement of the shoulder

Cr:

- R/o tumor from kidney, breast, lung, prostate when general exam is normal but pain severe
- Cervical spine disease: pain w cervical extension, C5 weakness of shoulder adduction (deltoid, supraspinatus), C6 weak extension carpus radialis, C7 weakness elbow extension (triceps); neck extension and lateral bending toward affected side closes neural foramina
- Adhesive capsulitis: initial pain phase 2–4 mo, followed by limited shoulder mobility 4–8 mo, then gradual return to nl ROM 18 mo–3 yr; at 7 yr 30% restricted mobility, 50% stiffness

Cmplc: Stage III after age 40: inflammation, permanent scarring, rotator cuff tendonitis tear, bone alterations, ruptured biceps

Xray:
- A-P and axillary views; adhesive capsulitis: nl xray, no degenerative bone loss
- Subacromial bursitis: calcific deposits on xray

Rx:

Therapeutic:
- Long head biceps tendonitis: rx bid w exercise; should improve in 3 wk; if not better in 6 mo, consider surgery
- Rotator cuff tendonitis exercises: pendulum, walk fingers up wall, exercises w arms close to body to avoid impingement, long stretches help to regain motor function; arthroscopic surgery for decompression impingement
- Heat before, ice after more strenuous exercise (when ready)
- Subacromial bursitis: 75% improve with steroid injections (Ann Rheum Dis 1984;43); 1 mL depot steroid mixed w 1% lidocaine
- Calcific tendonitis: may need closed lavage w lidocaine or surgical removal; regional anesthesia w interscalene block
- Adhesive capsulitis: 6–12 mo, gradual return to nl w physical therapy; use analgesics and NSAIDs

NSAID Use and Interactions
See Table 10-5.

Table 10-5. Duration and Adverse Effects of NSAIDs

	Half-life		
	Short	**Intermediate**	**Long**
Least side effects	Ibuprofen (Motrin)	Sulindac (Clinoril)	Nabumetone (Relafen)
Mid	Fenoprofen (Nalfon) Indomethacin (Indocin)	Naproxen (Naprosyn) Ketoprofen (Orudis) Tolmetin (Tolectin)	Piroxicam (Feldene)
Most side effects	Meclofenamate (Meclomen)		

Reproduced by permission from Henry D, et al. Variability in risk of gastrointestinal complications with individual non-steroidal anti-inflammatory drugs: results of a collaborative meta-analysis. BMJ 1996;312:1563–6.

1. Antacids make NSAIDs more tolerable, but decrease absorption; GI toxicity reduced by misoprostol 100 µg qid (limited by diarrhea), assessment and possible treatment of *Helicobacter pylori* infection before commencing long-term course NSAIDs in pts w h/o recurrent PUD
2. With anticoagulation interactions, GI bleed risk; decrease anticoagulant to achieve same PT or PTT; ibuprofen (Motrin), tolmetin (Tolectin), sulindac (Clinoril, Vioxx, Celebrex) have least GI adverse effects
3. Antirheumatic agents: watch WBC, platelets
4. Diuretics: adjustment may be necessary to maintain antihypertensive effects
5. Lithium: decreased clearance so monitor level 7 d after beginning NSAID, indomethacin (Indocin), piroxicam (Feldene) in particular
6. Methotrexate: displacement from protein-binding site increases its toxicity
7. Oral hypoglycemics: displacement from binding leads to sulfonylurea toxicity, particularly with fenoprofen (Nalfon), naproxen (Naprosyn), naproxen sodium (Anaprox)
8. Phenytoin: naproxen and fenoprofen (Nalfon) will displace, leading to phenytoin toxicity
9. Probenecid: increases plasma levels of most NSAIDs—can reduce levels of some NSAIDs (ketoprofen, meclofenamate [Meclomen], indomethacin [Indocin])
10. Renal insufficiency relative contraindication; ASA alternative and can monitor w drug levels

11 Gastrointestinal Disorders

11.1 ESOPHAGEAL PROBLEMS AND PEPTIC ULCER DISEASE

Clin Ger Med 1999;15:439,457; Jama 1996;275:622; Sci Am 1995;4:1; Surg Clin N Am 1994;74:93,113

Esophageal Problems—See Tables 11-1 and 11-2

Petic Ulcer Disease
Cause: Smoking, aspirin, NSAIDs (greatest risk within first 3 mo); *Helicobacter pylori* (50% seropositive by age 60) grows in mucus

Table 11-1. Common Esophageal Problems in Elderly

Type	Characteristics	Rx
Achalasia	2nd peak in elderly Failure of lower esophageal sphincter relaxation	Nitrates, calcium channel blockers Botulinum toxin injection Pneumatic dilatation
Esophageal Spasm		Nifedipine, diltiazem, sedatives, anticholinergics
Scleroderma		Can Rx reflux with proton pump inhibitors (PPI)
Rings	Intermittent dysphagia when diameter is less than 12–13 mm	Proton pump inhibitors (PPI) dilation with single large bougie
Gerd	Aspiration, cough, asthma, vocal cord infection, polyps, sore throat, eustachian tube, dysfx, dental enamel loss, chest pain	Elevate head of bed, stop smoking, calcium channel, anticholinergics, Reglan, cisapride

Table 11-2. Dysphagia

	OROPHARYNGEAL (Can't initiate swallowing or transfer food bolus from mouth to upper esophageal sphincter)	ESOPHAGEAL (Can't transfer from esophagus to stomach) ACHALASIA—failure to relax lower esophageal sphincter
CAUSE	Neurological—brainstem, anterior cortical stroke ALS, Parkinson's neoplasm, Alzheimer's Muscular—Myasthenia, Gravis, Eaton-Lambert, dermatomyositis, polymyositis Anatomic—neoplasm, Zenker's diverticula, cervical spurs, strictures, pemphigoid Iatrogenic—antipsychotics → tardive dyskinesia, radiation	
EPID		40s–50s 2nd peak in elderly
SX		30–50% Retrosternal chest pain, gradual solid liquid food dysphagia, 60–90% regurgitate undigested food ac If weight loss → 15 lbs/1 yr suspect malignancy
COURSE		R/O scleroderma, sarcoid
TESTS	Speech evil Modified Ba swallow with fiberoptic endoscopic exam	X ray "bird beak" narrowing at gastroesophageal junction "sigmoid esoph"—very dilated Endoscopy to R/O malignancy
RX	Correct underlying disorder Speech rx → turn head toward damaged side, strengthening tongue	Botulinum toxin injection into sphincter muscle lasts 24 mo— needs to be repeated Pneumatic dilatation (90% success rate), surgical myotomy laparoscopic (80–90% success)

overlying antral gastric mucosa cells in 95% of pts w duodenal ulcers and 60–75% of pts w gastric ulcers; 1st-degree relative = 3 times risk

Epidem: Mortality duodenal ulcer 2–5%/100,000 elderly/yr; 29–60% mortality from PUD in patients >65 yrs old; relapse 90% in 10 yr, quiescent after 10–15 yr; incidence increased in COPD, RA, cirrhosis, hyperparathyroidism

Pathophys: Gastric acid secretion not decreased w aging in healthy individuals (Gastroenterology 1996;110:1043); mucosal prostaglandin decreased, gastric bicarbonate decreased, and integrity of gastric mucosa decreased because of gastric blood flow; gastritis may be completely explained by *H. pylori* (Clin Ger Med 1999;15:439); gastric ulcers more often proximal in elderly

Sx: Only 35% of elderly have pain; less pain w NSAID usage; duodenal ulcer: deep epigastric pain relieved by food or antacids; hunger experienced 2 h after meals; vomiting indicates ulcer within pyloric channel; melena from erosion at the base of the ulcer is an unusual complication; occasionally present w anemia, MI, CVA

Crs: Gastric (bigger, bleed more in elderly) less common than duodenal

Cmplc: R/o:

1. Ischemic pain not relieved by food but may respond to vasodilator
2. Carcinoma: anorexia, nausea, weight loss
3. Acute cholecystitis: lancinating pain, fever, weight loss
4. Acute pancreatitis: nausea, emesis
5. Acute appendicitis
6. Other causes of upper GI bleeding (sources in order of decreasing prevalence): gastric ulcer, duodenal ulcer, gastric erosions, esophagitis, esophageal varices, neoplasm, Mallory-Weiss tears (J Am Geriatr Soc 1991;39:402)
7. GE reflux: rx w H_2 antagonist and prokinetic agent (metoclopramide [Reglan]) if sx persist, and decrease dose by 50% in elderly

Half of pts over the age of 70 have complications, higher mortality related to comorbidity, mortality rate 29–60%

- Bleeding ulcers: mortality rate 10–15%; 10–20% have no sx; re-bleed if hypotension or visible vessel or sentinel clot on endoscopy
- Obstruction from edema or fibrosis in the region of the ulcer: distension or fullness before meal completed; >300 mL gastric contents 4 h after meal completed
- Perforation (5–10% mortality): highest mortality/morbidity in the elderly; duodenal perforation 5 times more common than gastric perforation but gastric perforation mortality 5 times greater (30–50%); severe progressive mid-epigastric pain, later localizing to right lower abdomen if gastric contents spill along surface of right colon; can get posterior ulcer penetrating into pancreas causing acute pancreatitis, which rarely becomes recurrent or chronic

Lab: Endoscopy if gross upper GI bleed, no response to therapy, or multiple ulcers or gastric ulcer on previous exam

Basal and stimulated acid secretion when intractable to medical therapy; recurrent disease rapidly develops; gastric ulcer might be caused by carcinoma (33% of pts with ulcerated gastric carcinoma have achlorhydria after acid secretion stimulation whereas pts w benign disease have some acid secretion)

Breath urea test for *H. pylori* or rapid serologic tests (Nejm 1996;333:984); antibody testing less specific than urease enzyme testing of bx specimen

Rx:

Therapeutic:

- Diets not effective, although pts may prefer to avoid foods that have troubled them; avoid caffeine; refrain from eating at night
- Antacids 1 and 3 h after meals and on retiring as good as H_2-receptor antagonists (Drugs 1994;47:305); MgOH—osmotic diarrhea; calcium carbonate–acid rebound; aluminum hypophosphatemia—good for renal failure; alternating magnesium, aluminum, and calcium antacids avoids side effects
- H_2 receptors: rigorous separation of H_2 receptors and antacids probably not necessary; cimetidine available generically and 30–50% less expensive; side effects: prolongs half-life of phenytoin, theophylline, coumadin, β-blockers, lidocaine, diazepam, chlordiazepoxide because interact w hepatic P450 microenzyme (ranitidine binds P450 less, and famotidine, nizatidine do not bind P450); cause mental confusion—big problem in hospital as extensively used postop; after 2–3 mo rx for gastric ulcer, reevaluate (UGI or endoscopy) to identify 5% who progress to gastric cancer; if sx of duodenal ulcer improve, no further study needed
- Sucralfate: 1 gm 1 h before meals 3 d and hs; works for multiple gastric erosions as well; affects aluminum absorption (use w caution in renal failure because of impaired excretion of aluminum); interferes w tetracycline absorption; constipation
- Anticholinergics: propantheline 30 min before meals; selective inhibitor gastric acid secretion
- Omeprazole: 20–40 mg strongly inhibits hydrogen ion secretion by the gastric parietal cells; for resistant PUD, erosive gastritis; better than ranitidine, misoprostol in ulcers associated w NSAIDs; healing in 4 wk; interference w drugs metabolized by P450 system; decrease in the acid-induced metabolism of ingested digoxin (Ann IM

Table 11-3. Treatment of *Helicobacter pylori*

Regimen	Dosing	Eradication Rate
Triple antimicrobial therapy		
Omeprazole	20 mg bid × 1 wk	~90%
Clarithromycin	500 mg bid × 1 wk	
Metronidazole	500 mg bid × 1 wk	
Omeprazole	20 mg bid × 1 wk	~90%
Amoxicillin	1 gm bid × 1 wk	
Clarithromycin	500 mg bid × 1 wk	

Reproduced by permission from Borum ML. Peptic-ulcer disease in the elderly. Clin Geriatr Med 1999;15:467.

1991;115:540); acute hepatic toxicity (Am J Gastroenterol 1992;87:523)

- Misoprostol: 200 mg qid; synthetic prostaglandin E_1 analogue for prevention of NSAID-induced gastric ulcers, also prevents duodenal ulcers; dose-related diarrhea 13–40%, abdominal pain 7–20% (Nejm 1992;327:1575)
- *H. pylori* treatment: 2-wk course of amoxicillin 500 qid or clarithromycin 500 tid along w omeprazole 20 bid (Am J Gastroenterol 1994;89:39); triple-drug therapy w metronidazole 250 plus tetracycline 500 mg plus bismuth 2 tabs (all three doses qid w meals and evenings) results in >90% eradication—much less expensive alternative (Am Fam Phys 1995;52:1717); see Table 11-3
- Sedation: oxazepam 10 mg tid
- Surgery: Billroth I or II for recurrent ulcers produces dumping syndrome in 10% of pts

11.2 CELIAC SPRUE

J Am Geriatr Soc 2000;48:1690; Gastroenterology 1998;114:424; Sci Am 2000; "Gastroenterology" in Mansbach, C.M. Malabsorption and Maldigestion; 11:3; Nejm 1991;325:1709

Epidem: Short stature; 25% childhood or family hx; genetic predisposition (HLA) leads to intestinal reaction to x-gliadin fraction of gluten

Pathophys: Saccharides degraded by luminal bacterial into two- and three-carbon fragments with increased osmotic effect leading to diarrhea; severe damage to villi; dietary CHO digested to monosaccharides by enzyme intestinal surface

Sx: Profound fatigue by midday, cannot even do sedentary activity; stool change subtle, diarrhea intermittent for periods of 4–6 months or less; anorexia after several months/years, glossitis, unexplained anemia (Gut 1999;55:65; Minn Med 1995;78:29); apathy, wasting, but not until severe

Si: Anterior and lateral margins of tongue smooth; petechiae, ecchymosis, abdominal distention, ↑ bowel sounds, ↓ intestinal transit with advanced disease

Crs: ↓ Vit A, vit D leading to osteoporosis; ↓ vit E may lead to spinal cerebellar degeneration; ↓ vit K, ↓ vit B$_{12}$ leading to ataxia—most common neurologic manifestation; ↓ Ca, ↓ Mg resulting in tetany, mental confusion (small percentage) (Arch IM 1997;15:1013); ulcer, colitis or Crohn may precede or follow sprue by months or years; 15–20% histiocytic lymphomas, adenocarcinomas

R/o sideroderma, dermatitis herpetiformis (pruritic red skin blisters on shoulder, buttocks, knees, elbows), diabetic autoimmune neuropathy, florid thyrotoxicosis; epilepsy in 3–5%; prolonged Q-T; tropical sprue: lymphocytic infiltration on bx, geographic location, severe megaloblastic anemia 20–25 hct; ischemic: bloody diarrhea and pain 15 min after eating; chronic radiation enteritis: may lead to stricture

Lab: ↓ Albumin <2.5 gm/dL (protein loss through damaged surface membrane); megaloblastic anemia (50%); ↓ cholesterol; liver—abnormal AST, ACT resolve with rx (Clin Gastroenterol 1995;20:90); ↑ antigliadin A, G, ↑ antiendomysial antibody titers corresponds to xray changes

Rx: Diet excludes wheat, gluten, rye, barley, oats (Hosp Pract 1993;28:41); avoid milk—pts develop lactose intolerance; prednisone 20–40 mg if pt does not respond to gluten free diet; if becomes refractory to diet, look for tumors

See Tables 11-4 and 11-5

Table 11-4. Drug-induced Diarrhea

Drug-induced diarrhea (Clin Ger Med 2000;8:67)

Decreased gastric acid: leads to pathogens that cause diarrhea (*Shigella*, *Salmonella*, *Giardia lamblia*, and *Clostridium difficile*)
• Cimetidine (J Am Ger Soc 1993;41:940)

Decreased motility: gastric: leads to pathogens (Gastroenterol Clin N Am 1994;23:313)
• Metoclopramide
• Cisapride
• Erythromycin
• Diazepam

Small bowel: leads to pathogens
• Cholinomimetics, eg, tacrine (diarrhea rarely occurs w hypermotility of small bowel)

Secretory diarrhea: interferes w ATP pump
• Misoprostol
• 5-ASA
• Digoxin (second most common cause of drug-induced diarrhea)
• Colchicine

Osmotic diarrhea:
• Lactulose
• Acarbose

Mucosal damage:
• Antineoplastics
• Gold
• Penicillamine
• Methyldopa
• NSAIDs

11.3 DIVERTICULITIS

Surg Clin N Am 1994;74:293

Cause: Lack of dietary fiber

Epidem: >50% prevalence in persons over 70 yr

Pathophys: 90% in sigmoid colon because narrow caliber results in higher intraluminal pressure; found in R colon in the Asian population (Br J Surg 1971;58:902)

Sx: Pain 75% and hemorrhage 25%; abrupt, persistent L lower quadrant (sometimes R lower quadrant or suprapubic) colicky pain

Table 11-5. Diarrhea

	Crohn	Ulcerative Colitis	Diverticulitis	Mesenteric Ischemia	Villous Adenoma
Si/Sx/Lab	Blood/mucus/pus abdominal pain (postprandial)	Not as much bleeding as w younger pts	+/– Constipation, fever, leukocytosis, peritoneal sis; bleeding resolves spontaneously; be alert to presentation w few sx	L crampy postprandial pain; h/o decreased cardiac output, eg, afib; may lead to diarrhea, distension, and 50% bleed within 24 h, and nausea and vomiting	Decreased K+; chronic diarrhea presentation
Xray/endoscopy/ complc	Ulcers on sigmoidoscopy; bx: transluminal granuloma; complc: obstruction, hemorrhage, perforation, fistula, malnutrition, weight loss large, arthritis, skin and oral lesions	Friable; avoid BE if fever; bleeding leads to toxic megacolon; 20% increase risk for colon cancer in 10 yr	Complc: obstruction, perforation, fistula, abscess, peritonitis from gram-neg and anaerobic organisms	BE thumbprinting (blue submucosal hemorrhage adjacent to pallor; heal 2 wk or 15% stricture; 20% persistent; 10% gangrene (w 90% mortality)	Colonoscopy
Rx	See 11.4	See 11.5	Surgical resection >2 episodes; early detection and rx w antibiotics important to prevent hospitalization	Rest bowel, parenteral fluids, NG tube, broad-spectrum antibiotics, surgery for gangrene or impending perforation, or if not resolved in 2–3 wk	Surgery

increasing in severity over time, exacerbated by meals, relieved by bowel movements; more often constipation than diarrhea or alternating; anorexia; vomiting; fever may be presenting complaint; peritonitis; elderly may not have pain or fever, so serial exams important

Si: Distended abdomen, tympanic to percussion; bowel sounds diminished; localized tender mass; rebound tenderness locally; occult rectal bleeding

Crs: 3–10 d; recurrence rate 25% in first 5 yr

Cmplc: Perforation, fistula, abscess; urinary frequency, dysuria may suggest bladder involvement; most common cause of lower intestinal bleeding except angiodysplasia; w bleeding r/o colon cancer, ischemic bowel, angiodysplasia (R colon in 66% of pts, usually in the setting of previously undiagnosed asx disease, 70–80% resolve spontaneously, 3–5% require transfusions); B_{12} malabsorption → deficiency

Lab: Leukocytosis; white or red cells on UA if ureteral inflammation

Xray: Saw-toothed pattern and thickening of muscular wall of colon considered prediverticular condition; adynamic ileus, mechanical obstruction

Perform sigmoidoscopy early without vigorous bowel preparation and minimal air insufflation; wait wks for full colonoscopy to r/o cancer proximal to rectosigmoid region

CT if suspect abscess

For continued bleeding: selective mesenteric arteriography to localize extravasation and distinguish from angiodysplasia; bleeding rate <1 mL/min technetium-tagged rbc scan w diverticular bleeding

Rx:

Therapeutic:
- Bowel rest w IV hydration
- Surgical consultation early
- Analgesics cautiously because they mask symptoms
- Broad-spectrum antibiotics to cover gram-pos, anaerobic and aerobic gram-neg organisms; tetracycline if no leukocytosis or fever
- β-Lactam antibiotic w activity against anaerobic and enteric gram-neg organisms; if no improvement, CT to r/o intra-abdominal abscess (pain may be lacking, may not have increased WBC, anemia, increased alkaline phosphatase, ESR may be only clues), fistula formation; surgical mortality 20%, try percutaneous drainage first

- Diet can be advanced over few days to normal diet
- If severe, hemicolectomy indicated for spreading peritonitis; should be done in two-stage procedure in the elderly unless can attain preoperative percutaneous drainage of isolated diverticular abscess
- For active bleeding, vasopressin for interarterial vasoconstriction, embolization; if pt exsanguinating, consider partial colectomy
- In pts with early diverticulitis in NH or home w support, antibiotics and oral fluids w careful frequent evaluation appropriate

11.4 INFLAMMATORY BOWEL DISEASE (CROHN)

Epidem: Less common than ulcerative colitis; 16% of pts w Crohn disease are >65 yr; bimodal population and involvement of different segments of the intestines (more distal) in later years suggest different disease entities (Med Clin N Am 1994;78:1303)

Pathophys: Transmural; more likely to be distal part of small bowel, narrowing ileal lumen

Sx: Usually indolent; diarrhea persistent w large-bowel disease; less bleeding than w ulcerative colitis; mucus, pus, and abdominal pain (postprandial) may resemble small-bowel obstruction if terminal ileum involved (Am Fam Phys Monograph 1995;198:19)

Si: Aphthous ulcer in rectum; tender mass R lower quadrant usually inflamed bowel, mesentery, lymph nodes, sometimes abscess (small sealed off perforations); gross blood in stool unusual

Crs: High (85%) postop recurrence (Med Clin N Am 1990;74;183); see Table 11-3

Cmplc: Obstruction, perforation, fistula; malnutrition, 25-lb weight loss; arthritis; skin lesions; anal lesions; renal stones from calcium oxalate if terminal ileum involved

R/o:
- Cholelithiasis, cholecystitis
- PUD
- Mesenteric vascular insufficiency: pain disproportionate to belly tenderness; usually followed by bloody diarrhea within hours; treat w resection or reestablishment of arterial flow to involved bowel; chronic mesenteric ischemia presents w triad of postprandial pain, fear of eating, weight loss
- Tumors

- Amebic colitis: associated w inanition, fatigue
- *Clostridium difficile*
- Irritable bowel: recurrent crampy pain, bloating, flatulence, diarrhea and constipation; pain associated w stress, relieved by passage of flatus or stool
- Diverticulitis: 3–6 cm of bowel, while Crohn 10-cm segment w transverse fissures
- Bowel obstruction: periumbilical pain waxes and wanes q 10 min in lower bowel
- NSAID-induced enteropathy (Gut 1992;33:887): occult blood pos, anemia, rx w misoprostol

Lab: Anemia secondary to iron deficiency, ↓ vit B_{12} metabolized in terminal ileum; folate deficiency from sulfasalazine inhibition of its absorption; mild leukocytosis >10,000/dL; can also see granulomas on bx in ulcerative colitis

Xray: Sigmoid ulceration on BE

Rx:
- Sulfasalazine supplemented w folic acid, azathioprine, 6-mercaptopurine, methotrexate (Am J Gastroenterol 1997;92:7703)
- Infliximab (tumor necrosis factor) not in general use yet (Br J Surg 1997;84:1051)
- Budesonide associated w reduced systemic side effects (Nejm 1998;339:370)
- Poor candidates for ileoanal anastomoses because of disease and recurrences
- Colonoscopic bx q 8–10 yrs

Team Management: In contrast to results in pts w ulcerative colitis, elemental diets and TPN w bowel rest improve symptoms, inflammatory sequelae and nutritional status in pts w Crohn (Nejm 1996;334:841)

See Table 11-4

Table 11-6. Inflammatory Bowel Disease in the Elderly

Ulcerative Colitis	Crohn
Slight male predominance	Female predominance
Severe initial attacks	Delays in dx
High mortality w severe attack	Mortality not increased
More frequent proctosigmoid	More colonic, less ileum involved
Lower relapse rate	Low postop recurrence rates
Good long-term prognosis	Good response med rx

11.5 ULCERATIVE COLITIS

Sci Am 2001; "Gastroenterology" in Hanauer S. Inflammatory bowel disease; 4:4

Cause: Alteration in mucosal immune system

Epidem: 12% of pts are >60 yr; 3 times more common than Crohn disease; M > F (Gastroenterol Clin N Am 1990;19:361)

Sx: Tenesmus; presents more w diarrhea than bleeding in the elderly

Crs:
- Mild (60%, distal colon and rectum); even when disease remains quiescent, mucosa has abnormal dull flat or granular appearance
- Moderately severe (25%, >5 stools/d gross blood, cramping pain, intermittent temperature to 100.4 degrees F, intermittent fatigue, increased sleep requirement)
- Severe (15%, extreme fatigue, weakness, prostration; distended abdomen, tympany, bowel sounds often absent); increased risk for colon cancer 20%/10-yr duration; cancer risk independent of disease activity

Cmplc: Toxic megacolon 3%, perforation 3%, stricture 10%, severe hemorrhage 4%, cancer 3% (as high as 40% in pts who acquired the disease before the age of 15 yr) (Nejm 1990;323:1228); erythema nodosum 3%, aphthous mouth ulcers 10%, iritis 5%, arthritic large joints 5%, fatty liver 40%, pericholangitis 5%, cirrhosis 3%, sclerosing cholangitis 2.5%, pyoderma gangrenosum, uveitis, spondylitis (HLA-B27)

R/o: bacterial gastroenteritis, ischemic colitis, diverticulitis, amebiasis, Crohn, irritable bowel

Lab: CBC, electrolytes, liver profile, blood cultures

Xray: Avoid BE if fever or tachycardia or increased rectal bleeding as may cause toxic megacolon; friable sigmoid and rectum (grades 1–4 ranging from friability after swabbing to unprovoked bleeding before swabbing); small bowel follow-through; pseudopolyps (nodules of regenerative mucosa); aphthous ulcer rectum; see Table 11-7

Rx:

Preventive: Serial colonoscopies q yr w bx q 10 cm for 8 yrs after onset

Table 11-7. Findings on BE

Ulcerative Colitis	Crohn
Loss of haustra; multiple 1-mm diameter "collar button" ulcers	"Rose thorn" ulcers w deep tracts; ileum involvement w skip lesions; "thumbprinting"; transmural involvement; fistulas

Therapeutic:

- Antidiarrhea agents: diphenoxylate, loperamide, tincture of opium
- Sulfasalazine and 5-aminosalicylates (5-ASA) derivatives (mesalamine) for remissions or mild sx: 0.5 gm bid 2–4 d, then 0.5–1.5 gm qid (10% epigastric sx)
- Olsalazine (Gut 1994;35:1282), mesalamine for mild flares; corticosteroid enemas for mild to moderately active, 4 gm/60 mL (Gut 1992;33:947)
- Azathioprine 50 to 100 mg/d for several months; when bone marrow depression occurs, 3 d off drug will allow parameters to return to nl; ACTH 40 units IV q 12 h 7–14 d for moderate to severe sx
- Add cyclosporine 4 mg/kg/day IV for fulminant colitis or toxic megacolon; response in 4 d
- Diet: watch for lactose intolerance; Fe po
- Erythropoietin (Nejm 1996;334:619), transfusion for anemia
- Indications for proctocolectomy:
  1. Failure of intensive drug therapy after 2–4 wk
  2. Failure of toxic megacolon to improve after 4 d of intensive therapy
  3. Cannot distinguish stricture from cancer
  4. Severe extracolonic manifestations, ileal-rectal anastomosis, or ileoanal pouch (Am J Gastroenterol 1998;93:166)
- Antibiotics of no help (Am J Gastroenterol 1994;89:43)

11.6 ISCHEMIC BOWEL

Clin Ger Med 1999;15:527; Med Clin N Am 1994;78:1303

Cause: Associated w artificial mitral valve, afib, surgical bypass

Epidem: Most common cause of noninfectious colitis in the elderly; 1% of all admissions for acute abdomen

Pathophys: Mucosal, then serosal involvement; L colon (splenic flexure); "watershed" area prone to ischemia because of poor circulation

Sx: Abdominal pain (left-sided cramps in 75%), bleeding (50% within 24 h), distension, diarrhea, nausea, vomiting

Si: Decreased cardiac output

Crs: Bloody diarrhea, weight loss, decreased albumin; generally complete healing in 2 wk

Cmplc: Pseudo-obstruction, 15% strictures, 20% persistent ischemic colitis, 10% gangrene; 90% mortality

Lab:

Xray: Supine abdomen: gas in portal vein—poor px; done primarily to exclude other causes; BE: thumbprinting; sigmoidoscopy: focal hemorrhagic lesions, ischemic ulcerations (dark blue submucosal ulcerations adjacent to areas of pallor); CT, MRI: nonspecific edema; duplex ultrasound: to dx chronic mesenteric ischemia early by arterial narrowing, decreased blood flow

Rx:

Therapeutic: Bowel rest, parenteral fluids, NG tube; broad-spectrum antibiotics; surgery if suspect gangrene or perforation impending or not resolved in a couple wks; pseudo-obstruction: colonic decompression if cecal diameter >9 cm; see Table 11-8

11.7 GI BLEEDING (ANGIODYSPLASIA)

Clin Ger Med 1999;15:511; 1994;10:1

Cause: NSAIDs and ASA cause gastritis, gastric and duodenal ulcers (epigastric pain); Malory-Weiss tear (usually h/o vomiting); ETOH; potassium, vit C, quinidine, tetracycline, alendronate cause esophagitis or ulcer; aortoenteric fistula (h/o AAA repair or bypass);

Table 11-8. Mesenteric Ischemia

	Epidem	Sx	Rx
Acute			
Arterial			
Superior mesenteric artery (SMA) embolus	*77 yr, 40–50%, cardiac origin, SMA not occluded explaining why proximal small bowel spared	Severe abd pn out of proportion to exam, gut emptying, severe cardiac disease, progresses to peritoneal irritation	Rx <12 h, heparin, antibx, resect necrotic bowel, 2nd look operation 24–48 h or thrombolytics? (Ann Vasc Surg 1998;12:187)
SMA thrombus	*77 yr, 18–25%, diffuse ASVD	Same as CMI, distention in 12–24 hr, bloody stool, electrolyte abn late, irreversible, occlusion at origin SMA, collateral formation limits ischemic injury	Revasc to achieve SMA patency, no percutaneous transluminal angioplasty because increased risk of thrombus
Nonocclusive mesenteric ischemia	*63 yr, 20%	Low flow states superimposed on ASVD, patchy diffuse involvement, colicky, periumb pn	Vasodilators, eg, papaverine x 24 h
Venous			
Mesenteric venous thrombosis	*66 yr, 5%	Mild distention, pn weeks, abd trauma, sepsis, portal HTN, hypercoagulability, OCPs, protein def	Revasc
Chronic			
Arterial			
Chronic mesenteric ischemia (CMI)	Younger women	Postprandial pn 4 h, weight loss (food fear), visceral angina, ASVD of mesenteric circ usually 2 ves occluded SMA, celiac, IMA less common	
Venous			
Chronic mesenteric venous thrombosis	*74 yr		

* Average.
Source: Med Clin North Am 1994;78:1303; Clin Geriatr Med 1999;15:527.

varices (portal HTN, gastropathy liver disease); Rendu-Osler-Weber (h/o epistaxis)

Epidem: Mortality in old–old correlates w severe bleeding, ulcer >2 cm, bili >2.0; early endoscopy w heater probe decreases mortality (Br J Surg 1998;85:121); *H. pylori* rx decreases risk of GI bleed

Angiodysplasia: one of the most common causes of GI bleeding in the elderly; 25% associated w aortic stenosis (Am J Surg 1979;137:57)

Pathophys: Increased intraluminal pressure in the R colon leads to decreased mucosal blood flow and mesenteric ischemia leading to AV shunting in the submucosal layer of the bowel (Am Fam Phys 1985;32:93)

Sx: Melena = UGI, or small bowel or proximal colon bleed

Hematochezia = UGI bleed or brisk UGI bleed

Si: Stigmata of liver disease commonly seen; bleeding from diverticular lesions (arterial source) more severe than from ectasias (venous source)

Crs: GI bleed: hematochezia, hct decreased 5 points = brisk UGI or lower GI bleed; mortality related to smoking; in 80 yr olds mortality is 35% related to underlying DM, HTN, CAD, meds

Angiodysplasias: Usually stop spontaneously

Cmplc: Resting tachycardia = 10% blood loss; P increased 20 or systolic BP decreased 20 points = 20–30% blood loss

Lab: BUN/Cr ratio 20:1 suggests UGI bleed (absorption in proximal small bowel of hemoglobin); also a sign of prerenal azotemia

Xray: Avoid barium enema; Gastrografin if contrast agent necessary

Colonoscopic findings: telangiectasias, surface erosions <5 mm cecum and ascending colon, tortuous veins

Rx:

Therapeutic: Vit K, fresh frozen plasma if on coumadin; O_2; angiodysplasia: vasopressin, chemical embolization, electrocoagulation, laser, segmental resection, hemicolectomy; hormonal therapy controversial

11.8 PANCREATITIS/CHOLECYSTITIS

Surg Clin N Am 1994;74:317; Clin Ger Med 1999;15:571,579

Cause: Pancreatitis: ETOH >12–15 yrs, gallstones (most common, 75% of cases of acute pancreatitis in patients >80 yrs), meds (ethacrynic acid, corticosteroids, metronidazole, thiazide, estrogen), metabolic (hypercalcemia, hypertriglyceridemia, uremia), surgery, ERCP, sphincter of Oddi dysfunction, tumors, ischemia, perhaps periampullary diverticula, hereditary (trypsinogen, cystic fibrosis)

Epidem:
- Biliary disease leading indication for acute abdominal surgery in elderly
- Pancreatitis: 200 times incidence in pts >65 yrs; acute mortality rate 20% (Am J Surg 1986;152:638)

Pathophys: *Escherichia coli* and *Klebsiella* most common organisms in cholecystitis; anaerobic infections also; larger common bile duct in elderly; change in biliary metabolism (cholesterol saturation of bile is increased); predispose pts to cholecystitis

Sx:
- Cholecystitis: peritoneal signs are seen in <50% of pts and some pts have no abdominal tenderness; frequently low-grade temp elevations, but may be toxic-appearing w pt disoriented and showing no abdominal signs; 40% of acutely ill pts have empyema, perforation, gangrene; 15% have subphrenic abscess or liver abscess; acalculous cholecystitis similar to acute calculous cholecystitis in presentation but most prevalent after surgery, trauma, repeated transfusions, burns, prolonged parenteral nutrition, cancer
- Pancreatitis: altered mental status may be only presenting sx; epigastric pain radiating to back, pt sits forward; tachycardia, nausea, vomiting, fever, ileus, shock; chronic pancreatitis presents w pain; nutritional deficiency w protein and fat malabsorption; glucose intolerance more common than in young people

Cmplc:
- Choledocholithiasis 10–20% of time: 75% present w pain and jaundice, 18% w pain, 6% w jaundice; endoscopic sphincterotomy if unfit for surgery; mortality rates for operative common duct exploration are 6–12%, usually cardiac cause

- Gall bladder perforation due to decreased vascularity of fundus of gall bladder w aging
- Pancreatitis: left-sided effusions, localized parenchymal infiltrates (pancreatic effects on pulmonary surfactant) (Gastrointest Endosc Clin N Am 1990;19:433); renal failure and ARDS early, infection late
- Underlying adenocancer of the gallbladder: especially in women in 6th and 7th decades w gallstones
- R/o appendicitis
- R/o: pancreatic cancer w CA 19-9 marker (Clin Ger Med 1999;15:579)

Lab:
- Cholecystitis: leukocytosis in 66% of pts
- Pancreatitis: elevation of enzymes not correlated w prognosis or severity of disease

Xray: If dx uncertain, obtain CT w contrast; ensure adequate renal function prior to contrast

Rx:
- 9.8% mortality from surgery for acute cholecystitis because of delayed dx and comorbidities; laparoscopic cholecystectomy preferred (Ann Surg 1991;213:665)
- Pancreatitis: ERCP, sphincterotomy for gallstone pancreatitis (Lancet 1988;2:979); npo; NSAIDs for pain; ICU if severe to monitor cardiac, fluid, and electrolyte status and start enteral or parenteral feeding; antibiotics if not better 5 days, or ascites, or pseudocyst, or pancreatic necrosis; imipenem, consider adding fluconazole; lexipafant (platelet activation factor receptor antagonist) decreases mortality in severe acute pancreatitis (Gastroenterology 1997;112:A453); pancreatin: 8 tabs w meal for malabsorption

Px:
- Pancreatitis: APACHE II better predictor than Ranson criteria (Clin Ger Med 1999;15:579)

11.9 ENTERAL FEEDING

Crit Care Clin 1997;13:669; Nejm 1997;226:41

Indications: Pts with a functional GI tract who are unable to sustain adequate caloric intake by mouth; significant muscle wasting occurs after npo 7–10 days; discussion of alternative feeds if no hope for resuming po; no increase in lean body mass, but attenuation in the rate of loss of LBM (especially muscle) (Nutrition 1999;15:158)
- Neurologic disorders: trauma, CVA, and disease
- Malignancy: especially head and neck
- Burns
- Psychological disorder, eg, depression, anorexia
- Chemotherapy and radiation therapy
- GI disorder, eg, IBD, enterocutaneous fistula

Caloric Requirements:
- Adult: 25–35 kcal/day
- Elderly: 15–20 kcal/day
- Resting energy expenditure (REE):
  Male REE = $(789 \times BSA) + 137$
  Female REE = $(544 \times BSA) + 414$
- Hospitalized patients need 20% in excess of REE; burn patients need 100% in excess of REE
- Use LR as first fluid when hospitalizing: 28 mEq/L lactate combats muscle wasting; D5 provides 50 gm dextrose (minimal caloric supply)

Types of Tubes:
- NG tube: 8–10 Fr with mercury-weighted tip, pliable
- Gastrojejunostomy tube: percutaneous endoscopic placement with conscious sedation at bedside by GI or intra-operative placement by surgeon; 1% major complication rate; wait 2–3 days after placement for use; clean dressing changes qd; secure tube to prevent dislodgment

Types of Formulas:
- Intact protein isolates, starches and long-chain fatty acids; fed to stomach or small bowel; pt must have normal proteolytic and lipolytic functions; minimally hyperosmolar, 1 kcal/mL, come premixed
- Osmolite
- Osmolite HN (high nitrogen): better for smaller people

- Jevity: equivalent to Osmolite HN with fiber added; good for diarrhea and constipation; tolerated well
- Magna Cal: 2 cal/mL (double that of standard formulas); good for fluid-restricted patients
- Elemental formulas: protein hydrolysates or amino acids, glucose, oligosaccharides, medium chain triglycerides; require minimal digestion; use in pancreatitis, ulcerative colitis, GI fistula; 1 kcal/mL, hyperosmolar
- Vivamax and Vivamax HN
- Vital: good for fluid-restricted patients
- Criticare: formulated for patients under stress
- Immunoenhanced: specific nutrients including glutamine, arginine, omega-3 fatty acids, and nucleotides improve infection rate and hospital length of stay; no effect on mortality (Crit Care Med 1999;27:2799)
- IMPACT
- Immun-Aid: adds glutamine for improved 6 months survival in critically ill patients (Nutrition 1997;13:752); branched-chain amino acids
- Modular feedings: elements individually mixed by pharmacy to specific patient needs; most expensive

Administration:
- Aspiration precautions: head up at 30 degrees, chest xray for tube placement prior to use, ongoing clinical vigilance for continuing bowel function
- Begin with 1/4 strength solution with 0.5 mL water per 1 mL of feeding to prevent hypernatremia; for gastric feeding, increase concentration first, then volume; for small bowel feeding, increase volume first
- Check residuals every 2 h for first 48 h of feeding
- Decrease rate (hold feeds for 2 h) for residuals >100 mL
- Continuous infusion (gravity or pump) during sleeping hours for small bowel feeding; bolus of 200–400 mL q 4 h for gastric feeding
- Flush tube with 25–100 mL water after each continuous feed or bolus
- Limit bacterial overgrowth by refrigerating tube feeds; no more than 4 h at room temperature

Complications:
- Gastrointestinal: cramping, bloating, diarrhea; may rx by changing formula concentrations of feeds or adding bulk agent

Table 11-9. Complications of Tube Feedings

Complication	Intervention
Aspiration pneumonia	Check tube placement before commencing feeding Elevate head properly while feeding Adjust feeding rate to minimize gastric distention
Diarrhea	Switch to a different formula or dilution Administer kaolin-pectin suspension, paregoric, diphenoxylate, or codeine
Hyponatremia	Decrease water flushes Add sodium chloride to the formula Switch to a nutrient-dense formula
Skin irritation around tube site	Use cleansing mechanical barriers Use H_2 blockers to decrease gastric acidity

- Mechanical: tube obstruction, dislodgment; GI obstruction and peritoneal leakage
- Fluid, electrolyte abnormalities: hyperglycemia, hypernatremia, azotemia, hyperosmolar, nonketonic coma; daily electrolyte and glucose monitoring for first 48 h; may add insulin (N) to feeds to combat hyperglycemia; start with sliding scale; add approximate 24-h sliding scale requirement to feeds
- Aspiration: common, may be lethal; see above; a major cause of ARDS

Cmplc: See Table 11-9

11.10 HYPONATREMIA AND LIVER DISEASE

Hyponatremia—See Table 11-10
Liver Disease—See Table 11-11

$$\text{Fractional excretion of } Na^+ = \frac{\text{Urine } Na^+/\text{Plasma } Na^+}{\text{Urine Cr/Plasma Cr}} \times 100$$

- Prerenal <1%
- Renal (ATN) >1%

Table 11-10. Hyponatremia (<135 mEq/L; <120 mEq/L = seizures)

	Decreased Serum Osm (<275)		Nl Osm Hyperlipidemia	Increased Osm Hyperglycemia
Increased ECF	Nl ECF	Decreased ECF		
Urine Na <20 mEq/L	SIADH (CNS, lung, stress)	Urine Na >20 mEq/L	Hyperproteinemia	—
CHF	Dilutional hyponatremia	Renal		
Cirrhosis	Urine Na >20 mEq/L	Diuretic		
	Urine Osm >200	Addison's		
	Morphine, tricyclics, nicotine, NSAIDs, sulfonylureas, hyponatremia, adrenal insufficiency	Dehydration		
Rx: fluid restrict + furosemide; ?captopril	Water restrict; 0.9 or 3% saline + furosemide (increase Na 20 mEq/L/48 h)	Replace fluid; rx underlying disorder	—	—

ECF = extracellular fluid.
Reproduced by permission from Annals of Long-Term Care 98;6(suppl):4.

Table 11-11. Liver Disease in the Elderly

	Hep B/C	Pyogenic Liver abscess	Autoimmune Liver Disease	Hepatic Ischemia	PBC	Neoplasm
Cause		Direct extension from biliary tract, pancreatitis hematogenous from portal v. (divertic, appendicitis, Crohns), hematogenous from hepatic artery (endocarditis, prosthesis) malignancy		Results from hypertension and shock, ASCVD		Mets from colorectal CA most common 25% of colorectal CA pts have Mets on presentation. Abdomen, brain, lung, neuroendocrine mets to liver
Epid	Prevalence Hep B ↑ 3x in pts 64–74, 43% Hep C compared to younger group 7%	Primarily affects elderly	22% of pts with AH >65 yr, less severe (aminotransferase levels not as high) (Age Aging 1997;26:441)	6th, 7th decades	As many as 38% of new cases >65 yr (Gut 1997;41:430)	Pts >60 yr lower survival rates however tumor size most important prognostic factor
Sx	Mild, subclinical in Hep B & C			Critically ill or anorexic, fatigue	Extrahepatic disorders: hypothyroid, sicca syndrome, cutaneous xanthoma	
Si	5% Hep B lead to chronic hepatitis lead to HCC: the longer the infection exposure, the more the chance of HCC. Hep C ↑ mortality rate in elderly		Pts with AST >10x or Gamma globular >5x have 3-yr mortality rate of 50% (Med Clin NA 1996;80:973)		Once 5x of pruritus jaundice, hepatosplenomegaly and complications of cirrhosis develop adv age poor px (>90% die of liver disease)	
Lab		US, MRI not accurate, needle bx liver	Liver bx or might miss dx	Serum transaminase 25–250x nl during acute insult return to nl in 7–10 days, bili, alk phos 3–4x nl, PT nl		Difficult detect tumor Less than 1 cm radiologically and may not be assoc with alpha FP. Screen pts with Hep C with US and alpha FP of 6 mo

Source: Clin Geriatr Med 1999;15:559.

12   Dermatology

12.1 SKIN PROBLEMS (BENIGN AND MALIGNANT LESIONS)

Am J Med 1995;98:99S; Am Fam Phys Monograph 1995:193; Geriatrics 1993;48:30; J Am Acad Dermatol 1992;26:521; Nejm 1991;325:171

Epidem: The incidence of skin cancers increases exponentially with age and is thought to be related to UVB irradiation cumulated over a life span; worse in geographical areas of decreased ozone

Pathophys: Changes of aging skin

Epidermis:
- Flattening of dermal–epidermal junction leads to increased propensity to blister and erode w shear force
- Decreased moisture content of the stratum corneum; decreased secretion from sweat glands; xerosis
- Decreased epidermal turnover: slowed wound healing; increased secondary infection following minor trauma; hyperproliferative disorders such as psoriasis tend to improve
- Melanocytes decrease by about 10% every decade after age of 30 yr, leading to depigmentation; melanin normally functions to absorb carcinogenic UV light
- Cell-mediated immune response decreased (Langerhans cells or macrophages in the epidermis); more susceptibility to cutaneous tumors, but less potential for allergic contact sensitization

Dermis: The dermis decreases in density; relatively acellular, avascular, leading to poor insulation, pale skin, and hypo/hyperthermia; regression of subepidermal elastic fibers causes skin wrinkling; dermal clearance of foreign material decreased, prolonging contact dermatitis duration

Skin appendages:
- Sweat glands decreased causing dry skin, less body odor
- Pacinian and Meissner corpuscles decrease by approximately two-thirds, predisposing elderly to trauma, burns, and decreased ability to perform fine hand maneuvers
- Subcutaneous tissue volume decreased within weight-bearing surfaces such as feet, causing calluses, corns, ulcerations, and chronic pain

Rx:

Wrinkles: Rx topical tretinoin inhibits irradiation-induced matrix metalloproteinase (Nejm 1997;337:1419)

Prevention: Sunblock (15–30 SPF) applied daily each morning

12.2 ECZEMA

Appearance: Dry skin, fine fissuring, pruritic; lower legs; worsening in the winter

Rx: Of highest importance, increase hydration by applying emollients and bath oils, particularly after bathing; avoid excess exposure to water; increase use of room humidifiers; use steroid preparations only if severe or chronic
- Classes III–VI (triamcinolone 0.025%–0.1%–0.5%), class II (fluocinonide [Lidex]), class I (betamethasone dipropionate [Diprolene] 0.05%, cream 0.05%), class VII (hydrocortisone, nonfluorinated 0.1%)
- Lotion or gel for acute lesion (oozing, crusting, vesicles) to help drying; cream for subacute lesions (scales, patches); ointment for chronic lesions (dry skin, plaques, lichenification)

12.3 SEBORRHEIC DERMATITIS

Appearance: Greasy yellow scale w or w/o erythematous base on nasolabial folds, eyebrows, hairline, sideburns, posterior auricular, mid-chest

Rx: Hydrocortisone 1.0–2.5% after careful cleaning

12.4 ROSACEA

Cause: Facial mite (possibly)

Rx: Dermadex w metronidazole 0.75% gel bid for 6–9 wk; rx pustules w doxycycline 100 mg po, telangiectasias w electrodesiccation, rhinophyma w plastic surgery

12.5 PSORIASIS

Rx: Mild limited w topical corticosteroids; anthralin, tar 1–4% messy and irritating; recalcitrant cases w UV light, PUVA, topical vit D (calcipotriene) in limited doses because irritating; years of rx w UV light, methotrexate, cyclosporine, strong topical steroids may predispose pt to other health problems

12.6 SEBORRHEIC KERATOSIS

Appearance: Disseminated, pigmented, waxy, "stuck on"; may be very large or thickened

Crs: Benign

Rx: Electrocautery, particularly for large lesions; liquid nitrogen may work

Look-alikes: Bowen disease, superficial spreading melanoma

12.7 ACTINIC SENILE KERATOSIS

Appearance: Multiple, red/brown, flat/raised, with adherent scale, "sandpaper" feel

Crs: Most common precancerous lesion in whites, but frequency of overall conversion debated; 12%—squamous cell on lip

Rx: Liquid nitrogen—light 20-sec freeze; 5-fluorouracil 2–5% q d × 2–3 wk, may react w sun; warn pt of duration of sx of rx

12.8 BOWEN DERMATOSIS

Appearance: 66% solitary, 33% multiple, sharply demarcated, scaly, flat or raised

Crs: Not sun-induced; good prognosis

Rx: Curettage; electrodesiccation; deep excision if hair follicle; topical fluorouracil bid several weeks to larger lesions; Mohn surgery (serial layers excised until no microscopic evidence of cancer remains) and laser therapy also are options

Look-alikes: Eczema (palpable, thickened, red/brown w deepened skin lines), tinea, superficial basal cell carcinoma, irritated seborrheic keratosis

12.9 KERATOACANTHOMA

Appearance: Common in elderly men, dome-shaped, flesh-colored smooth nodule with depressed center filled with keratin plug; sun-exposed areas; backs of hands, arms, central face

Crs: Rapid growth 2 wk, stationary, involution

Rx: Hard to distinguish from squamous cell cancer, so excision or curettage; fulguration for lesions <2 cm

12.10 SQUAMOUS CELL CANCER

Cause: Sun, coal tar, creosote oil, paraffin oil exposures

Appearance: Head/forearm/neck/back; firm erythematous nodule with indistinct margins

Crs: Metastasize unpredictably to lymph nodes; most convert to malignant from actinic keratosis; ulcer indicates aggressive

Rx: Electrosurgery; chemotherapy; Mohn surgery; surgery—wide excision or Mohn dependent on location; radiation

12.11 LEUKOPLAKIA

Appearance: White plaque mucous membranes; hypertrophic
Crs: Precancerous; 10–17% develop into squamous cell carcinoma
(floor of mouth, ventral surface of tongue) 1–20 yr after initial onset
Rx: Excisional bx, electrodesiccation, liquid nitrogen, topical
fluorouracil, laser
Look-alikes: Candidiasis, secondary syphilis, vulvar atrophy; lichen
sclerosis et atrophicus (extends beyond mucous membrane to skin;
if does not respond to topical estrogen or corticosteroid, should bx,
although potential for malignancy small)

12.12 SCABIES

Appearance: Itching erythematous, papular eruption; excoriation,
secondary infection; axillary, waist, inner thigh, back, arm, leg;
burrows between fingers
Crs: Persists for decades untreated
Rx: Scrape skin parallel to surface of burrow deep enough to cause
pinpoint bleeding, use mineral oil and coverslip on slide to identify
mite, egg, or fecal material; Kwell (lindane) 1% or Eurax
(crotamiton) 10% or permethrin cream 5% 12 h, reapply in 1 wk,
itches for 2 wk; vacuum rugs, hot water wash, then heat-dry clothes;
treat close contacts
Look-alikes: Other bites (not in web spaces)

12.13 HERPES ZOSTER

Appearance: Usually unilateral tingling or pain 4–5 d; erythematous
grouped vesicles/crust; occasionally nodules, papules; may affect eye
(corneal ulceration); any dermatomes may be involved
Eye Findings:
1. Simplex—dendritic ulcers of cornea
2. Zoster—periphery of cornea with vascularization, ulceration,
   dendrites can happen (uncommon)

Crs: Often extended course of many weeks to several months w "postherpetic" pain; some communicability and best to avoid unnecessary exposure; NH staff require gloves if vesicles, crusting

Rx: If early, valacyclovir 1 gm tid × 7 d or famciclovir 750 mg tid × 7 d or acyclovir 800 mg 5 d 7–10 d or valacyclovir, 1 gm tid; if established for >3 d, antivirals probably not helpful (and are expensive); if no contraindication to corticosteroids (DM, HT, glaucoma), prednisone 60 mg tapered over 21 d (Nejm 1996;335:32); uveitis: topical corticosteroids w ophthalmologic consult, atropine to dilate pupils; pain management often a longer problem, as may require codeine or other opioids; for extended courses, long-term lower-dose antivirals can be helpful; cover acute lesions to decrease communicability

12.14 PEMPHIGUS VULGARIS

J Am Geriatr Soc 1998;46:92

Appearance: Oral mucosa and skin; IgG, C_3 deposits stratum malpighii; increased pemphigus antibody corresponds to severity of disease; px favorable for older people; 50% Jewish

Rx: Triamcinolone acetonide

12.15 BULLOUS PEMPHIGOID

Nejm 1995;333:1475

Appearance: Sudden-onset urticarial plaques or intact tense blisters; flexural blisters, rapid spread; immunofluorescent studies: C_3 along basement membrane

Rx: Untreated lesions may become extensive and highly symptomatic, resulting in death; early administration of prednisone 40–60 mg/d gives best response and begin tapering when no new lesions appearing; 2nd rx: azathioprine, cyclophosphamide, cyclosporine,

methotrexate, tetracycline, dapsone, sulfapyridine, gold; pulsed
corticosteroids, plasmapheresis, high-dose immune globulin
Look-alikes: Pemphigus vulgaris: no urticarial plaques; immunofluorescent studies: antibodies against intercellular cement

12.16 ONYCHOGRYPHOSIS

Appearance: Nails—patchy distal yellow discoloration; raised edge;
fragile; later thickening and curvature of nails due to chronic trauma;
more common in pts w atherosclerosis, fungi, or chronic paronychial
infection (usually secondary to candidal infection)
Crs: Chronic; rx expensive and of limited value in elderly w few
long-term cures
Rx: VoSol or rubbing alcohol to affected nail fold results in evaporation
of water in 10 min; if *Pseudomonas* present, use gentamicin ointment
or fluconazole; treat surrounding skin infections aggressively to
improve comfort; nail cutting, grinding to reduce mass of nail
important for foot comfort and injury prevention

12.17 MELANOMA

Appearance: Worrisome if asymmetric, irregular borders, >0.5 cm,
multiple colors white, red, blue, black
Lab: Pathology of bx specimen: Clark levels:
I—limited to epidermis, no invasion
II—into but not filling papillary dermis, 95% 5-yr survival
III—filling papillary dermis
IV—reticular dermis
V—subcuticular fat, 5-yr survival 40%
Rx: Full excision primary lesion

12.18 ORAL CANCER

Epidem: Squamous 95%; risk factors: age, male, previous oral malignancy, tobacco, alcohol, exposure to sunlight (lip)

Crs: Prognosis without lymph node involvement: 50% 5-yr-survival rate for tongue; 95% 5-yr-survival rate for lip

Rx:

Preventive: Quit smoking

Therapeutic: High morbidity from surgical resection, irradiation, cytotoxic chemotherapy: disfigurement, speech impediment, salivary gland hypofunction, osteomyelitis

12.19 PRESSURE SORES

J Am Geriatr Soc 1995;43:919

Epidem: 50–70% in pts older than age 70 in NH (J Am Geriatr Soc 1988;36:807); hospital prevalence 3–11%, with highest in coronary care unit; on admission to NH 11–35%

Pathophys: When pressure exceeds 32 mmHg, capillary blood flow is halted; prolonged hypoperfusion leads to hypoxia, acidosis, hemorrhage into the interstitium (nonblanchable erythema), toxic cellular wastes, cell death, and tissue necrosis (Med Clin N Am 1989;73:1511); pressure against the epidermis results in highest pressure nearest the bone, because pressure is more easily dissipated w deformation of the more superficial tissues

Pressure, friction, shear, chronic exposure to water (Ped Derm 1994;11:18); deficiencies in ascorbic acid, zinc, Fe (J Am Geriatr Soc 1993;41:357)

Si: See Table 12-1.

Complc: Offending organisms in sepsis: *Proteus mirabilis, Escherichia coli, Pseudomonas aeruginosa, Klebsiella, Bacteroides fragilis;* recurrence of pressure ulcer within 2 yr of surgical primary wound closure (Adv Wound Care 1994;7:40)

Lab: ESR to r/o osteomyelitis; serum albumin; CBC; serum glucose

Induced: Suspect osteomyelitis w elevated WBC, fever, and poor wound healing

Table 12-1. Staging of Pressure Sores

Stage I	Nonblanchable erythema of intact skin; early pressure sore may appear postoperatively as bruising
Stage II	Abrasion, opened blister, partial thickness involving epidermis and/or dermis
Stage III	Necrosis, undermining; full-thickness loss into the subcutaneous tissue
Stage IV	Sinus tracts, extension into the fascia, muscle, bone

Note: Most commonly scapula, iliac crest, sacrum, ischium, trochanter, lateral malleolus, heel, lateral edge of foot.

Rx:

Preventive: Braden scale predictive value 64–77% (Decubitus 1989; 2:44); Norton scale predictive value 0–37%; other similar scales (Am Fam Phys 1996;54:S1519)

Address risk factors for pressure sores in all patients: lymphopenia, immobility, dry skin, decreased body weight (Jama 1995;273:865)

Nonblanchable erythema is very important early sign (address immediately); turn sequentially from back to left to right side q 2 h; avoid direct pressure on the greater trochanter and lateral malleolus by positioning back at a 30-degree angle to the bed w pillows between knees and lower legs and along back and arms to maintain optimal positioning (AHCPR Pub No. 92-0047, 1992); reposition pts in chairs q 1 h; use trapezes, draw sheets; sitting on doughnut-type padding may cause ischemia (Ann IM 1986;105:337); education of multidisciplinary team decreased incidence of pressure sores by 63% (Arch IM 1988;148:2241)

Therapeutic: See Table 12-2.

1. Relieve pressure: mattresses and beds (list: J Am Geriatr Soc 1995;43:919); low-air-loss mattress cost-effective (J Gerontol 1995;141:6; Jama 1993;269:494); air-fluoridized beds for stages III–IV on two of the following areas: left hip, right hip, sacrum; or w recalcitrant wounds (J Am Geriatr Soc 1989;37:235); four-layer compression bandage more cost effective in persistent venous ulcers (BMJ 1998;316:1487)
2. Remove necrotic debris: chemical debridement w Granulex and Elase; dextrases may not be as effective
3. Control local infection: avoid systemic antibiotics unless there is an abscess or expanding cellulitis, then use clindamycin and

Table 12-2. Categories of Products and Devices Commonly Used in Wound Care

Category	Description	Characteristics	Concerns	Applications
Gauze, dry or wet	• Woven natural cotton fibers; non-woven rayon and polyester blends • Available in pads and rolls, sterile and non-sterile	• May be dampened with saline or water • Inexpensive • Facilitates wet-to-dry debridement • Non-adherent when used as wet-to-moist dressing • Minimally to moderately absorbent	• Wet-to-dry debridement painful, may damage healthy tissue • Woven variety is abrasive • May dehydrate wound • Requires frequent changes • Packing may harden, causing further pressure injury	*As primary dressing:* • Deep wounds; can be packed into undermined or tunneling areas *As secondary dressing:* • Can maintain a moist environment if kept moist, or under an occlusive secondary dressing • Can be used in large, necrotic wounds or presence of soft tissue infection
Impregnated gauze pads	• Woven or non-woven materials in which substances such as saline, water, iodinated agents, petrolatum, zinc compounds, sodium chloride, chlorhexadine gluconate, bismuth tribromophenate, or other materials have been incorporated	• Inexpensive • Non-adherent with specific product formulations	• Some impregnated material may be toxic to living tissue	• See above

Table 12-2. (cont'd)

Category	Description	Characteristics	Concerns	Applications
Transparent films	• Adhesive, transparent polyurethane membrane	• Occlusive and waterproof • Retains moisture • Impermeable to bacteria and contamination • Promotes autolysis, moist wound healing and epithelialization • Wound is visible • Non-absorbent • May be changed every 5–7 days	• Should not be used with moderate to heavy exudate • Risk of macerating surrounding skin	*As primary dressing:* • Open partial-thickness wounds, minimal exudate, clean wound base or intact skin (Stage 1) *As secondary dressing:* • May be used as secondary dressing over other more absorptive products
Hydrogels	• Glycerin- or water-based gel, amorphous or supported by fabric • Available as amorphous gels, wafers, sheets and impregnated gauze. • Available with or without adhesive borders	• Non-adherent • Fills dead space • Semi-occlusive • Promotes autolysis, moist wound healing • Easy to apply and remove • Minimally absorbent • Retains moisture and rehydrates wound	• Risk of macerating surrounding tissue • Secondary dressing required • Requires daily application (except when applied with adhesive borders) • Dries out easily • Risk of candidiasis	*As primary dressing:* • Full-thickness wounds with clean base and minimal or no exudate • Partial-thickness wounds with adherent necrosis or slough with minimal or no exudate
Hydrocolloids	• Adhesive wafers composed of gelatin, pectin and carboxymethyl-cellulose. • Available in wafers, sheets, paste or granules	• Occlusive and waterproof • Retains moisture • Impermeable to bacteria and contamination • Promotes autolysis and moist wound healing • Moderately absorbent • Easy to apply	• Should not be used with heavy exudate • Should not be used when soft tissue infection is present • May be difficult to remove; may have significant odor on removal, due to anaerobic colonization	*As primary dressing:* • Intact skin or a clean wound base with light to moderate exudate • Partial-thickness wounds with adherent necrosis or slough *As secondary dressing:* • Over wound fillers in deep wounds without undermining or tunneling

Alginates	• Non-woven fibers containing calcium sodium salts of alginic acid derived from seaweed • Available in pads or ropes	• Non-adherent • Highly absorbent • Promotes autolysis • Can be used on infected wounds	• Requires a secondary dressing • Should not be used on dry or low-exudate wounds; may desiccate wound • Requires daily application	*As primary dressing:* • Full-thickness wound with moderate to heavy exudate • Can be packed into areas of tunneling or undermining
Foams	• Hydrophilic polyurethane foam • Available in wafers, sheets, pillows with film covering	• Non-adherent • Easy to apply and remove • Highly absorbent	• Requires a secondary dressing (unless combined with an adhesive border)	*As primary dressing:* • Full-thickness wound with moderate to heavy exudate • May be used as "intermediate" dressing for absorbing excessive exudate over packing material
Wound fillers	• Copolymer starch, dextranomer beads or hydrocolloid paste that swells on contact with wound fluid to form a gel • Available in pastes, beads, powders, gels and fiber layers	• Non-adherent • Easy to apply and remove • Moderately to highly absorbent	• Usually requires a secondary dressing	*As primary dressing:* • Full-thickness wounds with moderate to heavy exudate, to fill dead space • Fiber layers can be packed into areas of tunneling and undermining
Composite dressings	• Combines various dressing categories in one product • Varies among manufacturers	• Provides multiple functions (such as bacterial barrier, absorptive layer, adhesive border, etc.)	• Use may be confusing	• Depends on components

DERMATOLOGY

Reproduced by permission from American Medical Directors Association. Pressure ulcer therapy companion: clinical practice guideline, 1999. Columbia, MD: American Medical Directors Association, 1999:21–22.

fluoroquinolones; avoid topical antiseptics such as hydrogen peroxide, potassium hypochlorite (Dakin solution), acetic acid, povidone-iodine (Betadine), may inhibit fibroblast growth (J Trauma 1993;35:8; Clin Ger Med 1992;8:835); povidone-iodine may be more beneficial than saline dressings for short periods of time, eg, 4–5 d for purulent, odoriferous wounds (Postgrad Med J 1993;69:S97); 1:100 strength of povidone-iodine not harmful to wounds; MRSA-infected wound: topical mupirocin (Bactroban); malodorous pressure sores: metronidazole gel (Am Fam Phys 1996;54:S1519)

4. Protect healthy tissue: stages II and III w little exudate; use petroleum gauze, or semipermeable or occlusive dressing q 2–3 d

5. Promote granulation: moist environment hastens healing w increased migration of fibroblasts and growth factor; hydrocolloid dressing q 3–5 d for stages III and IV, better than wet to dry, watch for infection; deep wound packing w space-occupying (eg, calcium alginates) or salt-impregnated dressings (Mesalt) for stages III and IV (J Am Geriatr Soc 1995;43:919)

6. General condition: high-protein diet (24% protein) enhances wound healing (J Am Geriatr Soc 1993;41:357); ascorbic acid 500 mg bid (J Gen IM 1991;6:81); zinc 200–600 mg qd (Adv Wound Care 1996;9:8; Ann IM 1986;105:342); nitro paste 2% for vasodilation (J Am Geriatr Soc 1997;45:895)

Future Treatment Options: Fibroblast growth factor (J Clin Invest 1993;92:2841), hyperbaric oxygen (Nejm 1996;334:1642; Jama 1990;263:2216)

13 Ethics

13.1 COMPETENCY

Arch IM 1995;155:502; Clin Ger Med 1994;10:403
See Tables 13-1, 13-2

"Informed consent" depends on competency, a legal definition
(J Am Geriatr Soc 2000;48:913); pt must demonstrate:
1. Ability to evidence a choice about treatment
2. Capacity to have factual understanding of the information that
the average pt would consider material to making the health care
decision in question
3. The ability to manipulate information rationally
4. The capacity to appreciate the nature of the specific situation
(Am J Psychiatry 1977;134:3)
Mini-Mental State Exam (MMSE) not good for predicting
competency scores <7 incompetent, score 27-competent, scores
7-27 not helpful; decision-making capacity in elderly does not
compare well to MMSE and should be assessed by direct methods
(J Am Geriatr Soc 1990;38:1097; Am J Psychiatry 1977;134:3);
autonomy assumes that persons possess the capacity to decide, to
carry out decisions, and to manage and be accountable for the
consequences of their decisions (J Am Geriatr Soc 1995;43:1437)

Table 13-1. Competency Profile

Name: SS#:   Date:

Decision to be made:

Criterion	Independent	With Assistance	Unable
1. Receives information			
2. Recognizes relevant information as information			
3. Remembers information			
4. Relates situation to oneself, values, and circumstances			
5. Reasons about alternatives			
6. Ranks alternatives in order of preference			
7. Resolves situations (dilemmas)			
8. Resigns self to the decision			
9. Recounts one's decision-making process			
10. Organizes effort to implement the decision			

From Nurs Home Med 1996;4:49A.

Table 13-2. Mnemonic for Evaluating Competency

"C"—consistent	Consistent on serial Mini Mental State Exam (MMSE); consistent decision on serial questioning; and consistent w life values
"O"—other alternatives to therapy	Understands other care alternatives, which, in turn, requires ability to understand factual material and manipulate information rationally
"M"—malleable	Physician must remain malleable; pts and families change their minds about end-of-life decisions in different settings and decisions should be reviewed w a change of setting
"P"—particulars	Pt must be able to appreciate the nature of the particular situation; physician must be particular about what pt is competent to do, eg, can decide health care but not run a household; degree of competence (supramaximal, full, limited) may differ depending on the domain (civil, personal, financial, health care) (Nurs Home Med 1996;4:81); least restrictive guardianship is the goal (partial capacity)

13.2 ADVANCE DIRECTIVES

Jama 1997;277:1854

Provide answers to the following treatment decisions:
1. Cardiac arrest
2. Acute, reversible, life-threatening event
3. Acute, nonreversible, life-threatening event
4. Nutrition (including fluids)
5. Routine blood work (J Am Geriatr Soc 1991;39:396,1221)

Directives completed at higher rates w physician-directed intervention (Arch IM 1994;154:2321); pre-hospital code status can be effectively made in the NH setting; has no effect on the short term but decreases use of hospital in the last months of life (J Am Geriatr Soc 1995;43:113)

Pts overemphasize benefit of CPR (J Gen IM 1993;8:295), but prognostic information influences decisions and most elderly do not want CPR (Nejm 1994;4:330,545); 14% of elderly will change opinion based on more information (Jama 1995;274:1775); doctors inaccurate in predicting survival of most terminally ill patients, perhaps why continued low rate of hospice referrals (BMJ 2000;320:469)

Medical futility: physiologic intervention no plausible effect on disease; quantitative: extremely unlikely to have effect on disease; qualitative: not improved, possibly diminished quality of life

APACHE (Acute Physiology and Chronic Health Evaluation) predictors of mortality depend on severity of illness and not age; age alone does not predict survival (Am J Emerg Med 1995;13:389; J Am Geriatr Soc 1995;43:520,1131; Jama 1990;264:2109); decreased survival in hospitalized pts >70 yr old probably due to underlying medical problems; predictors of poor outcome following CPR: hct <35, creatinine >1.5, BUN >65, albumin <2.7 gm/dL (J Am Geriatr Soc 1990;38:1057; Ann IM 1989;7:199); success rate of CPR in elderly >70 yr old so low may not be worthwhile (Arch IM 1993;153:1293; Ann IM 1989;111:193,199); poor outcome in NH facilities (J Am Geriatr Soc 1993;41:163,384)

Life values and resuscitation preferences are related; therefore important to discuss together (J Am Geriatr Soc 1996;44:958)

Nutrition: Basic human need vs extraordinary medical intervention (Clin Ger Med 1994;10:475); survey of NG tube feeds in elderly pts in a community hospital found that 53% of the time restraints were needed, and 24 of 29 pts were judged to be incompetent (Clin Ger Med 1994;10:475; Arch IM 1989;149:1937)

- States have various statutes regarding when tube feeding can be stopped or not started (Clin Ger Med 1994;10:475)
- Complete starvation associated with euphoria and analgesia (Clin Ger Med 1994;10:475; J Gen IM 1993;8:220)
- Hypernatremia, hypercalciuria, hyperosmolarity, azotemia all produce sedation during dying process (P. Rousseau. Hospice: Ethical issues in end-of-life care. March 1998, San Antonio, TX, American Medical Directors Association Conference)
- Feeding tubes do not prevent aspiration; patients w dementia who are fed by tube vs by hand have same survival rates; long-term rates of complications from tube feeding 32–70% including retraining patient; patients cannot enjoy eating w feeding tube; most patients change their mind about tube feeding when told they might have to be restrained (Nejm 2000;342:206)

13.3 SUBSTITUTED JUDGMENT

Competent pt can leave advance directives (living will, durable power of attorney for health care); cannot infer CPR decision on basis of pt having a "living will" (Arch IM 1995;155:171)

Majority directives to carry out CPR are made by pts; the majority of do-not-resuscitate (DNR) orders are made by families (Arch IM 1992;152:561; Jama 1985;253:2236); physicians and families are not good at predicting pt preferences (Arch Fam Med 1994;3:1057)

Long-term care residents at NH do not have long-term survival from CPR (J Am Ger Med 1993;41:163)

Poor survival in NH patients w unwitnessed arrest or asystole, electrical mechanical dissociation (J Am Geriatr Soc 1995;43:520); NH medical directors are more likely to support withholding rx in terminally ill pts, but are generally not in favor of mandatory DNR orders (J Am Ger Med 1995;43:1131; Ann Emerg Med 1994;23:997; J Am Board Fam Pract 1993;6:91)

If no appropriate surrogate can be found, then group of individuals who care for the pt may determine treatment (multidisciplinary health care team) according to American Geriatric Society (AGS) Ethics Committee Position 3 (J Am Geriatr Soc 1996;44:986)

Terminal patients request aggressive treatment when physicians have not given them realistic assessment of their px (Jama 1998;279:1709); families more likely to be accurate when have spoken w patient about end-of-life decisions, when patient has private insurance, when either have high school diploma; less accurate when surrogate has personal experience w life-sustaining therapy, attended religious services, or when patient anticipated living >10 yrs (Ann IM 1998;128:621)

Prior competent choice vs best interest standards moving focus to patient's subjective experience at time of therapy (J Am Geriatr Soc 1998;46:922)

13.4 REFUSAL OF TREATMENT

ETHICS

Competent Patients: Have the right to refuse rx; rx against pt wishes can be construed as assault and battery and has been prosecuted as such (Clin Ger Med 1994;10:475)

Incapacitated Patients: Rigid criteria such as permanent unconsciousness or poorly defined categories such as terminal condition inadequate alone to determine whether surrogate should have authority to refuse life-sustaining rx for pt because often substantial uncertainty about prognosis and most pt preferences are based on projected quality, not quantity, of life (AGS Ethics Committee Position 8, J Am Geriatr Soc 1996;44:986)

Physician-Assisted Suicide (Euthanasia): More ethical solution might be rx of pain, especially in dying patients, and compassionate care; pts unduly influenced by physical suffering, impairment, abandonment, financial bankruptcy (J Am Geriatr Soc 1995;43:553); treatment of mild-to-moderate depression does not necessarily result in increased desire for life-sustaining measures (Palliat Med 1998;12:255; Nejm 1997;337:1234; J Gerontol 1994;49:M15)

Assess cognitive status; assess how support people and family feel about suicide plan; explore unresolved religious, spiritual concerns (Ann IM 2000;132:209)

Withdrawing of Therapy: Not obligated to continue a therapy that is not accomplishing any of the predefined goals of therapy if the following conditions apply:
- Pt has irreversible loss of cognitive function
- No goal other than sustaining organic life is accomplished by therapy
- No other goals of therapy can be achieved
- Pt has not previously expressed preferences about being sustained in organic life (Clin Ger Med 1994;10:475); position supported by AMA council on ethical and judicial affairs

Withholding treatment vs withdrawing treatment may or not be morally equivalent (J Am Geriatr Soc 1995;43:716,696; U.S. President's Commission for the Study of Ethical Problems in Medicine and Biomedical and Behavioral Research. Summing up, final report on studies of the ethical and legal problems in medicine and biomedical and behavioral research. Washington, DC: The Commission, 1983); distinction exists between withholding and withdrawing very low-burden interventions in chronically ill pts, eg, pacemaker: changing timing of death, not killing (Jama 2000;283:1061)

Truth Telling (eg, Alzheimer): When pt decision-making capacity and ability to cope w medical information is impaired enough to warrant withholding information vs withholding information that deprives pt of opportunity to act on important medical and nonmedical (financial planning) life decisions

Index

DATE DUE

Demco, Inc. 38-293